# OSCE Stations
# for Medical Finals
# Book 2

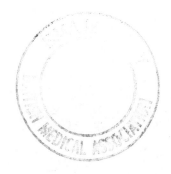

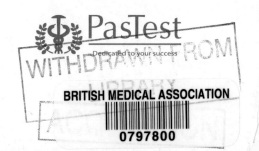

PasTest
Dedicated to your success

# OSCE Stations
# for Medical Finals
# Book 2

**Adam Feather FRCP**
Senior Lecturer in Medical Education,
St. Bartholomew's and the Royal London School of Medicine and Dentistry,
Consultant Geriatrician
Newham University Hospital NHS Trust

**Ashling Lillis BA (Cantab) MB BS  MRCP(UK)**
Acute Medicine Registrar,
King George Hospital,
Essex

**Tony Joy MBChB MRCS(Eng) DCH**
'Darzi' Fellow in Clinical Leadership
Registrar in Emergency Medicine
North East Thames Rotation
London

**John S P Lumley MS FRCS**
Emeritus Professor of Vascular Surgery,
St Bartholomew's and the Royal London
School of Medicine and Dentistry

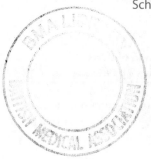

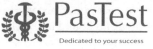

Dedicated to your success

PasTest Revision Books and Intensive Courses

PasTest has been established in the field of undergraduate and postgraduate medical education since 1972, providing revision books and intensive study courses for doctors preparing for their professional examinations.

Books and courses are available for:

Medical undergraduates, MRCGP, MRCP Parts 1 and 2, MRCPCH Parts 1 and 2, MRCS, MRCOG Parts 1 and 2, DRCOG, DCH, FRCA, Dentistry.

For further details contact:
PasTest, Freepost, Knutsford, Cheshire WA16 7BR
**Tel: 01565 752000  Fax: 01565 650264**
**www.pastest.co.uk  enquiries@pastest.co.uk**

Text prepared by Carnegie Book Production, Lancaster
Printed and bound in the UK by Page Bros, Norwich

# Contents

# About the authors

**Dr Ashling Lillis BA (Cantab) MB BS  MRCP(UK)**
Ashling is a trainee in Acute Internal Medicine in North East London. Having completed medical school and foundation training in Cambridge and then the East End of London she left for sunnier climbs with a year of medical practice in New Zealand. She returned to the East End to complete acute care core training at the Royal London Hospital, Whitechapel, at which time she became a clinical skills tutor at Barts and The London School of Medicine and Dentistry. She is now starting out on dual training in Acute Internal and General Medicine.

**Dr Tony Joy MBChB MRCS(Eng) DCH**
Tony is a Registrar in Emergency Medicine on the Northeast Thames Rotation in London. He is currently working as a 'Darzi' Fellow in Clinical Leadership at Newham University Hospital. Having qualified from the University of Sheffield in 2004, he worked briefly in Sri Lanka following the Boxing Day tsunami. After moving to London in 2005 he became interested in trauma and emergency medicine when working at the Royal London Hospital. He aims to become an Emergency Medicine Consultant, with particular interests in pre-hospital care, medical education and clinical leadership. In 2011 he married Amanda, and recently celebrated the arrival of a beautiful daughter, Madeleine.

**Dr Adam Feather FRCP**
Adam Feather is a Geriatrician at Newham University Hospital Trust and a Senior Lecturer in Medical Education at Barts and The London School of Medicine and Dentistry. He is the Lead for Clinical Skills and the Head of Final Year, and as such has responsibilities in supporting and preparing final year students in their transition to qualified doctors. He has been involved with the finals assessment both as a major contributor and lead for the past ten years. He is passionate about undergraduate medical education and has diverse interests including assessment, student support and curriculum design. He is perhaps best known for being the father of the soon-to-be-famous Jack Barney Feather.

**John S P Lumley MS FRCS**
John Lumley was formerly Honorary Consultant Surgeon to St Bartholomew's Hospital, the National Hospital for Neurology and Neurosurgery, Queen Square and the Hospital for Sick Children, Great Ormond Street, London. He has been World President of the International College of Surgeons, and Council Member, Journal Editor and Chairman of the Primary Fellowship Examiners of the Royal College of Surgeons. He has authored/edited over 50 texts, including one on conducting, having founded and conducted the Barts Academic Festival Choir and Orchestra (BAFCO) for over 40 years.

# Preface

OSCEs for Finals are based on clinical cases, each assessing you on the sequential management of a clinical problem. This form of scenario-based assessment is more akin to your future clinical practice than the more common independent OSCE format. We also give emphasis to the critical thinking, diagnostic reasoning and other aspects of professionalism that are essential for a practising doctor: these features are highlighted by icons and summary boxes throughout the text. Case-based assessment is widely used in postgraduate examinations, and is increasingly being introduced into the undergraduate curriculum and into finals.

The first two volumes of the series cover general medicine and surgery. The third volume is devoted to the specialities commonly included in the foundation programmes. Each clinical problem assesses history taking, examination, communication and data interpretation, and where appropriate, procedural and prescribing skills. The three volumes cover all of the procedures required by Tomorrow's Doctors (2009) and the Foundation Programme Application System (FPAS), and are the first set of books covering the skills and knowledge to be assessed in the new national prescribing skills assessment (PSA).

If successive tasks (stations) provide unwanted clues, they are placed on separate pages, as are the answers and patient prompts. Possible navigation difficulties are overcome by clear numbering and the use of icons. Uniform timing of stations can be a problem in a clinical examination; a text has no such limitations, and appropriate times are given for each question.

We advise working through the scenarios in student pairs, one of you being the examinee and the other the 'patient' and examiner (or a third member can take on one of these tasks): the separation of the patient history, examination and investigations of each scenario facilitates this approach. Marking is against a defined protocol, with grades from A-E: involvement in clinical practice and discussions with your teachers will indicate the required level of competence at each stage of your training. As you approach finals, your professional competence should be A or B, even if there are still gaps in your knowledge of specific diseases.

The texts are intended to refine your diagnostic approach, but they can also serve to revise the clinical features and investigation of specific conditions – this is facilitated by the refection and consolidation sections that bring together the salient features of each problem. Use the index to find the condition, and the icons in each scenario to locate individual stations for abnormal symptoms, signs and investigations. Consider how these abnormalities relate to the severity of the problem and how you would treat the patient at each stage of their disease.

Most stations refer to the reader as an FY1 doctor, rather than a medical student: this emphasises that the qualifying examination is to ensure that you are well trained and safe to progress to this level. The finals examiner expects fluency of your diagnostic approach, a reasoned differential diagnosis, and a caring and complete understanding of patient management.

# Acknowledgements

Thanks to Rebecca Spendiff, Consultant Radiologist at Colchester General Hospital

# How to use this book

The OSCEs in this text are based on 19 clinical problems (scenarios), and follow their management through diagnosis and treatment: thus reflecting the typical process used in clinical practice. In this case-based format, you need information for each station, but it must not give clues that could pre-empt subsequent questions and answers. To facilitate this, you are advised to work in pairs, one acting as a candidate and the other as the examiner – if you are the examiner, use the grey shaded patient instructions to respond to the candidate's questions, and then use the examiner's questions to assess and mark the candidate's performance. The patient/carer scripts state what information should be volunteered and areas that should be left for the candidate to actively explore. A third member can act as the patient for the **History** and **Examination** stations. Rotate the roles so that you all experience the various components of the OSCE format.

Each scenario is made up of a number of stations: the questions for these are sequential, followed by the answer section. The type of station content is indicated by a specific icon, so that they can be quickly identified in the question and answer sections. Cases do not necessarily have all types of station, but each begins with a **History**, followed by an **Examination** station. The **History** station starts with an instruction to the candidate, specifying their role and what is expected of them, eg whether you should take a full history or concentrate on a specific aspect – **read all OSCE instructions very carefully**. If not specified, take a full history of the presenting complaint and question the patient's past – drug use, allergies, social and family history – and undertake a systemic enquiry (by finals this should be a rapid review, and it is the examiner's job to ensure that you do not miss important information, as this could be detrimental in your subsequent clinical practice).

As you approach finals, you are expected to be competent in patient management, particularly in taking a history and examining a patient. You will probably have revised the factual content of clinical problems, but this series also gives prominence to the professionalism, the diagnostic process, your **Clinical communication skills** and the **diagnostic reasoning** that must underpin your answers. All participants must read the paragraphs on each history page to understand the meaning of the previous sentence. Icons are used to both emphasise these features in the examiner's assessment and to avoid writing them out again in full.

When assessing the history taking and presentation, the examiner gives a mark for content, professionalism, the diagnostic process, communication skills and, when questioned, the candidate's diagnostic reasoning, followed by a global mark for the whole – be aware that the examiner is taking into account all these elements of your history taking.

Marking is not further discussed in this section, but for more information on the subject go to page xxii. Similarly go to page xv for discussion on timing – examination circuits have to run to a schedule, and the time allowed for a station is usually more than adequate for a fair assessment. Be aware of the suggested times in the text, but you can be fluid in their use, as between you, you should cover and discuss all aspects of each station.

Your examination can be carried out, and assessed, on a model or a mannequin. Although abnormal signs are absent, with your partners, you can talk through the clinical features you are looking for and the techniques you are using, as you would in an observed examination station in finals. One of you acting as the model, or the examiner, can indicate the abnormal findings present as the examination proceeds. Again read the instructions with icons on the initial examination sheet and make sure they are taken into account in your presentation and assessment. An alternative approach is also given – the examination findings are provided, to be read and then presented (pages 379–390). Take enough time to take in this material, but be aware that a time may be suggested in finals. (The difficulty of avoiding pre-emptive clues in a text has already been mentioned – **avoid reading these pages before examining a model**.)

**Clinical communication skills** are essential in clinical practice and a number of these stations have been included to assess your approach to difficult explanations, such as surgical consent and terminal illness. Read the instructions thoroughly, including the additional icon linked material: be aware that, as with the **History** and **Examination** stations, the examiner is assessing your skills and training in all these areas.

**Data interpretation** is a key domain in your final assessment. Normal values are usually embedded in the question, but commit normal values of common investigations to memory. The questions in some of these stations are extended beyond the single case of the scenario, to expand their educational and assessment value.

The assessment of **Prescribing skills** is a mandatory part of finals (page xxi): as the NHS does not have a standard prescription chart, use either that of your local trust, or photocopy the chart(s) at the back of this book (page 391). In view of the potential harmful effect on patient safety, you must spend time to ensure competency in this area: marking must be stringent. Compare your answers with those in the text to ensure their accuracy in every detail.

**Procedural skills** cannot be assessed on patients in finals, but models or mannequins may be appropriate, or the candidate's understanding of the relevant apparatus can be tested. The text follows the same pattern and covers the competencies that are expected of a qualifying doctor (page xxi).

The **Consolidation and Reflection** section summarises the case and its components, and can serve as a reminder of these facts on completion of the scenario or at a later date. This information can be expanded and reinforced by use of the **Further reading** section.

# Introductory chapter

## Diagnostic medical graduates

Professor Sir George Paget introduced clinical assessments into the graduating finals at Cambridge University in the 1840s. Some may suggest that little changed until Harden and Gleason introduced the Objective Structured Clinical Examination (OSCE) in 1975. OSCEs, a derivation from the traditional approach of clinical short cases, and the 'bell day' or 'steeplechase' used in many anatomy examinations, introduced and reinforced several educationally important concepts. Perhaps most importantly, each student taking a formal clinical examination underwent a similar, objective and structured assessment. Their performance was observed by multiple examiners who marked the candidates' performance against a validated set of criteria, recorded on an itemised checklist.

Despite their 'educational excellence' it was not until the 1990s that they were fully embraced and developed further by the UK Medical Schools. However, like the 'Pagetoid' Final Examinations of the 19th and 20th century, over the last 10 years (both nationally and internationally) OSCEs have largely stagnated, and their reliability and defensibility, so important in an era of increasing litigation, have come to totally dominate other psychometric aspects, in particular face and content validity.

OSCEs are made up of a circuit of 'stations', each station being a self-contained area (a room or cubicle) in which the candidate is asked to perform a given clinical task. The tasks are largely independent of one another and the knowledge and skills utilised in one are neither required nor utilised in subsequent stations. The tasks may vary in duration but are often artificially remodelled and time limited by the practicalities of the examination.

As the candidate proceeds around the circuit they are asked to perform tasks in multiple and varying contexts and roles, each task observed by a different assessor. Whilst these multiple clinical 'biopsies' are the strength of the OSCE, this format poorly reflects the reality of working in the clinical environment, and students move from task to task with little or no testing of the linked diagnostic process required when seeing a single, 'real' patient.

In the earlier phases of the course, ie until such time as a student can demonstrate minimal competence, students and the assessments rightly concentrate on the content and to a far lesser extent the process, of the tasks. Sadly the 'what' (content), rather than the 'how' (process) has become the priority for the majority of students and has resulted in the modern phenomenon of the 'OSCE performance'; students enacting a performance to gain the necessary pass marks. This is sadly repeated in all station-based examinations, including final MB graduating examinations, and latterly has been creeping into the PACES assessment of the MRCP.

At graduation candidates should be expected to function at a more sophisticated level, being challenged and assessed around the 'how, when and why' and not simply the 'what.' In short our assessments need to encourage and test the **clinical diagnostic process and reasoning**.

## Clinical diagnostic process

In its simplest form the diagnostic process consists of taking a history from a patient, examining them, formulating a diagnosis, and then planning appropriate investigation and the subsequent therapeutic interventions. This involves a complex interaction between knowledge and skills, and is difficult to define, teach and perhaps most importantly, learn and assess.

## Diagnostic history + diagnostic examination = diagnostic clinical assessment

Imagine you are a clinician in the middle of nowhere, for example on an arctic expedition, on board a 747 mid Pacific, or in the outback of Australia or rural Africa. There are no triage teams, no monitoring machines or near patient testing, and CRP is the local beer. Given the limited clinical resources you may have at your disposal you must formulate an action plan based on the severity of the presentation. In the 'middle of nowhere' this may mean asking a plane with 400 fellow passengers on board to land, calling in the flying doctor service, rescue vessels or even an extraction team, so you had better be right! Now one begins to understand the potential importance of a diagnostic clinical assessment. By taking a history and performing a full, appropriate examination, one derives a working diagnosis and differentials. From these arise the management plan, including investigations and therapeutic interventions

*The history* should be well structured, appropriate to the severity of the presentation, and should include all important and relevant information. This process can only be achieved if supported by the necessary background knowledge. One must also be able to present this history in a logical, coherent and appropriate manner so that others can assist and intervene as required.

The subsequent *clinical examination* should confirm or refute the initial list of differentials from the history, and include such things as supporting evidence, eg associated risk factors. Thus the history and examination are intimately related and together form the '*clinical assessment*'. This assessment needs to acknowledge the '**severity of the presentation**', and should be used to target / focus the '*action plan*', ie the subsequent investigations and management, including procedures and other therapeutic interventions: but above all, this assessment must lead to a working diagnosis. Whether one is learning the process as a novice or taking a history as a senior clinician, the focus must be diagnostic. This diagnostic focus is perhaps the thing that separates doctors from many other clinicians.

How do we teach and learn these processes, knowledge and skills? There is a definite pathway of maturation from the competent FY1 to the experienced senior clinician. However, the way a working FY1 assesses a patient and formulates an action plan, increasingly bears less resemblance to that of our graduating finalists, and is almost unrecognisable in our novice clinical students. It is difficult to identify where this disjunction arose. Some may say it has ever been thus, but if so, it may reflect our over-reliance and underdevelopment of the OSCE: our over-dependence on this single clinical assessment format has reinforced and even exaggerated these differences. It is time for our teaching, the clinical learning environment we create, and the assessments we use, to promote and recognise this maturation process, and reverse the trend away from simple 'performance' and back towards focussed, diagnostic assessment and management.

## Back to the future

Most undergraduate OSCE stations utilise detailed, itemised checklists. These checklists and the duration of stations, mean students have become 'performance' orientated. The format of the objective checklist encourages students to work their way through the items on the list, gaining the necessary marks to pass the task, but failing to think about the clinical meaning and importance of their findings. Rarely are students required to act upon the clinical information they have gathered. Unchallenged and untested decisions and conclusions have no impact on the care of simulated patients and manikins.

## Scenario (case/patient)-based assessment

This series of books promotes a new approach to the OSCE, developing a scenario-based assessment for the 21$^{st}$ century. Circuits consist of a series of clinical cases or scenarios. We suggest three or four cases be used in a major summative assessment, reflecting realistic and deliverable circuits, but the number may vary with cohort numbers and available resources. Each case / scenario is subdivided into a number of sequential, interdependent tasks (typically five or six), always starting with a history taking station and progressing through stations on the relevant examination, data interpretation, procedures and clinical therapeutics. **Linking** the tasks together promotes clinical diagnostic reasoning, and the application and utilisation of knowledge and skills, requiring candidates to think and act on the clinical information they have gathered in previous stations. As the stations and tasks are linked, the candidate must start at station 1, and move through each of the subsequent stations in the given order. In real life, each task is performed with or on the same patient and their carers. But to retain the OSCEs' strength of multiple reviews by multiple people each task is performed at a separate station, observed by a different person.

## Domain based checklists

We have also promoted a more clinical approach to the tasks by removing the detailed itemised lists. Each station is subdivided into **DOMAINS**, and these are marked globally from Grade A (Excellent) to Grade E (Clear Fail). The items within each of the generic domains are considered below, and repeated (both boxed and with unique **icons**) at the start of the history and examination stations. The CONTENT ('what you did') domain differs between cases and is retained full.

We hope through use of these domain based prompts you will think about what you are doing and the relevance of the clinical findings, rather than simply your 'performance'. In the following paragraphs we have indicated the typical percentage of the total marks that each domain represents within a given station. This reinforces their relative importance, not only in each station but in the examination overall – reflecting the significant contribution these areas make to the care of patients, their carers and to effective team working.

We have reintroduced a number of important generic tasks that need reinforcement at an undergraduate level. These include assessment of (a) clinical diagnostic reasoning through a structured viva voce at the end of most stations, and (b) presentation skills – including presenting diagnostic summaries and interpretation of histories and examination findings. The 'ideal' presentation of history and examination can be found at the end of each case, along with weblinks and further reading.

**Mixing observed and unobserved stations** – purists may suggest that many of the unobserved stations we have included are simply written assessments, and argue that these have no place in an OSCE. However, they assess contextualised knowledge that occurs in real life – interpreting clinical data, challenging knowledge around differentials, therapeutics and completing relevant forms, eg a death certificate. With the increasing sophistication and utilisation of computer-based assessment, the often arbitrary division 'written' and 'clinical' assessment will probably blur and even merge in the near future.

## OSCEs for finals

The OSCEs for Finals Series aims to prepare you for finals with common case-based scenarios that provide you with a broad cover of the curriculum. Early in your course you can work slowly through these cases, learning how to approach a clinical problem, while later you can use the cases to manage problems that you are likely to encounter in finals, and under examination conditions.

The following paragraphs consider the design of the scenario-based OSCE, the domains we have chosen and the scoring system: these are of interest to both teachers and students. If, however, you are already conversant with these aspects of the assessment and just want to get on with it, go to 'How to use this book' on page ix, and proceed.

## Scenarios

This text contains 19 clinical scenarios; each is subdivided into five or six tasks, starting with taking a history from a patient or relative / carer, and progressing to the relevant diagnostic examination, data interpretation, procedures, therapeutic interventions and explanation stations. Unlike traditional OSCE circuits, students must all begin at a history station at the start of a given scenario, and thus the subsequent stations remain empty until such time as each student has passed through their starting history station and moved on sequentially through the tasks.

In the book we have tried to make all stations ten minutes in duration, but some are divided into two or three tasks: these timings are guestimates and you may find them too short or too long, depending on your year and level of skills. In a real examination this needs careful consideration and matching. We have also largely ignored the resources (especially trained examiners) required to run such examinations, but feel assessment teams may mix and match stations and scenarios to take account of such important issues.

You should work your way sequentially through each scenario before attempting a second. This allows the instructions of each station within a given scenario to give confirmatory findings regarding the preceding station, eg after completing the history, the examination instructions may confirm the working diagnosis and ask you to examine for additional diagnostic evidence. The data interpretation and therapeutic stations may give further confirmatory information, allowing all students to start the stations on equal footing, regardless of how they performed and the conclusions they reached in the preceding station. Although this 'double jeopardy' is true of real life working, ie if you get the diagnosis wrong all your subsequent actions, including investigations and interventions, are likewise wrong (double jeopardy), in an assessment where one is interested in the task as much as the correct answer, this needs to be avoided.

The **answer section** of each scenario is made up of several key elements:
(a)  **Patient, relative/carer scripts** (with shaded background) – these are paired with the appropriate histories and clinical communication stations. They facilitate a student role play of the various characters involved in the scenario
(b)  **Content** – this contains the icons of the three or four **constituent domains** within the larger itemised contents box. This content box is principally for the benefit of student learning and revision. In summative OSCEs, appropriately trained clinicians act as examiners, and as with other domains, in an examination, this box is simply presented as an icon or space. The repetition of the icons should prompt you to think about important clinical issues such as professionalism, diagnostic reasoning, process, presentation and communication skills.
(c)  The succinct '**presentation**' to colleagues of key, diagnostic findings is an essential skill that is rarely taught, and poorly learnt in the busy clinical areas of today's NHS. In each of the examination question stations we have provided a list of 'key' clinical findings (pages 379–390). Study these lists and present them to a colleague as if they are in the named clinical area.

**Presentation** is not an easy skill to master. However, as you approach graduation it is essential that you progress from merely being able to complete a history or examination in the correct order, as a novice clinician, to a more diagnostic appreciation and holistic approach. Through practice using these books with colleagues, and in the clinical areas to senior clinical colleagues, such presentations become second nature. Take note of how different clinical contexts allow for different presentations. Think how you might present cases to colleagues, on teaching rounds, business rounds, over the phone or written in the medical records or a referral letter. Each has its own skills and nuances and can only truly be learnt experientially within the clinical environment.

Keeping good medical notes is also an essential skill required of all graduating students, and although this is beyond the scope of these books, we recommend you think about how you would write up these cases in the medical notes.

(d) **Clinical diagnostic reasoning** – these boxes are set out as a structured viva voce; several questions are included towards the end of each station allowing assessment of diagnostic reasoning, data interpretation and therapeutic intervention.

(e) **Reflection and consolidation** – At the end of each scenario there is a diagnostic summary box that should prompt you to reflect on your performance, knowledge and skills. The case presentations are examples of an A-grade requirement. They are also a rapid reference for consolidating knowledge in the lead up to examinations.

(f) **Further reading and web links** – These direct you to key, up to date guidelines and other useful reading.

## Domains

If one looks at a typical itemised checklist used in undergraduate OSCEs it contains several generic items that are common to many stations, eg hand cleaning, introduction, gaining consent, formal completion, demonstrating a caring and professional attitude and a logical approach. These can be grouped together under common themes, or domains. Each domain is similar whatever the focus of the station. By including the domains, rather than the individual items, we hope students who have mastered the basic knowledge and skills of a given task will refocus away from the 'tick box mentality' and back towards a more holistic and diagnostic approach.

The following section explains each of the domains contained in these volumes. They are an amalgamation of our own observations, and domains used in other formal clinical assessments, eg PACES (MRCP). The explanations include typical items that are included in these domains with the icons as they appear within the book. Within these explanations there is also an indication of the percentage of marks that each domain might represent in a given station, and this in turn should guide you as to the proportion such domains represent of the total exam marks. For examiners and students this potentially allows for more meaningful and focussed feedback. When viewed in such a strategic light, you will appreciate how these essential but often disregarded components differentiate the excellent from the competent, and the competent from the failing student.

It remains almost impossible to define what makes a good doctor. The heterogeneity of the various specialities and the characteristics of their specialists exclude a simple, unifying answer. However, if you ask the general public what they want from their doctor, common, essential characteristics emerge, including professionalism, demonstrating a caring and empathetic manner, and being knowledgeable and skilful. These are reflected in the domains we and others include in our stations.

## Domain – Professionalism

**What is being assessed?** These are the holistic skills and attributes that are implicit in being a good doctor. Individually they are easily defined and effects are often far more than their sum. In the clinical arena they include NHS or locally regulated dress code, cleanliness, punctuality, caritas, reliability, trustworthiness, honour and attitude. These are extremely difficult to measure in an OSCE situation and so we rely on such items as hygiene, appearance / dress code, and elements of communication and process (checking patient identity, explanation of role) as proxies of true professionalism. Despite this use of proxies in exams, all clinicians should think about how they present themselves to their patients and how they interact with them.

Typical percentage
of a station
5 – 10%

**Typical items included from checklists**
- Professional appearance (NHS dress code) – including general appearance, hair and jewellery
- Maintains patient and personal safety
- Polite introduction; identifies patient or interviewee correctly; confirms patient's date of birth from name band or other source
- Obtains informal consent; maintains patient's privacy
- Displays empathetic and caring attitudes and behaviours throughout.

## Domain – Process

**What is being assessed?** Process is 'how' one completes a task. Whilst the majority of undergraduates concentrate on the content items on the checklists, many are unaware or disregard the process, ie how they achieve the end result. At the novice stage this approach may be quite appropriate but as one clinically matures, process becomes increasingly important, ensuring clinical acceptability (as defined by patients' expectations, colleagues, guidelines and professional standards), and a clinically relevant, appropriate and functional outcome. Whilst simulation has an important role in learning and practising clinical skills, low fidelity manikins cannot tell a student they are hurting them, have poor technique or are uncaring. Students often define OSCE tasks by the title of the station, eg in a phlebotomy station, students regard the task as ending up with blood in a blood bottle regardless of **how** they obtain that blood. It may be suggested that in real life, the process is the part that keeps you and the patient safe, and defines defensible practice. Ignoring these important factors often increases the likelihood of complication and harm.

Typical percentage
of a station
10 – 20%

### Typical items included from checklists

### In the History
- Good organisation and structure; appropriate use of open and closed questions
- Appropriate fluency / rhythm / pace to the interview – this may change depending on environment and acute nature of problem
- Allows appropriate time for patient to respond / reply to questions
- Appropriately acknowledges difficult or emotional areas of the patient's history.

### In the Examination
- Appropriate fluency / rhythm / pace to the examination – this may change depending on environment and acute nature of problem
- Organisation and structure of examination; sensitive and empathetic approach
- Uses appropriate clinical techniques throughout
- Maintains privacy and dignity throughout.

## Domain – Content

**What is being assessed?** This domain makes up the majority of marks within any given station, and has been largely left as an itemised checklist in these new volumes. Although this goes against our move towards a holistic / diagnostic focus it cannot be avoided if these volumes are to be useful aids to facilitate students' learning. In post-graduate examinations (eg PACES) and at medical schools where they are using domain-based checklists, this domain, like all the others, is simply represented by a box with a grading system, and it is left to the 'expert' examiner to use their experience and judgement as to the coverage of the task by the candidate.

Typical percentage of a station
60 – 70%

Students will focus on this domain for examination purposes, but we once again remind you that it is often their 'overall' performance that influences an examiner's global mark, and their 'excellence' of content may be downgraded by poor hygiene, communication, appearance and attitudes. Although these are rarely considered or practised by students, they may lead to your downfall.

## Domain – Clinical communication
## (in History and Examination stations)

**What is being assessed?** This incredibly important part of the doctor–patient interaction has become increasingly rewarded within procedure and clinical examination stations. It is now common for manikins to be 'molded' to a simulated patient to facilitate a more realistic interaction during a procedure or examination, eg DRE, vaginal and breast examination, and phlebotomy, arterial blood gas sampling and insertion of an intravenous cannula. Newly qualified clinicians quickly realise how essential these elements can be in calming, instilling confidence and building rapport with acutely ill, frightened or emotional patients.

Typical percentage of a station
5 – 10%

**Typical items included from checklists for clinical communication**

**In the History**
- Demonstrates a caring and sympathetic attitude
- Asks open questions
- Invites patient to ask questions and answers them appropriately
- Addresses patient's ideas, concerns and expectations.

**In an examination or procedure**
- Explains purpose of examination / procedure; explains examination / procedure as it proceeds
- Offers information in a clear, structured and fluent manner; avoiding jargon
- Listens to patient and responds appropriately
- Demonstrates appropriate body language.

## Domain – Clinical diagnostic reasoning (CDR)

**What is being assessed? This domain assesses**
- The quality of the information the student has gathered from their interaction with the patient, and
- How they are able to apply and utilise this information to the patient in front of them.

Typical percentage of a station

20 – 25%

Typically you are asked to present your history or clinical findings to the examiner, and are expected to demonstrate how you arrived at your clinical diagnosis. Subsidiary questions are directed around the major differentials diagnoses, and the future management of the patient, including investigations and therapeutic interventions.

Unlike the novice clinician, the graduating student must develop a method of synthesising this information as they proceed through the history or examination process, and be ready to present and utilise it a short period after completing these tasks. It is a difficult skill to learn but one that is essential in the time-pressured atmosphere of the 21st century NHS.

## Other Stations and icons used in these books

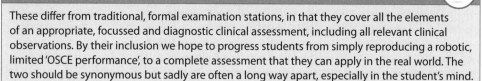

### Examination station

These differ from traditional, formal examination stations, in that they cover all the elements of an appropriate, focussed and diagnostic clinical assessment, including all relevant clinical observations. By their inclusion we hope to progress students from simply reproducing a robotic, limited 'OSCE performance', to a complete assessment that they can apply in the real world. The two should be synonymous but sadly are often a long way apart, especially in the student's mind.

### Clinical findings

The balloon icon denotes the clinical examination details for all scenarios given on pages 379–390. This is given separately to avoid prompting a candidate before he/she reaches the examination. When a model is available, they should read both the patient history and these examination details and act-out the findings, presenting them to the candidate at appropriate times in the examination. If no model is available, read this information carefully, organising it into systems so that it is easily recalled. No time limit is given for this task, as it is more important for the information to be fully understood, and the time needed varies between individuals; it reduces considerably with experience. We encourage you to listen to, read and reflect upon the way clinical information is presented in different clinical contexts. Presentation of information, verbal (face to face), verbal (telephone), written in the medical records, via email or referral letter all have particular nuances and skills and we hope these volumes challenge you to reflect upon and improve your own abilities in these areas. **[NB If you have a model do not read this section]**

## Data interpretation

These stations include interpretation of haematological, biochemical, microbiological, radiological and specialist investigation results. The majority of the data is directly relevant to the patient case (scenario) but we have used 'poetic license' to extend this to include data that is commonly assessed within final graduating examinations. Although it is common practice to allow candidates to use normal values embedded within the assessment, we encourage you to learn the normal ranges of common clinical data.

## Communication skills

This is an important part of history taking, as considered above: independent communication stations focus on specific, difficult areas such as consent and giving important or difficult news to a patient or carer.

## Prescribing

These (and other) stations cover all aspects of prescribing and in particular ensure you are confident in the types of skills and knowledge being assessed in the new national Prescribing Skills Assessment (PSA). These include:

- Prescription review
- Adverse drug reactions
- Drug calculations
- Communication with patients
- Data interpretation
- Drug monitoring
- Planning therapeutic management
- Prescribing.

We encourage you to use locally employed drug and fluid prescribing charts but have also provided copies that can be photocopied (page 391): use the Drug memo (page 396) to be sure you include all relevant data

## Procedure stations

The Foundation Programme Application System (FPAS) and Tomorrow's Doctors (2009) set out a series of 20 – 30 competencies that all graduating students must be proficient with before starting their FY1 employment. We have ensured that all of these competencies are fully covered through this series of books. We recommend that you are familiar with all the procedures included in these documents and are both competent and confident in your ability to perform them.
www.gmc-uk.org/static/documents/content/GMC_TD_09__1.11.11.pdf
www.foundationprogramme.nhs.uk/pages/home

> **Consolidation and reflection**
>
> This section, at the end of each scenario is to encourage you to reflect on your skills and knowledge in the key areas covered. You should find the section useful to direct your learning and examination preparation. The history and examination sections can be used as a guide to presenting the key diagnostic information in an appropriate manner for both clinical practice and graduating OSCEs.

> **Further reading and web links**
>
> This concluding section contains useful web links and reading that we have used when writing the scenarios.

## Setting the pass mark using domain-based lists

The standard setting of the pass / fail cut off, ie the pass mark in high stakes summative assessments (like finals) has become increasingly sophisticated and important over the past 20 years. The general public, the GMC, clinical colleagues and peers wish to know that newly graduating doctors have passed a robust set of assessments that are able to differentiate the competent from the incompetent. Likewise, students want to be certain that their performance can be quantified as a pass or fail with a reasonable degree of certainty.

Most UK undergraduate OSCE assessments utilise two methods to pass and fail candidates. The first is an absolute score. Each item on the checklist is given a value according to its perceived importance and contribution to the overall task. These are then summed to give a total for each station. The pass mark for each station is set by a given standard setting method (see Global score and borderline regression method) and the mean of all the station pass marks is used as the pass mark for the examination.

The second method is the requirement to pass a given number of stations within each part of the OSCE, and of the overall number of stations; eg if an OSCE is made up of a total of 17 stations, a candidate might have to pass a total of 12 or more stations, regardless of their absolute score. Typically these 17 stations would consist of five clinical examination stations, six 'communication skills' stations and six procedure stations. It may be deemed that a candidate has to pass a minimum of four examination stations, four communication skills and four procedure stations, irrespective of their absolute score. These slightly arbitrary divides are used to stop candidates compensating very poor performance in one area with very strong performance in another.

Previously **norm referenced** methods were commonly used, whereby the distribution of examination marks were drawn out and a set percentage of the cohort passed or failed. This was an arbitrary division and did not take into account the variation in cohort performance. The same number would pass or fail regardless of the candidates' performance. Today **criterion referenced** methods are preferred. These measure the performance of the cohort against a given set of criteria, setting the pass mark prior to the examination. There is no set number of passing and failing students but such methods rely on large numbers of experienced examiners being involved in setting the scores.

## The global score

The **borderline group** method is an '**on the day**' criterion referenced method whereby candidates are graded against the expected performance and each other. Candidates are given a global grade at the end of the station based on the examiner's expert opinion. This does not contribute to the overall score but is used to define the pass mark of the station and the overall examination. Each student is graded as Competent, Borderline or Fail, or variations thereof. The 'borderline' students' checklist scores are added together and the mean of these scores is used to define the pass mark of each station. These mean scores are then added together, and this gives the pass mark for the whole examination. More recently the **borderline regression method** has become increasingly employed. This involves two borderline grades, Borderline Pass and Borderline Fail. These in turn are used to derive the pass mark.

In keeping with a borderline regression method we have chosen to have five grades, A – E for both our domains and our global scores. Whilst peers may not be expert enough to differentiate passing and failing performances, we hope teachers and students alike will appreciate the inclusion of these grades.

**A – Excellent** – This applies to a candidate who in the opinion of the assessor gives a near perfect or perfect performance. Such students often receive every available (or very nearly every available) mark within the station or the domain. Their technique, their interaction with the patient and their professionalism are all excellent, and are perhaps above the standard expected of a student at this level of training.

**B – Good** – This applies to a candidate who in the opinion of the assessor gives a good, but not perfect performance. This type of student is often awarded the majority of the available marks but their interaction, communication, clinical technique or fluency may not be quite as good as the excellent student.

**C – Borderline Pass** – This is a candidate who in the examiner's opinion was just competent and demonstrated techniques, knowledge and skills that perhaps raise a few concerns.

**D – Borderline Fail** – This is a candidate who in the examiner's opinion demonstrated techniques, knowledge and skills that raised a number of concerns, and is deemed just below the standard required to pass the examination.

**E – Clear Fail** – This is a candidate who in the opinion of the examiner has clearly failed the examination. They often have poor examination technique, poor knowledge and skills, and their interaction with the patient or examiner may be poor or dangerous.

In this series of books we have produced a hybrid checklist containing elements of an itemised checklist and domain-based list. If a pure domain-based list were to be used, each candidate would need to get a C (borderline pass) or above in all the domains and the global rating to pass the station. If it were needed to quantify the grades obtained, each element of each domain would need to be assigned a score by an expert set of judges / examiners. This is unnecessary in examinations where a pass or fail grade is awarded but may be necessary in examinations of excellence.

# Glossary

| | |
|---|---|
| 5-ASA | 5-amino salicylic acid |
| 5-FU | 5-Fluoro-uracil |
| 5HT | 5-Hydroxy-tryptamine |
| A2RB | Angiotensin 2 receptor blocker |
| AA | Alcoholics Anonymous |
| AB | Apex beat |
| ABGs | Arterial blood gases |
| ABE | Actual base excess |
| ABPI | Ankle-brachial pressure index |
| AC | Abdominal circumference |
| ACE inhibitors | Angiotensin converting enzyme |
| ACTH | Adrenocorticotrophic hormone |
| ACS | Acute coronary syndrome |
| ADH | Anti-diuretic hormone |
| ADL | Activity of daily living |
| AF | Atrial fibrilation |
| AFP | Alpha-fetoprotein |
| aGBM | Anti-glomerular basement membrane |
| AGT | Angiotensin |
| AHBe/c | Anti Hepatitis B envelope/core |
| AIDS | Acquired immune deficiency syndrome |
| AKA | Also known as |
| AKI | Acute kidney injury |
| Alb | Albumin |
| Alk phos | Alkaline phosphatase |
| ALT | Alanine amino-transferase |
| AMA | Anti-mitochondrial antibody |
| AMTS | Abridged mental test score |
| ANCA | Anti neutrophil cytoplasmic antibody |
| Anti dsDNA | Double stranded deoxyribonucleic acid |
| Anti-Jo | Specific antigen |
| Anti-La | Specific antigen |
| Anti-RNP | Ribonucleic protein |
| Anti-Ro | Specific antigen |
| Anti-SCL70 | Specific antigen |
| Anti-TPO | Anti-thyroid peroxidase |
| Anti-TG | Anti-thyroglobulin |
| AP | Antero-posterior |
| APC gene | Adenomatosis polyposis coli |
| APTT | Activated partial thromboplastin time |
| APVU | Alert; Pain; Voice; Unresponsive |
| ARDS | Adult respiratory distress syndrome |

| | |
|---|---|
| ARM | Artificial rupture of membranes |
| AS | Aortic stenosis |
| ASH | Action on smoking and health |
| ASMA | Anti-smooth muscle antibody |
| ASO(T) | Anti streptolysin-O-titre |
| AST | Aspartate amino-transferase |
| ATLS | Advanced trauma life support |
| AV | Arterio-venous |
| AV | Atrio-ventricular |
| aVF | Augmented voltage lead left lower leg |
| aVL | Augmented voltage lead left arm |
| AVPU | Alert, voice, pain, unresponsive (scale) |
| aVR | Augmented voltage lead right arm |
| AVSD | Atrioventricular septal defect |
| AXR | Abdominal X-ray |
| AZT | Azidothymidine (generic name: Zidovudine) |
| BAL | Broncho-alveolar lavage |
| BBB | Bundle branch block |
| BCC | Basal cell carcinoma |
| BCG | Bacille Calmette-Guerin |
| bd | Twice daily (bis die) |
| BE | Base excess |
| Beta HCG | Beta human chorionic gonadotrophin |
| BHL | Bilateral hilar lymphadenopathy |
| BiPAP | Biphasic positive airway pressure |
| BM | Bone marrow |
| BM stix | Blood monitoring |
| BMA | British Medical Association |
| BMI | Body mass index |
| BMR | Basal metabolic rate |
| BNF | British national formulary |
| BP | Blood pressure |
| bpm | Beats per minute |
| BRCA | Breast cancer susceptibility genes |
| BXS | Base excess |
| C | Cervical |
| Ca | Cancer |
| CA | Cyclic AMP |
| $Ca^{++}$ | Calcium |
| CABG | Coronary bypass graft |
| CAP | Community acquired pneumonia |
| CAGE questionnaire | Cut down annoyed guilty eye-opener |
| CAPD | Chronic ambulatory peritoneal dialysis |
| CBD | Common bile duct |
| CBG | Capillary blood glucose |
| $CCa^{++}$ | Corrected calcium |

| | |
|---|---|
| CD4 | A surface antigen principally found on helper-inducer T-lymphocyte |
| CDR | Clinical diagnostic reasoning |
| CEA | Carcinoembryonic antigen |
| CEX | Clinical evaluation exercise |
| CK | Creatinine phosphokinase |
| Cl | Chloride |
| CLL | Chronic lymphocytic leukaemia |
| cm | Centimetre |
| CML | Chronic myeloid leukaemia |
| CMV | Cytomegalovirus |
| CN | Cranial nerve |
| CNS | Central nervous system |
| CNS | Clinical nurse specialist |
| CO | Complaining of |
| $CO_2$ | Carbon dioxide |
| COCP | Combined oral contraceptive pill |
| COMT | Catechol $O$-methyl transferase |
| COPD | Chronic obstructive pulmonary disease |
| CPA | Cerebellopontine angle tumour |
| CPAP | Continuous positive airway pressure |
| CPN | Community psychiatric nurse |
| CPR | Cardio pulmonary resuscitation |
| Cr | Creatinine |
| CRAG | Cryptococcal antibody (test) |
| CRP | C-reactive protein |
| CRT | Capillary refill time |
| CS | Caesarean section |
| CSF | Cerebro-spinal fluid |
| CSU | Catheter specimen of urine |
| CT | Computerised tomography |
| CTG | Cardiotocography |
| CTPA | CT-pulmonary angiogram |
| CVA | Cerebro-vascular accident |
| CVP | Central venous pressure |
| CVS | Chorionic villi sampling |
| CWD | Consistent with dates |
| CXR | Chest radiograph |
| DCCT | Diabetes control and complications trial |
| DDAVP | Desmopressin, synthetic vasopressin |
| DIC | Disseminated intravascular coagulopathy |
| DIP joints | Distal inter-phalangeal joints |
| DKA | Diabetic keto-acidosis |
| dl | Decilitres |
| DLCO | Diffusion lung capacity for carbon monoxide |
| DM | Diabetes mellitus |

| | |
|---|---|
| DMC | Diagnostic memory clinic |
| DMSA | Dimercaptosuccinic acid |
| DNA | Deoxyribonucleic acid |
| DNAR | Do not attempt resuscitation |
| DOB | Date of birth |
| DoPS | Directly observed procedural skills |
| DP | Dorsalis pedis artery |
| DPLD | Diffuse parenchymal lung disease |
| DRE | Digital rectal examination |
| DSN | Diabetic specialist nurse |
| DT | Delirium tremens |
| D&V | Diarrhoea and vomiting |
| DVLA | Driving vehicle licensing authority |
| DVT | Deep vein thrombosis |
| ECG | Electrocardiogram |
| ED | Emergency Department |
| EDV | End diastolic department |
| EEG | Electroencephalogram |
| eGFR | Estimated glomerula filtration rate |
| EMQ | Extended matching question |
| ENT | Ear, nose and throat |
| ERCP | Endoscopic retrograde cholangiopancreatography |
| ESR | Erythrocyte sedimentation rate |
| ET | Exercise test |
| ETEC | Enterotoxigenic *Escherichia coli* |
| ETT | Exercise tolerance test |
| EUA | Examination under anaesthesia |
| FBC | Full blood count |
| FDP | Fibrin degredation products |
| FEV1 | Forced expiratory volume in one second |
| FFP | Fresh frozen plasma |
| FH | Family history |
| FHx | Family history |
| fl | Femtolitres |
| F:M | Female:male (ratio) |
| FNA | Fine needle aspirate |
| FPIO | Family practice – prescription chart |
| FRC | Functional residual capacity |
| FRIVII/R | Fixed rate intravenous insulin infusion/rate |
| FROM | Full range of movement |
| fT4 | Free thyroxine |
| FTA | Fluorescent treponemal antibody |
| FVC | Forced vital capacity |
| FY1/2 | Foundation year 1/2 |
| G | Gram |
| G6PD | Glucose 6 phosphate dehydrogenase |

| | |
|---|---|
| GABA | Gamma-amino butyric acid |
| GCS | Glasgow coma scale |
| GFR | Glomerula filtration rate |
| gGT | Gama-elutamyl transferase |
| GI | Gastrointestinal |
| GIT | Gastrointestinal tract |
| GP | General Practitioner |
| GRACE | Global registry of acute coronary events |
| GTN | Glyceryl trinitrate |
| GU | Genito-urinary |
| HASU | Hyperacute stroke unit |
| HAV | Hepatitis A virus |
| Hb | Haemoglobin |
| HbA-1c | Measure of glycosylated haemoglobin |
| HBA-1c | Haemoglobin A-1c |
| HBD | Hepatobiliary disease |
| HBe | Hepatitis Be |
| HC | Hepatitis C |
| $HCO_3^-$ | Bicarbonate |
| HCV | Hepatitis C virus |
| HHS | Hyperosmolar hyperglycaemic syndrome |
| HIB | *Haemophilus influenzae* type B (vaccine) |
| HIV | Human immunodeficiency virus |
| HLA | Human leucocyte antigen |
| HOCM | Hypertrophic cardiomyopathy |
| HONK | Hyperosmolar-non-ketotic |
| HR | Heart rate |
| HRCT | High resolution computerised tomography |
| HS | Heart sound |
| ICP | Intra-cranial pressure |
| ICU | Intensive care unit |
| IDDM | Insulin dependent diabetes mellitus |
| Ig | Immunoglobulin |
| IgM | Immunoglobulin M |
| IGT | Impaired glucose tolerance |
| IHD | Ischaemic heart disease |
| Im | Intramuscular |
| IMCA | Independent mental capacity advocate |
| INR | International ratio |
| IPF | Idiopathic pulmonary fibrosis |
| ISMN | Iso-sorbide mono-nitrate |
| ITU | Intensive therapy unit |
| IU | International unit(s) |
| IV | Intravenous |
| IVI | Intravenous infusion |
| IVP | Intravenous pyelogram |

| | |
|---|---|
| IVU | Intravenous urogram |
| JPS | Joint position sense |
| JVP | Jugularvenous pressure |
| K⁺ | Potassium |
| kg | Kilogram |
| kPa | Kilopascals |
| KUB | Kidneys/ureters/bladder |
| L | Litre |
| LAD | Left anterior descending |
| LBBB | Left bundle branch block |
| LDH | Lactate dehydrogenase |
| LDL | Low-density lipoprotein |
| LFT | Liver function tests |
| LKM-1 | Liver, kidney, muscle |
| LMA | Laryngeal mask airway |
| LMN | Lower motor neurone |
| LMW | Low molecular weight |
| LMWH | Low molecular weight heparin |
| LOC | Loss of conciousness |
| LT | Light touch |
| LTOT | Long-term oxygen therapy |
| LV | Left ventricle |
| LVEF | Left ventricular ejection fraction |
| m | Metre |
| MAOI | Mono-amine oxidase inhibitor |
| MAU | Medical admissions unit |
| MC&S | Microscopy, culture and sensitivity |
| MCH | Mean corpuscular haemoglobin |
| MCV | Mean corpuscular volume |
| MDT | Multidisciplinary team |
| mg | Milligram |
| Mg⁺⁺ | Magnesium |
| MI | Myocardial infarction |
| mmol | Millimoles |
| MMSE | Mini-mental state examination |
| MPTP | 1-methyl 4-phenyl-1.2.3.6 tetrahydropyridine |
| MR | Mitral regurgitation |
| MRA | Magnetic resonance angiogram |
| MRI | Magnetic resonance imaging |
| MRSA | Methicillin resistant staphylococcus |
| MS | Multiple sclerosis or Mitral stenosis |
| MSU | Mid-stream urine |
| Na⁺ | Sodium |
| NAD | No abnormality detected |
| NEC | Necrotising enterocolitis |
| Neut | Neutrophilis |

| | |
|---|---|
| NFA | No focal abnormality |
| NG(T) | Nasogastric (tube) |
| NIDDM | Non-insulin dependent diabetes mellitus |
| NIPPV | Noninvasive positive pressure ventilation |
| NIV | Noninvasive ventilation |
| NKDA | No known drug allergy |
| NMDA | N-methyl d-aspartate (antagonist) |
| Non-STEMI | ST elevation myocardial infarction |
| NSAID | Non steroidal anti-inflammatory drug |
| $O_2$ | Oxygen |
| Obs | Observations |
| OCP | Oral contraceptive pill |
| od | Omni die (once daily) |
| OGD | Oesophagogastroduodenoscopy |
| ORIF | Open reduction internal fixation |
| OSCE | Objective structured clinical examination |
| PA | Postero-anterior |
| $PaCO_2$ | Arterial pressure of carbon dioxide |
| PAD | Peripheral arterial disease |
| PAN | Perinuclear anti-neutrophilic |
| $PaO_2$ | Arterial pressure of oxygen |
| PCA | Patient-controlled analgesia |
| PCI | Percutaneous coronary intervention |
| PCR | Polymerase chain reaction |
| PCV | Packed cell volume |
| PD | Parkinson's disease |
| PDA | Patent ductus arteriosus |
| PE | Pulmonary embolism |
| PEA | Persistent electrical activity |
| PEFR | Peak expiratory flow rate |
| PERL(A) | Pupils equal reactive to light (and accommodation) |
| PET | Positron emission tomography |
| pH | Puissance d'Hydrogen $= - \log (H^+)$ |
| PICA | Posterior inferior cerebellar artery |
| Plats | Platelets |
| PMH | Previous medical history |
| Pmol | Picomol |
| PMR | Polymyalgia rheumatica |
| PND | Paroxysmal nocturnal dyspnoea |
| PNS | Peripheral nervous system |
| PO | Per oral |
| $PO_4^-$ | Phosphate |
| PP | Pin prick |
| PPP | Palpable peripheral pulses |
| PR | Per rectum |
| PQRST | ECG complex |

| | |
|---|---|
| PRN | As required (*pro re nata*) |
| PSM | Pansystolic murmur |
| PT | Posterior tibial artery |
| PT | Prothrombin time |
| Q | ECG wave |
| Qds | Four times/day (quarter in die) |
| QRST | ECG complex |
| RBC | Red blood count |
| RCT | Randomised, controlled trial |
| Retics | Reticulocytes |
| ROM | Range of movement |
| RV | Residual volume |
| SACD | Subacute combined degeneration of the spinal cord |
| SAH | Subarachnoid haemorrhage |
| SARS | Severe acute respiratory syndrome |
| Sats | Saturation |
| SCLC | Small cell lung cancer |
| SDH | Subdural haemorrhage |
| SE | Side effects |
| S-FJ | Sapheno-femoral junction |
| SHx | Social history |
| SIADH | Syndrome of inappropriate antidiuretic hormone secretion |
| SL | Sublingual |
| SLE | Systemic lupus erythematosus |
| SOA | Swelling of ankle |
| SOCRATES | Site/Onset/Character/Radiation/Association/Times/ Exacerbations/relieving factors/severity |
| SOL | Space occupying lesion |
| SpO2 | Saturation percentage oxygen |
| SpR | Specialist registrar |
| SROM | Spontaneous rupture of membranes |
| SSRI | Selective serotonin reuptake inhibitor |
| ST | ECG interval |
| ST 1-4 | Specialist trainee (years 1–4) |
| Stat | Statim (immediately) |
| STEMI | ST elevation MI |
| SVT | Supraventricular tachycardia |
| SXR | Skull X-ray |
| T | ECG wave/temperature/tablet |
| T2DM | Type 2 diabetes melitus |
| T3 | Tri-iodo-thyronine |
| T4 | Tetra-iodo-thyronine (thyroxine) |
| TB | Tuberculosis |
| TBil | Total bilirubin |
| TBM | Tuberculosus meningitis |
| T cholesterol | Total cholesterol |

| | |
|---|---|
| tds | Ter die sumendus – (to be taken three times daily) |
| TED | Thrombo-embolic |
| Temp | Temperature |
| TFTs | Thyroid function tests |
| TIA | Transient ischaemic attack |
| TIBC | Total iron binding capacity |
| TLC | Total lung capacity |
| TOP | Termination of pregnancy |
| TPA | Tissue plasminogen activator |
| TPN | Total paraenteral nutrition |
| TSH | Thyroid stimulating hormone |
| TT | Thrombin time |
| TTA | To take away (medication) |
| TTO | To take out (medication) |
| TVF | Tactile vocal fremitus |
| U&Es | Urea and electrolytes |
| UGIB | Upper gastrointestinal bleed |
| UGT/UGIT | Upper gastrointestinal tract |
| UMN | Upper motor neurone |
| UO | Urine output |
| Ur | Urea |
| USS | Ultrasound scan |
| UTI | Urinary tract infection |
| UV | Ultraviolet |
| V 1-6 | ECG chest leads |
| VDRL | Venereal disease research laboratory |
| VF | Ventricular fibrillation/vocal fremitus |
| VIB | Vibration |
| VNS | Vascular nerve specialist |
| V/Q scan | Ventilation/perfusion scan |
| VSD | Ventricular septal defect |
| VTE | Venous thrombo-embolic |
| WBC | White blood cell |
| WCC | White cell count |
| YO | Type 1 purkinje cell cytoplasmic autoantibodies (PCA-1) |

# Scenario 1:
# 'No post today'

## Station 1

*History*                    *10-minute station*

**You are the FY1 doctor on call with the Acute Medical Team. The next patient is Mr Mohammed Iqbal, who has been brought into the Emergency Department by ambulance after suffering an episode of severe chest pain while at work.**

- **Please take a focussed history from the patient with a view to presenting the history and likely diagnosis to the Medical Registrar.**

*You will be assessed on the following areas, as well as the content and diagnostic reasoning of your history – take them into account in your presentation.*

### Professionalism

- Professional appearance (NHS dress code) – including general appearance, hair and jewellery
- Maintains patient and personal safety
- Polite introduction; identifies patient or interviewee correctly; confirms patient's date of birth from name band or other source
- Obtains informal consent; maintains patient's privacy
- Displays empathetic and caring attitudes and behaviours throughout.

### Process

- Good organisation and structure; appropriate use of open and closed questions
- Appropriate fluency/rhythm/pace to the interview – this may change depending on environment and acute nature of the problem
- Appropriate time for the patient to respond/reply to questions
- Appropriate acknowledgement of difficult or emotional areas of the patient's history.

### Communication skills

- Demonstrates caring and sympathetic attitude
- Asks open questions
- Invites patient to ask questions and answers them appropriately
- Addresses patient's ideas, concerns and expectations.

## Station 2

*Examination*  *10-minute station*

After completing and presenting the history, the Medical Registrar asks you to perform a focussed examination of the patient. Mr Iqbal has been seen by the nurse in the resus area, and is attached to a cardiac monitor. The nurse has recorded Mr Iqbal's observations on the chart. You may ask for these during your assessment.

■ Please present the relevant findings to your colleague in an appropriate manner for a busy medical on call (if you do not have a model, please read and present the information on page 379).

*You will be assessed on the following areas, as well as the content and skills of your examination – take them into account in your presentation.*

### Professionalism

- Professional appearance; maintains infection control standards, including hand cleaning and appropriate use of gloves and aprons
- Maintains patient and personal safety
- Polite introduction; identifies patient and confirms date of birth from name band or other source
- Obtains informal consent; maintains patient privacy and dignity
- Displays empathetic and caring attitudes and behaviours throughout.

### Process

- Appropriate fluency/rhythm/pace to the examination – this may change depending on environment and acute nature of the problem
- Organisation and structure of examination; sensitive and empathetic approach
- Uses appropriate clinical techniques throughout
- Maintains privacy and dignity throughout.

### Clinical communication

- Explains proposed examination/procedure: explains examination/procedure as it proceeds
- Offers information in a clear, structured and fluent manner, avoiding jargon
- Listens to patient and responds appropriately
- Demonstrates appropriate body language.

## Station 3

*Data interpretation*                    *10-minute station*

Mr Iqbal's ECG shows global T-wave inversion, and he is transferred immediately to the CCU for ongoing management. The Medical Registrar on call is one of the cardiology trainees and hands you five ECGs belonging to patients on the CCU.

■ Please indicate whether each of the statements are TRUE (T) or FALSE (F) regarding each of the ECGs shown below. You may assume all ECGs are running at 25 mm/s.

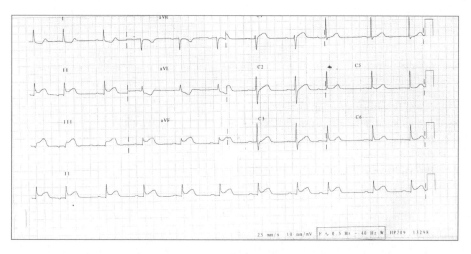

1

    A   The rhythm shown is sinus arrhythmia.

    B   There is evidence of first-degree heart block.

    C   There is anterior ST depression.

    D   There are inverted T waves in the lateral and high lateral leads.

    E   There are features to suggest an acute inferior STEMI.

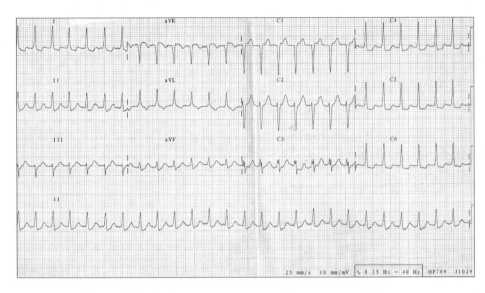

**2**

    A    There is left axis deviation.
    B    There is inferior ST segment depression.
    C    There is ST segment depression in the septo-lateral leads.
    D    There is evidence of poor anterior R-wave progression.
    E    The rhythm shown is atrial fibrillation.

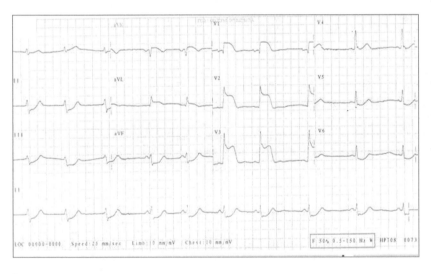

**3**

    A    There is both a nodal and sinus rhythm demonstrated.
    B    The axis is deviated to the right.
    C    There is ST depression in the infero-lateral leads.
    D    There is anterior ST elevation.
    E    This ECG pattern represents left main stem obstruction.

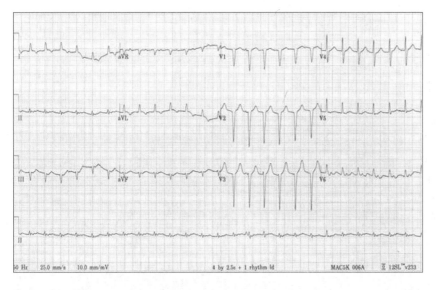

**4**

A   The rate is approximately 150 bpm.
B   There is left axis deviation.
C   There is T-wave inversion in the high-lateral leads.
D   There is normal anterior R-wave progression.
E   This patient is likely to have a normal LV ejection fraction.

SCENARIO 1

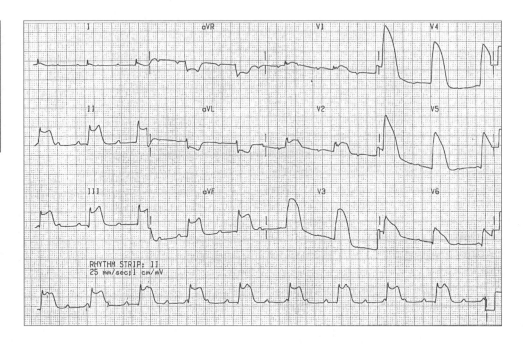

5

    A    This is Mobitz type I second-degree heart block.

    B    The axis is normal.

    C    There is anterior ST elevation.

    D    There is ST elevation in the infero-lateral leads.

    E    There is ST depression in the high lateral leads.

## Station 4

*Procedural skills*                        *10-minute station*

Mr Iqbal requires a second intravenous cannula inserted for his intravenous insulin infusion.

■ Please write up the fixed-rate intravenous insulin infusion on the chart provided.

   Mr Mohammed Iqbal; DOB 23/08/57; Hospital No. 5463721; Consultant
     Dr Westmore; Ward CCU; Bleep 332

**Procedure A**

■ Please make up the insulin infusion using the equipment provided, explaining the process to the examiner as you proceed.

**Equipment provided**

• 50 ml syringe, insulin (100 unit vial), 0.9% saline – 250 ml bag

• Needles to draw up medications, extension tubing

## Procedure B

■ Now please insert a cannula in the manikin arm, explaining the process to Mr Iqbal as you proceed. Connect the intravenous insulin infusion to the cannula.

### Equipment provided

- Gloves, alcohol swab to clean the skin, cannula, cannula dressing, tourniquet
- 0.9% saline flush, 5 ml syringe and needles

## Station 5

*Clinical communication skills*               *10-minute station*

Despite analgesia and other acute interventions, Mr Iqbal remains clinically too unstable to transfer to the local cardiac centre for acute percutaneous coronary intervention (PCI). The Cardiology Registrar on the evening CCU ward round decides that Mr Iqbal should receive terofiban and heparin, prior to transfer to the local 'heart centre'.

■ Please calculate Mr Iqbal's CRUSADE score using the admission data and the nomogram provided below and then explain to the Cardiology Registrar what this means, as if you were explaining it to the patient.

### Admission data

- o Investigations – FBC: Hb 12.9g/dl, MCV 87 fl, Hct (%) 43.6, WCC 14.3 x 109/l, platelets 223 x 109/l
- o eGFR 87 ml/min
- o Observations – HR 104 bpm, BP 183/98 mmHg (large cuff required), RR 18 bpm, $O_2$ sats 87% on air, temperature 36.5 °C, CBG 16.4 mmol/l
- o CV examinations – pulse 100 regular, low volume, normal character; no carotid or other bruits heard; BP 190/100, JVP not seen; heart sounds 1 + 2 + ? 3rd heart sound
- o Focussed examination – no ankle oedema; all peripheral pulses palpable; no ulcers or scars
- o RS examination: bibasal crackles to the midzones.

| Predictor | Range | Score |
|---|---|---|
| Baseline haematocrit (%) | <31 | 9 |
| | 31–33.9 | 7 |
| | 34–36.9 | 3 |
| | 37–39.9 | 2 |
| | ≥40 | 0 |
| Creatinine clearance (ml/min) | ≤15 | 39 |
| | >15–30 | 35 |
| | >30–60 | 28 |
| | >60–90 | 17 |
| | >90–120 | 7 |
| | ≥120 | 0 |

| Predictor | Range | Score |
|---|---|---|
| Heart rate (bpm) | ≤70 | 0 |
| | 71–80 | 1 |
| | 81–90 | 3 |
| | 91–100 | 6 |
| | 101–110 | 8 |
| | 111–120 | 10 |
| | ≥121 | 11 |
| Sex | Male | 0 |
| | Female | 8 |
| Signs of CHF at presentation | No | 0 |
| | Yes | 7 |
| Prior vascular disease | No | 0 |
| | Yes | 6 |
| Diabetes mellitus | No | 0 |
| | Yes | 6 |
| Systolic blood pressure (mmHg) | ≤90 | 10 |
| | 91–100 | 8 |
| | 101–120 | 5 |
| | 121–180 | 1 |
| | 181–200 | 3 |
| | ≥201 | 5 |

Note: heart rate is truncated at <70 bpm
CrCl: Cockcroft-Gault is truncated at >90 ml/min; prior vascular disease is defined as prior PAD or stroke

| The CRUSADE bleeding score to assess baseline risk of major bleeding in non-ST-segment elevation myocardial infarction | | |
|---|---|---|
| Risk group | CRUSADE score | Risk of major bleed |
| Very low | <21 | 3.1% |
| Low | 21–30 | 5.5% |
| Moderate | 31–40 | 8.6% |
| High | 41–50 | 11.9% |
| Very high | >50 | 19.5% |

# Answers

## Station 1 – History

**Patient script**

You are Mr Iqbal Mohammed (DOB 23 August 1957), a 54-year-old postal worker in the local post office depot. You were brought into the Emergency Department this morning at about 09:30 after having suffered a severe episode of chest pain.

Over the past 4–6 weeks you have been suffering with occasional episodes of chest pain that you initially thought was 'bad indigestion'. The first episode occurred while you were at work pushing some of the heavy trolleys around the depot. The pain was very tight and 'squeezing', 'like a band around my chest'. It only lasted about a minute but was really bad and took your breath away. You had to sit down for about 5 minutes before you felt OK again. Since then you've had two to three similar episodes, the last one while playing football with your grandson. This was a more severe and prolonged episode, lasting about 5 minutes or so, but you had to laugh it off as your grandson became frightened. The pain was severe, and central, radiating to your jaw and left hand. You were sweaty and felt sick but it went off by itself after you lay down on the ground after about 5–10 minutes.

Today's episode came on at the depot, just after you had finished your morning tea break. You were walking up a flight of stairs when the pain suddenly came on. This was different to all the other episodes.

The pain was severe (the worst you've experienced), 'squeezing and crushing the life out of me'. The pain was central, radiating to your jaw, left and right arms, but not through to your back. You collapsed down the stairs and your work colleague pulled you to safety and made a pillow for you with his jacket. Your colleague said 'it looked like all the life had drained out of me' and you were dizzy and faint but don't think you passed out. The pain continued for at least 10–15 minutes before the ambulance men arrived and gave you oxygen and some tablets up under your upper gums. You still feel as if you have a little chest discomfort but nothing like the pain you had earlier.

If asked you deny any symptoms of heart failure, eg peripheral oedema, orthopnoea, PND, shortness of breath, wheeze, dry cough or frothy white sputum.

Risk factors: your father and his parents all died of heart and stroke problems before the age of 70. You have two close cousins who have had heart attacks in the last few years. You smoked 20+ cigarettes/day until 4 or 5 years ago but stopped when your grandson was born. You do not drink any alcohol.

Your doctor told you recently that you were very overweight and this was putting you at risk for high blood pressure and diabetes. You are 5 feet 8 inches (1 m 72 cm) and 15 and a half stone. You don't know about your blood pressure. Your doctor told you to lose weight or he would have to start you on diabetes tablets. You do not know about your cholesterol and have never had symptoms suggestive of a stroke, peripheral vascular disease or IHD.

You have no significant previous medical history; you had an appendicetomy at 11 years old.

You are not on any regular medications, but do take the occasional 'zantac', Rennie tablets and paracetamol. You have no known allergies.

You are married with five children aged 26, 24, 21, 20 and 17 years. The youngest three still live at home, and two of them are unemployed. You work in the local post office depot and are the shop steward of the local postal union.

You think you may have had a heart attack this morning as the pain was so bad and you felt so unwell. You are hoping that it's nothing too serious, as you need to get back to work soon. You are the main breadwinner in the house, and everyone is reliant on you.

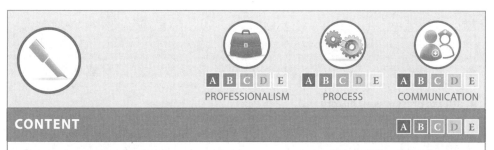

PROFESSIONALISM — A B C D E

PROCESS — A B C D E

COMMUNICATION — A B C D E

SCENARIO 1

## CONTENT

A B C D E

**Identifies key information**
- Pain: chronological progression; onset, frequency, duration, character, radiation, relieving and exacerbating factors
- Associated features: shortness of breath, nausea and vomiting, dizziness, presyncope and syncope, feeling unwell, washed out, palpitations.

**Includes important negatives, including systemic enquiry**
- No radiation to the back (thoracic aortic aneurysm)
- No features of heart failure: peripheral oedema, orthopnoea, PND, shortness of breath, wheeze, dry cough, frothy white sputum
- No features suggestive of gastrointestinal or hepatobiliary disease
- Excludes other systemic symptoms.

**Identifies key information from rest of history**
- Cardiovascular risk: family history, known IHD, stroke or PVD, diabetes mellitus, hypertension, smoking, alcohol, others
- Relevant facts about employment, housing, social support, life stressors.

**Completing the patient history**
- Drug and allergy history: Zantac and indigestion tablets; occasional paracetamol; no known drug allergies
- Previous medical history: nil known
- Social and occupational history: as above.

**Summarises important areas of the history back to the patient**

**Invites patient to ask questions and deals with them appropriately**

**Establishes patient's ideas, concerns and expectations**

11

## CLINICAL DIAGNOSTIC REASONING

- **Please present your history**
  - Candidate offers a logical, well-structured account of the history.

- **What is your diagnosis?**
  - Candidate offers the correct diagnosis and appropriate differentials
  - The patient has presented with ACS but the history suggests a severe episode: MI?

- **Can you describe how you would manage this patient? What three essential bedside (clinical) investigations would you perform?**
  - Nurse in high-dependency area, cardiac monitor, IV access, aspirin and clopidogrel, oxygen and some further pain relief, eg IV morphine and anti-emetic; full examination and further investigations
  - BP, CBG, ECG, oxygen sats ± ABGs.

**Demonstrates safe, sensible and appropriate management plan**

**Demonstrates clear and logical diagnostic reasoning**

## GLOBAL HISTORY MARK

# Station 2 – Examination

**Patient script (see also page 379)**

If you are an actor/patient, read the patient history and physical signs fully – when the candidate comes to an abnormal site in their examination, act out tenderness and/or volunteer the relevant physical sign.

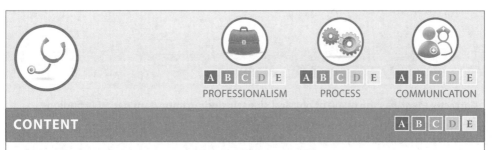

PROFESSIONALISM   PROCESS   COMMUNICATION

## CONTENT

A B C D E

**Exposes and positions patient correctly and maintains comfort**

**Comments on wellbeing of patient, ie well or unwell**

**'Feet to face'**
- Observes, and comments on patient and surroundings from foot of bed
- Evidence of previous cardiac surgery, eg sternotomy, JVP, anaemia, colour/perfusion.

**Asks for appropriate/relevant clinical observations**
- HR 104 bpm, BP 183/98 mmHg (large cuff required), RR 18 bpm, $O_2$ sats 87% on air, temperature 36.5 °C, CBG 16.4 mmol/l
- Urinalysis: WCC nil, protein 1+, blood negative, nitrites negative, glucose 3+.

**General/systemic examination**
- Hands and upper limbs: tar staining, perfusion of hands, anaemia, stigmata of hyperlipidaemia; comments on general signs, eg clubbing, leuconychia
- Face and neck: signs of anaemia, peri-orbital xanthelasma, central cyanosis.

**Focussed examination**
- Inspection: sternotomy scar, JVP – makes appropriate assessment, including correct positioning of patient, correct technique; comments correctly on JVP
- Palpation: carotid pulse – comments on character and presence of bruits
- Apex beat: position and character
- Assesses and comments on heaves and thrills
- Auscultation: listens in correct areas, assesses for radiation, manoeuvres patient correctly, appropriate use of stethoscope – bell and diaphragm.

**Completes examination by identifying relevant additional clinical signs**
- Signs of left and right heart failure: bibasal crackles, pleural effusions, peripheral oedema; hepatomegaly/ascites
- Signs of PVD and generalised atherosclerosis: AAA, peripheral pulses, abdominal bruits.

**Thanks patient, offers assistance, maintains patient's dignity and privacy until they are dressed**

## CLINICAL DIAGNOSTIC REASONING

Correctly identifies the relevant physical signs, including important negative findings

- **What does a third heart sound represent?**
  - Fluid overload in keeping with his heart failure

- **Given these clinical findings, can you name three acute therapeutic interventions you would arrange for this gentleman in the Emergency Department (he has already had oxygen, GTN spray and anti-platelet treatment)?**
  - Ongoing pain: further GTN or IV morphine and anti-emetics
  - Pulmonary oedema (bibasal crackles and hypoxia): oxygen to maintain sats between 94 and 98%, IV GTN infusion and IV furosemide; may require IV diamorphine (venodilator and analgesic, as above)
  - Hypertension: this would also be accounted for with the GTN infusion
  - CBG >11.0 mmol/l: IV insulin infusion (either sliding scale or FRIVII).

**Demonstrates safe, sensible and appropriate management plan**

**Demonstrates clear and logical diagnostic reasoning**

## GLOBAL EXAMINATION MARK

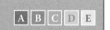

## Station 3 – Data interpretation

1    A True
     B True
     C False
     D False
     E True

This ECG demonstrates a large inferior STEMI with high lateral (I and aVL) ST depression. The antero-lateral leads are normal. There is sinus arrhythmia with first-degree heart block.

2    A False
     B True
     C True
     D True
     E False

This ECG demonstrates atrial flutter with 2 : 1 block. This is commonly seen in older patients who are acutely unwell with chest pathology, eg chest infection or pulmonary embolism, especially if there is underlying ischaemic heart disease. The axis is moving towards the left but because leads I and II are both very positive, this means the axis will remain within normal limits. There is septo-lateral (V3–V6) ST depression extending into the high lateral (I and aVL) leads. There is relatively absent R-wave progression in leads V1–V3.

3      A True
       B False
       C True
       D True
       E True

This ECG demonstrates a large anterior STEMI with deep ST depression in the infero-lateral leads. The rhythm is unstable owing to the acute ischaemia and starts as a nodal rhythm but progresses into sinus arrhythmia. The axis is neutral as all three leads are almost isoelectric. As all three territories of the heart demonstrate acute ischaemia, this would suggest there is left main stem disease with a dominant left circumflex artery.

4      A True
       B True
       C True
       D False
       E False

This ECG demonstrates atrial flutter with 2 : 1 block, giving the classical regular appearance at a rate of 150 bpm. There are several features of underlying ischaemic heart disease including left axis deviation, partial left bundle branch block and poor anterior R-wave progression. There is T-wave inversion in the high lateral leads (I and aVL). Given the rate and the features of the IHD, this patient will rapidly develop acute heart failure. They are unlikely to have a normal LV ejection fraction.

5      A False
       B True
       C True
       D True
       E True

This ECG demonstrates a massive STEMI involving the antero-lateral and inferior territories. There is also ST depression in lead aVL. There is third-degree (complete) heart block with a normal axis. This again may well represent left main stem disease with a dominant circumflex artery. This patient needs urgent coronary intervention.

## GLOBAL DATA INTERPRETATION MARK

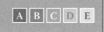

## Station 4 – Procedural skills

**SCENARIO 1**

| Allergies, sensitivities and adverse drug reactions | | | | | Patient details/addressograph | |
|---|---|---|---|---|---|---|
| No known allergies ☐ | | Initials | | Gender Ⓜ/ F | NHS/ Hospital No:  5463721 | |
| Not possible to ascertain ☐ | | Date | | Weight (kg)          Date | | |
| Medicine/substance | Reaction & Severity | Initials & Date | | 100 kg | Surname:  IQBAL | |
| | | | | Height | First name:  Mohammed | |
| Alerts | | | | Surface area (m²) | Date of birth:  23.08.57 | |

| Infusion prescriptions continued | | | | | | | | | | SC = subcutaneous | | IVC = intravenous central IVP = intravenous peripheral | | |
|---|---|---|---|---|---|---|---|---|---|---|---|---|---|---|
| Date & time | Route | Infusion Fluid | | | | Duration | Rate | Prescriber's signature & bleep no. | Date given | Given by / Added by | Check by | Start time | Finish time | Pharmacy |
| | | Name & strength | Volume | Approved name with expiry / unit number | Dose | | | | | | | | | |
| 07/05 | IV | 0.9 % saline Exp: Batch/unit no: | 50 ml | ACTRAPID INSULIN | 50 UNITS | TO RUN IV AT 0.1 UNITS/=10u/kg/hr kg/hr | | AF 622 | | | | | | |
| 07/05 | IV | Exp: Batch/unit no: | | 50 UNITS OF ACTRAPID INSULIN IN 50 mls OF 0.9% SALINE | | | | | | | | | | |
| | | Exp: Batch/unit no: | | TO RUN IV ACCORDING TO SLIDING SCALE CBG                        UNITS/HOUR | | | | | | | | | | |
| | | Exp: Batch/unit no: | | 0–4.0                        0 4.1–7.0                     1.0 | | | | | | | | | | |
| | | Exp: Batch/unit no: | | 7.1–11.0                   2.0 11.1–15.0                 3.0 | | | | | | | | | | |
| | | Exp: Batch/unit no: | | 15.1–21.0                 4.0 21.1–28.0                 5.0 | | | | | | | | | | |
| | | Exp: Batch/unit no: | | >28.0                        6.0 Please call DR if CBG >28.0 | | | | AF 622 | | | | | | |
| | | Exp: Batch/unit no: | | | | | | | | | | | | |
| | | Exp: Batch/unit no: | | | | | | | | | | | | |
| | | | | | | | | | | | | | | |
| | | | | | | | | | | | | | | |

## Procedure A: Intravenous insulin infusion

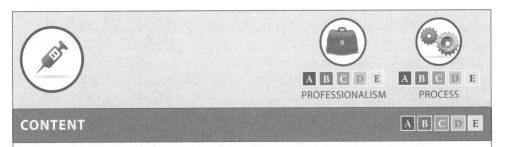

**CONTENT**  A B C D E

**Identifies and sets out equipment correctly; maintains aseptic technique throughout**
- Insulin vial (100 units)
- 250 ml bag of 0.9% saline
- Syringes
- Needles
- Medication label (sticker) to be completed by candidate.

**Correctly performs the procedure**
- Identifies patient from hospital bracelet (one cannot verbally confirm patient's name and DOB as he is confused)
- Puts on gloves
- For both drugs (0.9% saline and insulin): checks vial/bag for correct name of drug and expiry date
- Checks correct patient identity against prescription on the chart
- Breaks open 0.9% saline and draws up 50 ml into 50 ml syringe using 'green' needle
- Draws up 50 units of insulin using the appropriate needle and syringe
- Using a second needle adds the insulin to the normal saline
- Ensures insulin is adequately mixed with saline
- Correctly completes medication label and applies it to the syringe.

**Obtains an acceptable/appropriate result**

**Disposes of all sharps and other items correctly**

**Ensures patient receives correct advice about what to do next and follow-up**

**Ensures nursing staff or other healthcare professionals receive correct information about the consequences/outcome of the procedure/task**

**SCENARIO 1**

## Procedure B: Cannulation

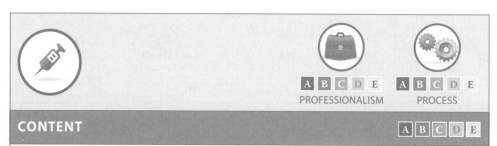

PROFESSIONALISM     PROCESS

A B **C** D E     A B **C** D E

### CONTENT

A B **C** D E

**Exposes and positions patient correctly and maintains comfort**

**Exposes forearm and assesses for appropriate vein**

**Identifies and sets out equipment correctly; maintains aseptic technique throughout**
- Gloves
- Alcohol swab to clean the skin
- Appropriate cannula (G14 or G16)
- Cannula dressing
- Tourniquet
- Extension tubing for cannula
- 0.9% saline flush
- 5 ml syringe and needles
- Labelled insulin infusion
- Sharps bin.

**Correctly performs the procedure**
- Puts on gloves
- Identifies patient's ID from patient, against hospital bracelet and the prescription chart
- Checks correct details of the infusion against prescription chart
- Primes extension tubing using 0.9% saline flush
- Connects tubing to insulin infusion syringe
- Applies tourniquet to manikin arm
- Identifies appropriate vein to site cannula
- Cleans skin with alcohol swab
- Inserts cannula using appropriate technique: needle held at 45° to skin, smooth insertion under skin into vein
- Acknowledges flashback of blood
- Withdraws introducer to a degree, then inserts cannula to hub
- Releases tourniquet, presses on proximal vein while withdrawing introducer, connects cap
- Applies dressing
- Flushes the cannula using prepared 5 ml, 0.9% saline flush
- Connects primed extension tubing and insulin infusion.

**Obtains an acceptable/appropriate result**

**Disposes of all sharps and other items correctly**

**Ensures patient receives correct advice about what to do next and follow-up**

**Ensures nursing staff or other healthcare professionals receive correct information about the consequences/outcome of the procedure/task**

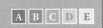

## GLOBAL PROCEDURE MARK

A B C D E

## Station 5 – Clinical communication skills

**Patient script**

You have been told that you are very unwell and need to be transferred to the 'heart attack centre' as soon as possible. However you need to be 'a bit better' and as such need to first go to the heart ward to make sure you are safe to travel.

You have also been told that you will need to be on lots of medicines to keep your heart safe and that these have all been shown to help people like you when they are having a heart attack.

However, one of the doctors has told you that many of the medicines may make you bleed and that someone will be coming to explain this to you.
You have been told that aspirin stops the blood forming clots that in turn cause heart attacks, but you don't really know about the other medicines.

When told you have a 1 : 8–1 : 9 risk of having a major bleed, you tell the 'doctor' that this is TOO HIGH a RISK and that you don't want the medicines. However, if the candidate is sympathetic, calm and reassuring, you will be convinced that this is a worthwhile risk. If the candidate is unsympathetic, bullying or aggressive, you should not change your mind.

If the candidate uses medical jargon or terms that you don't think an intelligent lay person would know or understand you should challenge them to explain these to you.

You expect the doctors 'know best' but are very worried about the risk of the bleeding.

SCENARIO 1

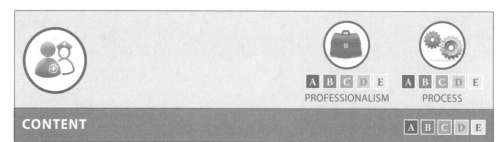

PROFESSIONALISM | A B **C** D E

PROCESS | A B **C** D E

## CONTENT · A B C **D** E

**Confirms reason for discussion – to talk to patient about the new medications and their risks and benefits**

**Establishes what patient wishes to know; gains agreement/informal consent to participate in the discussion**

**Reviews patient's current understanding of clinical situation and summarises what has happened so far**

**Establishes patient's ideas, concerns and expectations**

**Explains the key, important information; invites patient to ask questions and is able to deal with them appropriately**
- Explains the aims of treatment and their benefits: to stop further clot progression and possible myocardial damage
- Introduces the idea of possible risks: may cause significant bleeding, eg from the bowel or possibly inside the brain
- Introduces idea of objective scoring system and how it can be used to calculate risk
- Shows patient that calculated CRUSADE score is 41
- Correctly explains the relative risk (11.9%, ie approx 1 : 8–1 : 9 risk) using clear, jargon-free and understandable language
- Deals sympathetically and appropriately with patient's initial response ('If it's that high doctor I don't want it')
- Revisits ideas, concerns and expectations and deals with them appropriately
- Avoids giving wrong or disinformation
- Avoids aggressive or judgemental language.

**Summarises important areas of the consultation back to the patient**

**Clarifies patient's final position**
- If patient is willing to take treatment, records this in the medical notes and prescribes the medications
- If patient is NOT willing to take the treatment, records this in the notes BUT may ask one of his/her seniors to come and revisit the issues once the patient has had time to think about them.

**Formally ends the consultation and ensures appropriate follow-up has been discussed**

## CLINICAL DIAGNOSTIC REASONING

A B C D E

**Correctly calculates CRUSADE score (41)**

**Correctly identifies and explains what a relative risk of 11.9% means**

**Successfully negotiates a satisfactory, safe management plan**

**Demonstrates clear and logical diagnostic reasoning**

## GLOBAL CLINICAL COMMUNICATION MARK

A B C D E

# Scenario 1: Reflection and consolidation

| History |
| --- |

Mr Iqbal is a 54-year-old British-born Asian man. He was brought into the Emergency Department at about 09.30 after having suffered a severe episode of chest pain. Over the past 4–6 weeks he has been suffering with occasional episodes of chest pain that he initially thought was 'bad indigestion'. The first episode occurred while he was at work pushing some of the heavy trolleys around the postal depot. The pain was very tight and 'squeezing', 'like a band around his chest'. It only lasted about a minute but was really bad and took his breath away. He had to sit down for about 5 minutes before he felt OK again. Since then he's had two to three similar episodes, the last one while playing football with his grandson. This was a more severe and prolonged episode, lasting about 5–10 minutes. The pain was severe, and central, radiating to his jaw and left hand. He was sweaty and felt sick but it went off by itself after he lay down on the ground.

Today's episode came on at the postal depot just after his morning tea. He was walking up a flight of stairs when the pain came on suddenly. This was the most severe pain he'd ever experienced and he described it as 'squeezing and crushing the life out of me'. The pain was central, radiating to his jaw, left and right arms. He collapsed down the stairs but a work colleague pulled him to safety and made a pillow for him with a jacket. He was dizzy and faint but didn't pass out. The pain continued for at least 10–15 minutes before the ambulance men arrived and gave him oxygen and some buccal nitrate. On arrival he still had a little chest discomfort. He had no symptoms of heart failure.

Risk factors:

- Strong family history of IHD and CV disease. including his father and grandparents dying of heart and stroke problems before the age of 70; Mr Iqbal also has two close cousins who have had MI in the last few years
- Probable pre-diabetes
- Ex-smoker: 20+ cigarettes/day until 4 or 5 years ago
- No known hypertension, stroke or PVD
- Alcohol: nil
- Weight: grossly overweight, being 5'8" and 15 and a half stone
- No regular medications; no known allergies
- PMH – no significant history
- Married with five children aged 26–17 years; the youngest three still live at home, two of them are unemployed
- Works in the local post office depot; shop steward of the local postal union and is the main bread-winner.

## Examination

On examination, Mr Iqbal is an obese, middle-aged Asian man. On arrival in the Emergency Department he looked unwell, pale and clammy and still had slight chest discomfort.

- Vital observations were: HR 104 bpm, BP 183/98 mmHg (large cuff required), RR 18 bpm, $O_2$ sats 87% on air, temperature 36.5 °C, CBG 16.4 mmol/l
- Feet to face: very overweight but nil else of note
- General examination: fingers of right hand heavily tar stained; no anaemia, no stigmata of hyperlipidaemia
- No carotid or other bruits heard
- CV examination: pulse 100 regular, low volume, normal character; BP 190/100 mmHg, JVP – not seen; HS 1 + 2 + ? 3rd heart sound
- RS examination: bibasal crackles to the midzones
- No ankle oedema
- All peripheral pulses palpable.
- Abdomen: obese, no organomegaly or masses
- Neurology: not formally assessed.

In summary, this is a 64-year-old Asian man with features suggestive of obesity, T2DM, ACS, LVF and poorly controlled hypertension.

## Investigations

Blood tests including FBC, U&Es, RBG, lipids, troponin (at 12 hours)
CXR: to confirm the features of heart failure; other features to look for include calcified valves, cardiomegaly and signs of respiratory disease eg features of COPD (chronic smoker)
ECG: to confirm or exclude signs of:
- Acute or chronic IHD, eg ST segment changes, T-wave changes, left bundle branch block
- Arrhythmia and signs of heart block

Hypertensive changes, eg left axis deviation, voltage criteria of LVH.

## Management

Acute ACS protocol, including LMWH or fondaparinux, aspirin and clopidogrel, anti-anginals – beta blockers, nitrates
Mr Iqbal has ongoing pain and therefore requires further anti-platelet and anticoagulants (see NICE guidelines below)
Treatment of LVF: IV nitrates and furosemide
IV insulin infusion
Secondary prophylaxis: statin, anti-platelets, anti-hypertensives
Further investigation according to GRACE or similar score – once stabilised Mr Iqbal will need PCI and possible stenting
Will need dietitian and diabetes specialist nurse review and will require a sensible but effective weight-loss programme.

## Further reading and web links

http://www.crusadebleedingscore.org/index.html
http://www.nice.org.uk/nicemedia/live/11552/33013/33013.pdf
NICE guidelines of ACS and NSTEMI
http://www.nice.org.uk/nicemedia/live/12947/47918/47918.pdf
NICE guidelines on the management of cardiac chest pain of recent onset

# Scenario 2: 'Collapse'

## Station 1

*History*                                     *10-minute station*

You are a FY1 doctor on the Medical Admissions Unit (MAU). A young man, Mr Thomas Appleby, has been referred to the MAU with shortness of breath and chest pain.

■ Please take a history from Mr Appleby and present it to your Registrar with a differential diagnosis and management plan.

*You will be assessed on the following areas, as well as the content and diagnostic reasoning of your history – take them into account in your presentation.*

### Professionalism

- Professional appearance (NHS dress code) – including general appearance, hair and jewellery
- Maintains patient and personal safety
- Polite introduction; identifies patient or interviewee correctly; confirms patient's date of birth from name band or other source
- Obtains informal consent; maintains patient's privacy
- Displays empathetic and caring attitudes and behaviours throughout.

### Process

- Good organisation and structure; appropriate use of open and closed questions
- Appropriate fluency/rhythm/pace to the interview – this may change depending on environment and acute nature of the problem
- Appropriate time for the patient to respond/reply to questions
- Appropriate acknowledgement of difficult or emotional areas of the patient's history.

### Communication skills

- Demonstrates caring and sympathetic attitude
- Asks open questions
- Invites patient to ask questions and answers them appropriately
- Addresses patient's ideas, concerns and expectations.

## Station 2

*Examination*                    *10-minute station*

■ After presenting your history, you have 10 minutes to complete a respiratory examination of Mr Appleby and present it to your Registrar (if you do not have a model, please read and present the information given on page 380).

*You will be assessed on the following areas, as well as the content and skills of your examination – take them into account in your presentation.*

### Professionalism

- Professional appearance; maintains infection control standards, including hand cleaning and appropriate use of gloves and aprons
- Maintains patient and personal safety
- Polite introduction; identifies patient and confirms date of birth from name band or other source
- Obtains informal consent; maintains patient privacy and dignity
- Displays empathetic and caring attitudes and behaviours throughout.

### Process

- Appropriate fluency/rhythm/pace to the examination – this may change depending on environment and acute nature of the problem
- Organisation and structure of examination; sensitive and empathetic approach
- Uses appropriate clinical techniques throughout
- Maintains privacy and dignity throughout.

### Clinical communication

- Explains proposed examination/procedure: explains examination/procedure as it proceeds
- Offers information in a clear, structured and fluent manner, avoiding jargon
- Listens to patient and responds appropriately
- Demonstrates appropriate body language.

SCENARIO 2

## Station 3

*Data interpretation*                    *10-minute station*

Mr Appleby has gone to the X-ray department to have a chest X-ray. Whilst you are waiting for him to return, the on-call Registrar asks you to review the chest X-ray of other patients admitted on the medical take.

■ Please indicate whether each of the statements are TRUE (T) or FALSE (F).

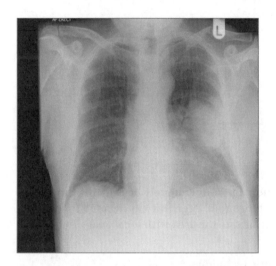

1
A   Shows pulmonary oedema
B   Shows a cavitating lesion
C   Is most likely a squamous cell carcinoma
D   Should be treated with broad spectrum antibiotics
E   Should be investigated with a CT

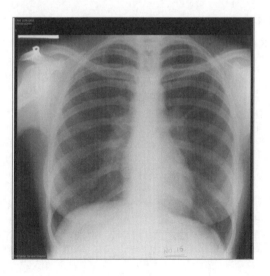

2
A   Shows pulmonary oedema
B   Shows a widened mediastinum
C   May be associated with a high serum ACE level
D   Can be seen in lymphoma
E   Should be investigated with percutaneous biopsy

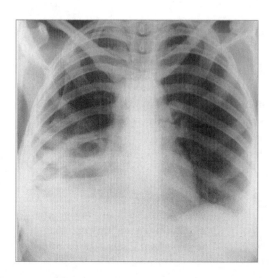

3

A   Shows a right lower lobe pneumonia
B   Shows a right pneumothorax
C   Requires an intercostal drain insertion
D   May be associated with mediastinal injuries
E   Shows subcutaneous emphysema

## Station 4

*Procedural skills*                    *10-minute station*

Mr Appleby has had an attempt at aspiration, but unfortunately he remains short of breath with complete collapse of his right lung. Your Registrar has decided to insert an intercostal drain. He has asked you to infiltrate the area with local anaesthetic.

**Procedure**
- Please complete the task using an aseptic technique.

**Equipment provided**
- Sterile dressing pack
- Local anaesthetics – not exceeding 3 mg/kg lidocaine
- ChloraPrep®
- 10 ml syringe
- Drawing-up needle
- 18 G green needle
- 22 G orange needle

## Station 5

*Prescribing skills*                    *10-minute station*

Mr Appleby's chest drain has been successfully inserted and attached to an underwater seal chest drain. It is bubbling and swinging appropriately. He has had paracetamol 1 g po so far but still rates his pain as 6 out of 10.

- Please prescribe an appropriate analgesia regime for Mr Appleby's admission. The regime should include regular analgesia including anti-inflammatories and also breakthrough PRN analgesia.

### Details

- ○ Mr Thomas Appleby
- ○ DOB 23/2/1987
- ○ Hospital number: 2346547
- ○ Ward: MAU
- ○ Consultant: Dr Hadley
- ○ No known drug allergies

**Remember: DRUG DRs Don't Forget Signing Off (page 396)**

# Answers

## Station 1 – History

**Patient script**

You are Mr Thomas Appleby (DOB 23 February 1987). You went to your GP today after developing sudden right-sided chest pain when you were out jogging. The pain is sharp and stabbing in nature and 'catches me every time I take a breath.' It doesn't move anywhere and you would rate it as 4/10 in severity. You were concerned that when you tried to continue running you became short of breath, but this settled when you were not exerting yourself. You are currently feeling somewhat breathless just sitting and talking.

You have had no cough, fever or blood in your sputum. If asked you have no leg swelling and have had no recent period of immobility or long flights.

You are a fit and healthy young man who has no medical problems, no family history of clotting problems or respiratory disease. You are a non-smoker; you work as a photographer and often travel abroad for work. You have no allergies and no regular medications.

You are concerned that you have a clot on your lung, as you had a close friend who died recently from a pulmonary embolism and he had described chest pain and being short of breath shortly before he died.

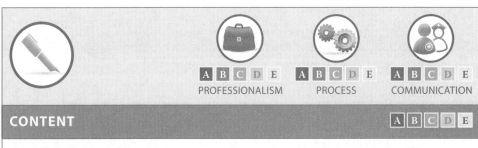

PROFESSIONALISM PROCESS COMMUNICATION

SCENARIO 2

## CONTENT

A B C D E

**Identifies key information**
- Establishes presence of sudden onset pleuritic chest pain (including site, onset, radiation)
- Presence of progressive shortness of breath.

**Includes important negatives, including systemic enquiry**
- Establishes absence of cough, fever, wheeze or haemoptysis.

**Completing the patient history**
- Drug and allergy history: nil regular and no allergies
- Previous medical history: nil of note; no similar episodes
- Social and occupational history: non-smoker
- Family history: no family history of respiratory disease or thromboembolism.

**Summarises important areas of the history back to the patient**

**Invites patient to ask questions and deals with them appropriately**

**Establishes patient's ideas, concerns and expectations**
- Patient believes that the pain is due to a pulmonary embolism and is concerned that this may be fatal.

## CLINICAL DIAGNOSTIC REASONING

A B C D E

- **Please present your history**
  - Candidate offers a logical, well-structured account of the history.

- **What is your differential diagnosis?**
  - Candidate offers the correct diagnosis and appropriate differentials
  - Pneumothorax
  - Pulmonary embolism
  - Musculoskeletal chest pain.

- **What initial investigations would you request after your examination?**
  - Chest X-ray
  - ECG
  - Oxygen saturations
  - FBC.

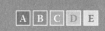

| GLOBAL HISTORY MARK | A B C D E |
| --- | --- |

## Station 2 – Examination

**Patient script (see also page 380)**

You are a young man who is breathless at rest, breathing at 20 breaths per minute. You find it painful to take deep breaths.

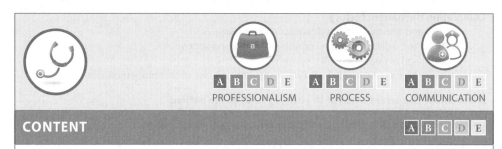

| | | | |
| --- | --- | --- | --- |
| | A B C D E | A B C D E | A B C D E |
| | PROFESSIONALISM | PROCESS | COMMUNICATION |

| CONTENT | A B C D E |
| --- | --- |

**Exposes and positions patient correctly and maintains comfort**

**Comments on wellbeing of patient, ie well or unwell**

**Asks for appropriate/relevant clinical observations**
- Observations: HR 103 bpm, BP 115/75 mmHg, RR 20 bpm, $O_2$ sats 90% on air, temperature 37.1 °C.

**Focussed examination**
- Inspection: assesses hands and nails for signs such as clubbing, palmar erythema; assesses trachea
- Palpation: assesses chest expansion anteriorly and posteriorly
- Percussion: in all zones including apices; examines for an any change in tactile vocal resonance
- Auscultation: auscultates in all areas, no breath sounds audible on the right side.

**Thanks patient, offers assistance, maintains patient's dignity and privacy until they are dressed**

## CLINICAL DIAGNOSTIC REASONING

**Correctly identifies the relevant physical signs, including important negative findings**

■ **A patient with a similar clinical history presents to you in the Emergency Department: what clinical signs would suggest a tension pneumothorax?**
  - Hyper-resonant percussion note on one side
  - Deviation of the trachea away from the hyper-resonant side
  - Low oxygen saturations, tachycardia and hypotension.

■ **What emergency management would you instigate?**
  - Emergency needle decompression (thoracocentesis)
  - A wide-bore cannula inserted into the second right intercostal space in the midclavicular line.

## GLOBAL EXAMINATION MARK

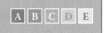

# Station 3 – Data interpretation

**1. A: F, B: F, C: T, D: F, E: T**

This X-ray shows a left middle lobe mass lesion. The most likely diagnosis is that of a bronchial carcinoma, most commonly a squamous cell carcinoma. The investigation of choice in the first instance could a CT of the thorax and then most likely a bronchoscopy and biopsy to obtain a tissue sample for histopathology.

**2. A: F, B: F, C :T, D: T, E: F**

This X-ray shows bilateral hilar lymphadenopathy. The mediastinum is otherwise normal. The finding of BHL is seen in sarcoidosis, lymphoma, tuberculosis as well as extrinsic allergic alveolitis. It should be investigated with bronchoscopy and bronchial alveolar lavage.

**3. A: F, B: T, C: T, D: T, E: F**

This X-ray shows a right side hydro-pneumothorax, that being a right pleural effusion and associated pneumothorax. The most likely cause of this appearance is a traumatic injury resulting in a haemothorax and collapse of the right lung. The priority in management of these patients is to insert a wide bore intercostal drain and exclude any associated mediastinal injuries.

## GLOBAL DATA INTERPRETATION MARK

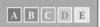

## Station 4 – Procedural skills

### Procedure: local anaesthetic infiltration

SCENARIO 2

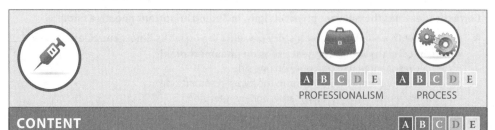

PROFESSIONALISM | A B C D E

PROCESS | A B C D E

### CONTENT | A B C D E

**Exposes and positions patient correctly and maintains comfort**

**Identifies and sets out equipment correctly; maintains aseptic technique throughout**

**Correctly performs the procedure**
- Confirms the area identified for chest drain insertion by Registrar, ensuring that the area is just superior to the rib edge in order to avoid the neurovascular bundle
- Washes hands and applies sterile glove
- Cleans area with a ChloraPrep® and leaves to dry for at least one minute
- Draws up the local anaesthetic into a 10 ml syringe with a 23 G needle; removes air
- Changes the needle to a 25 G needle and infiltrates 1–2 ml lidocaine under the skin as a 'bleb'
- Uses a 21 G needle and inserts it into the skin at 90 degrees to the skin aspirating whilst advancing the needle to ensure the needle is not in a vessel
- Infiltrates the area in an 'umbrella' along the rib edge
- Notes that it would take 5–10 minutes for the local anaesthetic to take effect before starting the procedure
- Removes the needle.

**Obtains an acceptable/appropriate result**

**Disposes of all sharps and other items correctly**

**Ensures patient receives correct advice about what to do next and follow-up**

**Ensures nursing staff or other healthcare professionals receive correct information about the consequences/outcome of the procedure/task**

**Thanks patient, offers assistance, maintains patient's dignity and privacy until they are dressed**

### GLOBAL PROCEDURE MARK | A B C D E

## Station 5 – Prescribing skills

| Allergies, sensitivities and adverse drug reactions | | | Patient details/addressograph | |
|---|---|---|---|---|
| No known allergies ✓ | Initials  AF | Gender (M)/ F | NHS/ Hospital No:  2346547 | |
| Not possible to ascertain ☐ | Date | Weight (kg) | Date | |
| Medicine/substance | Reaction & Severity | Initials & Date | | Surname:  APPLEBY |
| | | | Height | First name:  THOMAS |
| Alerts | | | Surface area (m²) | Date of birth:  23.02.1987 |

### IN-PATIENT MEDICATION PRESCRIPTION AND ADMINISTRATION RECORD

PasTest HOSPITAL

| Consultant HADLEY | Trainee Dr. Name and Bleep no. FEATHER 622 | Date of admission 7/05 | Date chart reboarded | Estimated date of discharge |
|---|---|---|---|---|
| This chart is no. 1 ............ of ............ 1 | Transcribing Check by Pharmacy Sign ............ Date ............ | Ward 1. ........MAU........ | | 2. ............ |

### Regular prescriptions continued

**Regular medications**

| | Dose | | | Date | 7 | 8 | 9 | 10 | 11 | 12 | | | | | Signature and bleep no. | Pharmacy |
|---|---|---|---|---|---|---|---|---|---|---|---|---|---|---|---|---|
| Date 7/05 | | | | Medication PARACETAMOL | | | | Instructions | | | | | | AF 622 | | ☐ |
| Route PO | | | | | | | | | | | | | | | | |
| Signature | | | | | | | | | | | | | | | | |
| 06 | | | | | | | | | | | | | | | | |
| ⑨ | 1g | | | | | | | | | | | | | | | |
| ⑫ | 1g | | | | | | | | | | | | | | | |
| ⑱ | 1g | | | | | | | | | | | | | | | |
| ㉒ | 1g | | | | | | | | | | | | | | | |
| 24 | | | | | | | | | | | | | | | | |

### Regular prescriptions continued

**Regular medications**

| | Dose | | | Date | 7 | 8 | 9 | 10 | 11 | 12 | | | | | Signature and bleep no. | Pharmacy |
|---|---|---|---|---|---|---|---|---|---|---|---|---|---|---|---|---|
| Date 7/05 | | | | Medication IBRUPROFREN | | | | Instructions | | | | | | AF 622 | | ☐ |
| Route PO | | | | | | | | | | | | | | | | |
| Signature | | | | | | | | | | | | | | | | |
| 06 | | | | | | | | | | | | | | | | |
| ⑨ | 600mg | | | | | | | | | | | | | | | |
| ⑫ | 600mg | | | | | | | | | | | | | | | |
| ⑱ | 600mg | | | | | | | | | | | | | | | |
| ㉒ | 600mg | | | | | | | | | | | | | | | |
| 24 | | | | | | | | | | | | | | | | |

'COLLAPSE'

### Regular prescriptions continued

**Regular medications**

| | Dose | | | Date | | | | | | | | | | Signature and bleep no. | Pharmacy |
|---|---|---|---|---|---|---|---|---|---|---|---|---|---|---|---|
| | | | | 7 | 8 | 9 | 10 | 11 | 12 | | | | | | |
| Date 7/05 | | | | Medication | | | | Instructions | | | | | | Signature and bleep no. | Pharmacy |
| Route PO | | | | CODEINE PHOSPHATE | | | | | | | | | | AF 622 | |
| Signature | | | | | | | | | | | | | | | |
| 06 | | | | | | | | | | | | | | | |
| ⑨ | 30mg | | | | | | | | | | | | | | |
| ⑫ | 30mg | | | | | | | | | | | | | | |
| ⑱ | 30mg | | | | | | | | | | | | | | |
| ㉒ | 30mg | | | | | | | | | | | | | | |
| 24 | | | | | | | | | | | | | | | |

### As required medications

| Medication | | | | Date | | | | | | | | | | | | | | | | |
|---|---|---|---|---|---|---|---|---|---|---|---|---|---|---|---|---|---|---|---|---|
| TRAMADOL | | | | | | | | | | | | | | | | | | | | |
| Indication | | | | Time | | | | | | | | | | | | | | | | |
| Dose | Route | Maximum frequency / dose | Start date | Dose | | | | | | | | | | | | | | | | |
| 50 mg | PO | TDS | 7/05 | | | | | | | | | | | | | | | | | |
| | | | Stop date | Route | | | | | | | | | | | | | | | | |
| Signature | | | | | | | | | | | | | | | | | | | | |
| AF | | | Bleep no. 622 | Given | | | | | | | | | | | | | | | | |
| Additional instructions: | | | | | | | | | | Pharmacy | | | | | | | | | | |

### As required medications

| Medication | | | | Date | | | | | | | | | | | | | | | | |
|---|---|---|---|---|---|---|---|---|---|---|---|---|---|---|---|---|---|---|---|---|
| OROMORPH | | | | | | | | | | | | | | | | | | | | |
| Indication | | | | Time | | | | | | | | | | | | | | | | |
| Dose | Route | Maximum frequency / dose | Start date | Dose | | | | | | | | | | | | | | | | |
| 25 mL | PO | As Req± | 7/05 | | | | | | | | | | | | | | | | | |
| | | | Stop date | Route | | | | | | | | | | | | | | | | |
| Signature | | | | | | | | | | | | | | | | | | | | |
| AF | | | Bleep no. 622 | Given | | | | | | | | | | | | | | | | |
| Additional instructions: | | | | | | | | | | Pharmacy | | | | | | | | | | |

## GLOBAL PRESCRIBING MARK

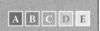

A  B  C  D  E

# Scenario 2: Reflection and consolidation

## History

Mr Appleby is a fit and well 25-year-old man who presents with sudden onset of right-sided pleuritic chest pain. This occurred whilst out running this morning. It was accompanied with progressive shortness of breath. He has had no swelling of his legs, and denies any trauma to the chest. He denies any respiratory symptoms and has no risk factors for venous thromboembolism. He has no family history of VTE or respiratory disease and is a non-smoker. The most likely diagnosis is that of a spontaneous pneumothorax.

## Examination

On examination, this young man is breathless at rest with a RR of 20 bpm at rest. He has oxygen saturations of 95% on air. He has a tachycardia of 104 bpm and a blood pressure of 115/75 mmHg. He has reduced chest expansion on the right side of the thorax with a central trachea. This is associated with a hyper-resonant percussion note on the right side and absent breath sounds. This clinical picture is suggestive of large right-sided pneumothorax with no evidence of cardiovascular compromise.

## Investigations

A pneumothorax is defined as air in the pleural space (between the lung and the chest). It can be spontaneous or occur after an injury to the thorax (for example after chest trauma or central line insertion). Spontaneous pneumothoraces can be defined as either primary or secondary. Primary pneumothoraces arise in otherwise healthy people without any lung disease. Risk factors for spontaneous pneumothorax are due to rupture of small subpleural bursae, and are more common in tall thin men aged 20-40; often occurring in smokers and those with a family history.

Secondary pneumothoraces occur in subjects with underlying lung disease, such as COPD, when the lung tissue has been damaged and bullae (large air-filled pockets) within the lung tissue.

It is important to define pneumothoraces as primary or secondary as they are managed differently.

## Management

The management of spontaneous pneumothoraces depends on their size and the symptoms asscociated with them. If the rim of air is greater than 2 cm or the patient is breathless then treatment is required. Initially with aspiration and if two attempts at aspiration failed then chest drain insertion with an underwater seal drain is indicated.

However, if the patient is asymptomatic and the rim of air is less than 2 cm then a conservative approach can be adopted. Most of these pneumothoraces will resolve spontaneously and a follow-up chest x-ray to ensure this has occurred.

**Further reading and web links**
*BTS guidelines on management of spontaneous pneumothoraces*:
http://thorax.bmj.com/content/58/suppl_2/ii39.full.pdf
*Patient.uk information on flying with medical conditions*:
www.patient.co.uk/doctor/Flying-with-Medical-Conditions.htm

# Scenario 3:
# 'One too many'

## Station 1

*History*                                    *10-minute station*

You are the FY1 doctor on the Medical Admissions Unit (MAU). Mr Connor Mackay is a 61-year-old man. He has been found by his brother on the floor of his flat after not coming to the pub as usual for the last 3 days. He is drowsy and your Registrar is making an initial physical assessment.

■ **Please obtain further information regarding Mr Mackay's medical history and of this presentation from his brother.**

*You will be assessed on the following areas, as well as the content and diagnostic reasoning of your history – take them into account in your presentation.*

### Professionalism

- Professional appearance (NHS dress code) – including general appearance, hair and jewellery
- Maintains patient and personal safety
- Polite introduction; identifies patient or interviewee correctly; confirms patient's date of birth from name band or other source
- Obtains informal consent; maintains patient's privacy
- Displays empathetic and caring attitudes and behaviours throughout.

### Process

- Good organisation and structure; appropriate use of open and closed questions
- Appropriate fluency/rhythm/pace to the interview – this may change depending on environment and acute nature of the problem
- Appropriate time for the patient to respond/reply to questions
- Appropriate acknowledgement of difficult or emotional areas of the patient's history.

### Communication skills

- Demonstrates caring and sympathetic attitude
- Asks open questions
- Invites patient to ask questions and answers them appropriately
- Addresses patient's ideas, concerns and expectations.

# Station 2

*Examination*                                           *10-minute station*

■ **After presenting the history to your Registrar please make a clinical assessment of Mr Mackay. Your Registrar will observe you and ask you to present your findings after your examination along with an initial management plan (if you do not have a model, please read and present the information given on page 380).**

*You will be assessed on the following areas, as well as the content and skills of your examination – take them into account in your presentation.*

## Professionalism

- Professional appearance; maintains infection control standards, including hand cleaning and appropriate use of gloves and aprons
- Maintains patient and personal safety
- Polite introduction; identifies patient and confirms date of birth from name band or other source
- Obtains informal consent; maintains patient privacy and dignity
- Displays empathetic and caring attitudes and behaviours throughout.

## Process

- Appropriate fluency/rhythm/pace to the examination – this may change depending on environment and acute nature of the problem
- Organisation and structure of examination; sensitive and empathetic approach
- Uses appropriate clinical techniques throughout
- Maintains privacy and dignity throughout.

## Clinical communication

- Explains proposed examination/procedure: explains examination/procedure as it proceeds
- Offers information in a clear, structured and fluent manner, avoiding jargon
- Listens to patient and responds appropriately
- Demonstrates appropriate body language.

## Station 3

*Data interpretation*                    *10-minute station*

You have requested your initial investigations, and they show deranged liver function tests. Your Registrar has results for a number of patients who have deranged liver functions.

■ Please match the diagnoses with the clinical scenarios below.

    A   Autoimmune hepatitis
    B   Budd-Chiari syndrome
    C   Ischaemic hepatitis
    D   Wilsonian crisis
    E   Drug-induced hepatic toxicity
    F   Acute hepatitis A infection
    G   Alcoholic hepatitis
    H   Non-alcoholic steatohepatitis
    I   Acute hepatitis C infection

1.   A 27-year-old man presents with a past medical history of depression and a 3-day history of right upper quadrant discomfort and jaundice and is now confused. His blood tests show an alanine amino-transferase (ALT) of 650, bilirubin of 165 and alkaline phosphatase (ALP) of 115.

2.   A 57-year-old woman presents with a 6-month history of lethargy, myalgia and itching. She has now developed increasing jaundice. Her only medical history is that of Sjögren's syndrome. Her initial liver function tests (LFTs) demonstrate a raised ALT, aspartate amino-transferase (AST) and total protein.

3.   A 62-year-old man is on intensive care after an out of hospital cardiac arrest 2 days ago. He was successfully resuscitated after 15 minutes but has now developed grossly elevated LFTs and coagulopathy with an ALT of 1245 and an ALP of 350.

4.   A 64-year-old man presents with a 2-week history of diarrhoea and fever after returning from backpacking in Turkey. He is obviously jaundiced but his examination is otherwise normal.

5.   A 32-year-old woman presents with a 3-day history of abdominal pain, abdominal distension and now a deep jaundice. She is tender in the right upper quadrant. Her LFTs show a mixed transaminitis and obstructive picture. Her only medical history is that of a deep vein thrombosis 6 years ago.

# Station 4

*Procedural skills*                    *10-minute station*

### Procedure A
■ Your Registrar has asked you to perform a supervised ascitic fluid tap to exclude the diagnosis of spontaneous bacterial peritonitis. Mr Mackay's blood results show platelets of 134 and a prothrombin time (PT) of 11.4 with an activated partial thromboplastin time (APTT) of 28.2.

### Equipment provided
- Sterile dressing pack and gloves
- 2 × ChloraPrep®
- 1 vial 1% lidocaine for infiltration
- 10 ml syringe
- 20 ml syringe
- 3 needles: one 21 G, one 23 G and one 25 G
- Gauze and dressing for site
- 3 sterile pots for specimen collection

### Procedure B
■ You have aspirated 20 ml straw-coloured fluid. Please complete laboratory requests for the cytology, biochemistry and microbiology tests you feel are appropriate.

### Details
- Mr Connor Mackay
- DOB 16/11/1950
- Hospital number: 97867564
- Ward: MAU
- Consultant: Dr Evans

SCENARIO 3

| PasTest Hospital | | Patient Details | |
|---|---|---|---|
| Laboratory Department | | Name | |
| Date | | D.O.B | |
| | | Hospital Number | |
| Clinical Details | | Ward | |
| Tests required | | Consultant | |
| Person requesting tests | | | |
| Contact details | | Signature | |

## Station 5

*Prescribing skills*                      *10-minute station*

Your patient is being admitted to the Medical High Dependency Unit.

- Please prescribe the appropriate medications for Mr Mackay, as given below.
    1. Pabrinex vitamin solution
    2. PRN benzodiazepines for withdrawal symptoms
    3. Empirical antibiotics for spontaneous bacterial peritonitis (SBP)
    4. Terlipressin
    5. Three doses of vitamin K.
- You may be asked the properties of these medications.

**Details**

- o Mr Connor Mackay
- o DOB 16/11/1950
- o Hospital number: 97867564
- o Ward: MAU
- o Consultant: Dr Evans
- o Weight: 76 kg
- o Drug allergies: nil known

---

**Remember: DRUG DRs D**on't **F**orget **S**igning **O**ff (page 396)

---

SCENARIO 3

# Answers

## Station 1 – History

**Patient script**

You are Mr Michael Mackay, brother of Mr Connor Mackay (DOB 16 November 1950). You do not live with your brother but you see Connor most days at your local pub. You became worried when he had not come to the pub for 3 days and was not answering his telephone. You went into the flat and found him on the floor in the bathroom. He was drowsy and 'talking nonsense'. There were some very dark faeces in the toilet. He was much more yellow in his skin and eyes than he has been before.

Your brother has drunk excessive alcohol for over 30 years. He used to drink up to two bottles of whisky per day until about 6 months ago, when he first became jaundiced. At that time he was admitted to hospital and diagnosed with liver cirrhosis. He was in hospital for 10 days and his jaundice and the swelling in his abdomen improved. His was abstinent for approximately 2 months but has been drinking again since then but 'just 2 or 3 pints of lager per day'.

You are unsure if your brother has ever vomited blood before. The last time you saw him was 3 days ago, when he was much less jaundiced.

Connor has been a smoker of 10–15 cigarettes per day for 40 years. He is supposed to be taking vitamins and 'some other' medications but you don't believe he has been taking these. He has no known drug allergies. He has no other medical problems. He was working as a postal worker up until 15 years ago, when his marriage broke down and his alcohol intake increased significantly. You are unsure if he has been drinking more heavily at home but you do know that he gets tremors if he doesn't drink every day. You do not think he has ever had a seizure related to stopping drinking.

A B C D E    A B C D E    A B C D E

PROFESSIONALISM    PROCESS    COMMUNICATION

**SCENARIO 3**

## CONTENT

A B C D E

### Identifies key information
- Establishes patient found on the floor today, drowsy and speaking incoherently; patient last seen 3 days before
- Establishes presence of jaundice and possible bleeding from the gastrointestinal tract
- Establishes alcohol history: 30 years of excess alcohol; drinking up to 50 units of whisky per day; probable reduction of intake for last 6 months
- Establishes presence of previous withdrawal symptoms on discontinuing alcohol.

### Includes important negatives, including systemic enquiry

### Completing the patient history
- Drug and allergy history: medications unknown and no allergies
- Previous medical history: known cirrhosis diagnosed 6 months ago with episode of decompensated liver failure; no other known medical conditions
- Social and occupational history: lives alone; smoker with 20 pack year history
- Family history: no relevant family history known.

### Summarises important areas of the history back to the patient

### Invites patient to ask questions and deals with them appropriately

### Establishes patient's ideas, concerns and expectations

## CLINICAL DIAGNOSTIC REASONING

A B C D E

- **Please present your history**
  - Candidate offers a logical, well-structured account of the history.

- **This patient is known to have cirrhosis: what are three common causes of cirrhosis?**
  - Alcoholic liver disease
  - Chronic hepatitis (B and C)
  - Non-alcoholic steatohepatitis
  - Primary biliary cirrhosis.

## GLOBAL HISTORY MARK

A B C D E

# Station 2 – Examination

Patient script (see also page 380)

You are Mr Connor Mackay (DOB 16 November 1950). You are drowsy and only open your eyes when you are subjected to a painful stimulus. You are breathing deeply and slowly and mumble incoherently when spoken to. You will localise to any painful stimuli.

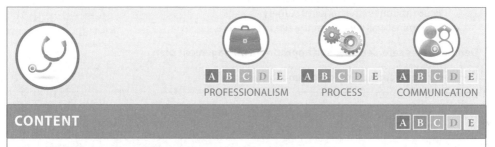

PROFESSIONALISM  PROCESS  COMMUNICATION

## CONTENT    A B C D E

**Exposes and positions patient correctly and maintains comfort**

**Comments on wellbeing of patient, ie well or unwell**
- Patient drowsy with GCS of (12) E3V3M5, maintaining his airway
- Patient icteric with distended abdomen.

**'Feet to face'**
- Observes and comments on patient and surroundings from foot of bed.

**Asks for appropriate/relevant clinical observations**
- Observations: HR 110 bpm, BP 115/65 mmHg, RR 10 bpm, $O_2$ sats 95% on air, temperature 37.1 °C, BM 5.2.

**Focussed examination of gastrointestinal system**
- Inspection: assesses hands, identifying leuconychia, palor, erythema, asterixis; examines face, identifying deep jaundice; examines chest, identifying gynaecomastia, and multiple spider naevi; examines abdomen, identifying caput medusa and gross distension
- Palpation: assesses for organomegaly and shifting dullness
- Percussion: assesses for pertitonism
- Auscultation: auscultates for bowel sounds.

**Completes examination by identifying relevant additional clinical signs**
- Requests a rectal examination, to assess for malaena
- Examines for peripheral oedema.

## CLINICAL DIAGNOSTIC REASONING

Identifies correct physical signs, including important negative findings; does not identify signs that are not present

- You have noted the ascites present in the examination of this patient. If you were to perform a paracentesis or diagnostic 'tap' of this fluid, what are three contraindications to this procedure?
  - Uncooperative patient
  - Uncorrected significant coagulopathy
  - Acute abdomen that requires surgery
  - Abdominal wall cellulitis at the site of puncture.

Demonstrates safe, sensible and appropriate management plan

Demonstrates clear and logical diagnostic reasoning

## GLOBAL EXAMINATION MARK

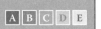

# Station 3 – Data interpretation

1    E

2    A

3    C

4    F

5    B

## GLOBAL DATA INTERPRETATION MARK

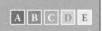

## Station 4 – Procedural skills

**Procedure: ascitic fluid aspiration**

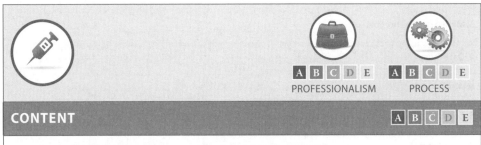

PROFESSIONALISM     PROCESS

### CONTENT     A B C D E

**Exposes and positions patient correctly and maintains comfort**
- Appropriately positions patient supine with arms by side, and exposes the abdomen.

**Identifies and sets out equipment correctly; maintains aseptic technique throughout**

**Correctly performs the procedure**
- Identifies area for safe aspiration, ideally in the left iliac fossa
- Cleans area with a ChloraPrep® and leaves to dry for at least one minute
- Draws up the local anaesthetic into a 10 ml syringe with a 23 G needle; removes air
- Changes the needle to a 25 G needle and infiltrates 1–2 ml lidocaine
- Uses a 20 ml syringe and 21 G needle and inserts it into the skin at 90 degrees to the skin, aspirating whilst advancing the needle
- Aspirates 20 ml fluid
- Removes the needle quickly afterwards and applies dressing to site
- Places fluid in three sterile pots.

**Obtains an acceptable/appropriate result**

**Disposes of all sharps and other items correctly**

**Ensures patient receives correct advice about what to do next and follow-up**

**Ensures nursing staff or other healthcare professionals receive correct information about the consequences/outcome of the procedure/task**

**Thanks patient, offers assistance, maintains patient's dignity and privacy until they are dressed**

SCENARIO 3

| Requesting tests | |
|---|---|
| 1. Name of patient | Connor Mackay |
| 2. Date of birth | 16.11.1950 |
| 3. Medical record number | 97867564 |
| 4. Date today | 7.05.2012 |
| 5. Ward | MAU |
| 6. Consultant | Evans |
| 7. Tests requested<br><br>(a) Biochemistry – glucose, protein, LDH, amylase<br><br>(b) Cytology – to exclude a malignant cause of ascitic fluid<br><br>(c) Microbiology – samples for both microscopy, culture and sensitivity (MC&S) | |
| 8. Concise clinical details<br><br>Ascitic fluid ?SBP | |
| For each request: | |
| 9. The request is signed/signature<br><br>10. Contact details of person requesting test | A FEATHER<br>Bleep 622 |

**GLOBAL PROCEDURE MARK**

## Station 5 – Prescribing skills

1. Pabrinex vitamin solution: this a parenteral preparation of vitamins B and C in those who are likely to be deplete, such as those with alcoholism or in those who have been malnourished for other reasons. It should be given as a pair of vials at two to three times per day for 3–5 days to replenish stores of these vitamins and decrease the likelihood of developing Wernicke's encephalopathy.

2. PRN benzodiazepines for withdrawal symptoms: those who are dependent on alcohol are very likely to develop symptoms of withdrawal when admitted to hospital for any reasons and abruptly discontinue their alcohol intake. In those who are already drowsy there is no requirement for benzodiazepines, but they should be available on the 'as required' side in case the symptoms of withdrawal develop. An appropriate prescription would be diazepam 10–20 mg po every 2-4 hours for symptoms of withdrawal. In those who present with symptoms of withdrawal, a weaning regimen of a longer acting benzodiazepine such as chlordiazepoxide would be more appropriate.

3. Empirical antibiotics for spontaneous bacterial peritonitis (SBP): those patients who have chronic ascites are at a significant risk of SBP (the presence of bacterial infection in ascitic fluid without an obvious source of infection). The pathogenesis is thought to be related to the intrahepatic shunting of colonised blood and reduced host defences in the ascitic fluid related to cirrhosis. The usual pathogens are *E. coli*; however, antibiotics should have cover for Gram-positive pathogens, as these make up at least a quarter of infections. Therefore a sensible antibiotic choice would be Co-amoxiclav 1.2 g tds or a piperacillin and tazobactam (Tazocin) 4.5 g.

4. Terlipressin: this is an analogue of vasopressin (a vasoactive agent), which is used in the treatment of bleeding from oesophageal varices. It is thought to act by reducing splanchnic vasodilatation. The dose is 2 mg IV every 4-6 hours for 72 hours.

5. Three doses of vitamin K: in cirrhosis a hypocoaguable state may develop owing to decreased hepatic synthesis of vitamin K-dependent clotting factors (II, VII. IX and X) and reduced liver activation of these products. In those who are coagulopathic, vitamin K should be supplemented to aid clotting factor production and function. The dose is 10 mg po/IV for 3 days.

SCENARIO 3

**SCENARIO 3**

| Allergies, sensitivities and adverse drug reactions | | | | | Patient details/addressograph | |
|---|---|---|---|---|---|---|
| No known allergies ✓ | | Initials *AF* | | Gender (M) F | NHS/ Hospital No: *97867564* | |
| Not possible to ascertain ☐ | | Date | | Weight (kg) | Date | |
| Medicine/substance | Reaction & Severity | Initials & Date | | *76kg* | | Surname: *MACKAY* |
| | | | | Height | | First name: *CONNOR* |
| Alerts | | | | Surface area (m²) | | Date of birth: *16.11.50* |

## IN-PATIENT MEDICATION PRESCRIPTION AND ADMINISTRATION RECORD

PasTest HOSPITAL

| Consultant *EVANS* | Trainee Dr. Name and Bleep no. *FEATHER 622* | Date of admission *7.05.12* | Date chart reboarded | Estimated date of discharge |
|---|---|---|---|---|
| This chart is no. .................... of .................... | Transcribing Check by Pharmacy Sign ............ Date ............ | Ward 1. ...*MAU*................................................ 2. ............ | | |

Supplementary Medication charts in use: Other (please specify): 1 .................................................... 2 ....................................................

| Epidural/PCA ☐ | Syringe driver ☐ | | TPN ☐ | Chemotherapy ☐ | Insulin sliding scale ☐ |
|---|---|---|---|---|---|

**Once only medications – loading doses, pre-medication, PGDs or surgical antibiotic propylaxis**

| Date | Time to be given | Medicine (approved name) | Dose | Route | Signature and bleep no. | Pharmacy | Time given | Given by | Checked by |
|---|---|---|---|---|---|---|---|---|---|
| 7/05 | Stat | PABRINEX I + II | vials | IV | AF 622 | | | | |
| 7/05 | Stat | VITAMIN K | 10mg | IV (slowly) | AF 622 | | | | |
| 7/05 | Stat | CEFOTAXIME | 2g | IV | AF 622 | | | | |
| 7/05 | Stat | TERLIPRESSIN | 2mg | IV | AF 622 | | | | |
| | | | | | | | | | |

**Thromboprophylaxis please prescribe treatment regimens in the regular medications section**

| Choice of mechanical prophylaxis and leg(s) to be applied to | | | | | | Enter Time | Enter details below |
|---|---|---|---|---|---|---|---|
| Graduated elastic compression stockings | Intermittent pneumatic compression device (IPC) | Leg | | | | | |
| | | Left | Right | Both | | | |
| ✓ Start Date: 7/05 | ☐ End Date: | Signature and Bleep No. | ☐ | ☐ | ✓ | | |
| ☐ Start Date: | ☐ End Date: | Signature and Bleep No. AF | ☐ | ☐ | ☐ | | |

| Medication NOT FOR HEPARIN | Dose | Dose Change | Enter Time | Enter details below | | |
|---|---|---|---|---|---|---|
| Please ensure you have completed the VTE risk assessment form | Date | *INR > 2.0* | | | | |
| | Route | | | | | |
| | Signature | | Instructions | | Pharmacy | ☐ |
| | Bleep no. | | | | | |

## Regular prescriptions continued

**Anti-infectives prescription**  *prescribe long term prophylaxis and anti-tuberculosis medications in regular medications section*

| For 7 Days | Dose | | | Date | 7 | 8 | 9 | 10 | 11 | 12 | 13 | | | | | |
|---|---|---|---|---|---|---|---|---|---|---|---|---|---|---|---|---|
| Date | 7/05 | | | **Medication** CEFOTAXIME | | | | **Indication** SBP | | | | **Signature and bleep no.** AF 622 | | | **Pharmacy** ☐ | |
| Route | IV | | | | | | | | | | | | | | | |
| Signature | AF | | | | | | | | | | | | | | | |
| 06 | | | | | | | | | | | | | | | | |
| (09) | 2g | | | ✕ | | | | | | | | | | | | |
| 12 | | | | | | | | | | | | | | | | |
| 18 | | | | | | | | | | | | | | | | |
| (22) | 2g | | | | | | | | | | | | | | | |
| 24 | | | | | | | | | | | | | | | | |

## Regular prescriptions continued

| | Dose | | | Date | 7 | 8 | 9 | 10 | 11 | 12 | | | | | | |
|---|---|---|---|---|---|---|---|---|---|---|---|---|---|---|---|---|
| Date | 7/05 | | | **Medication** PABRINEX vials I + II | | | | **Indication** SBP | | | | **Signature and bleep no.** AF 622 | | | **Pharmacy** ☐ | |
| Route | IV | | | | | | | | | | | | | | | |
| Signature | AF | | | | | | | | | | | | | | | |
| 06 | | | | | | | | | | | | | | | | |
| (09) | I + II | | | ✕ ——— | | | | | | | | | | | | |
| 12 | | | | | | | | | | | | | | | | |
| (18) | I + II | | | ✕ ——— | | | | | | | | | | | | |
| 22 | | | | | | | | | | | | | | | | |
| 24 | | | | | | | | | | | | | | | | |

## Regular prescriptions continued

| | Dose | | | Date | 7 | 8 | 9 | 10 | | | | | | | | |
|---|---|---|---|---|---|---|---|---|---|---|---|---|---|---|---|---|
| Date | 7/05 | | | **Medication** VITAMIN K | | | | **Indication** SBP | | | | **Signature and bleep no.** AF 622 | | | **Pharmacy** ☐ | |
| Route | IV | | | | | | | | | | | | | | | |
| Signature | AF | | | | | | | | | | | | | | | |
| 06 | | | | | | | | | | | | | | | | |
| (09) | 10mg | | | ✕ ——— | | | | | | | | | | | | |
| 12 | | | | | | | | | | | | | | | | |
| 18 | | | | | | | | | | | | | | | | |
| 22 | | | | | | | | | | | | | | | | |
| 24 | | | | | | | | | | | | | | | | |

## Regular prescriptions continued

| | Dose | | | Date FOR 72 HOURS | | | | | | | | | | | | |
|---|---|---|---|---|---|---|---|---|---|---|---|---|---|---|---|---|
| Date | 7/05 | | | **Medication** TERLIPRESSIN | | | | **Indication** SBP | | | | **Signature and bleep no.** AF 622 | | | **Pharmacy** ☐ | |
| Route | IV | | | | | | | | | | | | | | | |
| Signature | AF | | | | | | | | | | | | | | | |
| (06) | 2mg | | | | | | | | | | | | | | | |
| 09 | | | | | | | | | | | | | | | | |
| (12) | 2mg | | | | | | | | | | | | | | | |
| (18) | 2mg | | | | | | | | | | | | | | | |
| 22 | | | | | | | | | | | | | | | | |
| (24) | 2mg | | | | | | | | | | | | | | | |

| As required medications | | | | | | | | | | | | | | | | | | | |
|---|---|---|---|---|---|---|---|---|---|---|---|---|---|---|---|---|---|---|---|
| **Medication** DIAZEPAM | | | **Date** | | | | | | | | | | | | | | | | |
| **Indication** | | | **Time** | | | | | | | | | | | | | | | | |

| Dose | Route | Maximum frequency / dose | Start date | Dose | | | | | | | | | | | | | | |
|---|---|---|---|---|---|---|---|---|---|---|---|---|---|---|---|---|---|---|
| 10 mg | PO | | 7/05 | | | | | | | | | | | | | | | |
| | | 4 Hourly | Stop date | Route | | | | | | | | | | | | | | |
| **Signature** AF | | | Bleep no. 622 | Given | | | | | | | | | | | | | | |

Additional instructions: AS REQUIRED     Pharmacy ☐

| Infusion prescriptions continued | | | | | | | | | | SC = subcutaneous | | IVC = intravenous central IVP = intravenous peripheral | |
|---|---|---|---|---|---|---|---|---|---|---|---|---|---|
| Date & time | Route | Infusion Fluid | | Medication | | Duration | Rate | Prescriber's signature & bleep no. | Date given | Given by / Added by | Check by | Start time / Finish time | Pharmacy |
| | | Name & strength | Volume | Approved name with expiry / unit number | Dose | | | | | | | | |
| 7/05 | IV | 5% DEXTROSE Exp: Batch/unit no: | 1L | | | | 8° | AF 622 | | | | | |
| 7/05 | IV | 5% DEXTROSE Exp: Batch/unit no: | 1L | + 20mmol KCL | | | 8° | AF 622 | | | | | |
| 7/05 | IV | 5% DEXTROSE Exp: Batch/unit no: | 1L | + 20mmol KCL | | | 8° | AF 622 | | | | | |
| | | Exp: Batch/unit no: | | | | | | | | | | | |
| | | Exp: Batch/unit no: | | | | | | | | | | | |
| | | Exp: Batch/unit no: | | | | | | | | | | | |
| | | Exp: Batch/unit no: | | | | | | | | | | | |
| | | Exp: Batch/unit no: | | | | | | | | | | | |
| | | Exp: Batch/unit no: | | | | | | | | | | | |
| | | | | | | | | | | | | | |
| | | | | | | | | | | | | | |

**GLOBAL PRESCRIBING MARK**     A B C D E

# Scenario 3: Reflection and consolidation

## History

Mr Connor Mackay is a 62-year-old man who has a history of alcohol-related cirrhosis. The information gathered today is from his brother Michael, as Mr Mackay is drowsy and confused. He has drunk excessive alcohol for 30 years, drinking up to 50 units of alcohol per day. He was diagnosed with cirrhosis after his first episode of decompensated liver failure 6 months ago. It is unclear if he has had a previous gastrointestinal bleed or varices. He continues to drink up to 9 units of lager per day.

He presents today having been found by his brother having not been seen in 72 hours. He was found drowsy and confused with increased jaundice; there was evidence of altered blood in the toilet, suggesting possible gastrointestinal bleeding.

Mr Mackay has a 20 pack year smoking history. He had regular medications but does not take any of these; he is not known to have any allergies. He is an unemployed ex-postal worker and lives alone. He suffered from tremors when not drinking, but it is not known if he has had seizures or delirium tremens.

The history suggests decompensated alcoholic liver disease and the possible trigger is gastrointestinal bleeding.

## Examination

This middle-aged man is drowsy with a GCS of 12; he is maintaining his airway and has a respiratory rate of 10 with sats of 95% on room air, and his pupils are equal and reactive. He is tachycardic at 110 but not hypotensive. He has a normal temperature and his blood sugar level is 5.2.

He is obviously jaundiced with evidence of decompensated liver disease, including leuconychia, and palmar erythema on the hands. Many spider naevi and gynaecomastia are noted on examination of the chest.

Abdominal examination reveals caput medusa and a distended abdomen with shifting dullness suggesting ascites. The liver edge and spleen are not palpable. There is no evidence of peritonitis and bowel sounds are audible. There is no gross peripheral oedema but there is evidence of excoriation over the abdomen. Digital rectal examination reveals melaena.

The examination is suggestive of decompensated liver disease; there is evidence of gastrointestinal bleeding, which may be due to oesophageal varices caused by portal hypotension. He is encephalopathic and drowsy with tachycardia, which may be suggestive of hypovolaemia.

## Investigations

In patients with presumed cirrhosis there are a number of investigations:
- Ultrasound
- Baseline FBC, clotting, U&E, LFT, glucose.

If cirrhosis is seen on ultrasound then further investigations should be undertaken:
- Hepatitis B and C serology
- Autoantibodies and immunoglobulins (PBC and autoimmune hepatitis)
- Ferritin (haemochromatosis)
- Caeruloplasmin (Wilson disease)
- Alpha1-antitrypsin
- Alfa-feta protein (presence of hepatocellular carcinoma).

Assess synthetic function:
- International ratio (INR)/PT (acute function)
- Albumin (chronic function).

Liver biopsy

Consider endoscopic retrograde cholangiopancreatography (ERCP) to exclude primary sclerosing cholangitis in patients with risk factors.

## Management

The key to management of alcoholic liver disease is to prevent further insult to the liver. This means that abstinence from alcohol is vital. Community support and detoxification services exist throughout the country and have good efficacy.

The management of ascites related to cirrhosis is maintaining a low salt diet, and using diuretics (spironolactone has good evidence) and then paracentesis when required for symptomatic benefit.

Liver transplantation in alcoholic liver disease is a controversial area, and until recently transplantation has been reserved for those who have remained abstinent for 6 months. However liver centres are increasingly considering transplantation for acute decompensated alcoholic liver disease.

## Further reading and web links

British Liver Trust: clear patient information on liver disease
www.britishlivertrust.org.uk/home/the-liver/liver-disease.aspx
BMJ best practice advice on assessment of ascites
http://bestpractice.bmj.com/best-practice/monograph/41/diagnosis.html

# Scenario 4:
# 'Lost for words'

## Station 1

*History*                                    *10-minute station*

You are the FY1 attending a GP practice as part of a 'career taster week'. The next patient, Mr Cameron Campbell-Smith, has been booked in to see the GP as an emergency and has agreed to talk to you first.

■ **Please take a focussed history from the patient with a view to presenting it to the GP as if you were in a busy GP surgery.**

*You will be assessed on the following areas, as well as the content and diagnostic reasoning of your history – take them into account in your presentation.*

**Professionalism**

- Professional appearance (NHS dress code) – including general appearance, hair and jewellery
- Maintains patient and personal safety
- Polite introduction; identifies patient or interviewee correctly; confirms patient's date of birth from name band or other source
- Obtains informal consent; maintains patient's privacy
- Displays empathetic and caring attitudes and behaviours throughout.

**Process**

- Good organisation and structure; appropriate use of open and closed questions
- Appropriate fluency/rhythm/pace to the interview – this may change depending on environment and acute nature of the problem
- Appropriate time for the patient to respond/reply to questions
- Appropriate acknowledgement of difficult or emotional areas of the patient's history.

**Communication skills**

- Demonstrates caring and sympathetic attitude
- Asks open questions
- Invites patient to ask questions and answers them appropriately
- Addresses patient's ideas, concerns and expectations.

## Station 2

*Examination*                                    *10-minute station*

Unfortunately Mr Cameron Campbell-Smith fails to keep his TIA clinic appointment and 3 weeks later is brought to the Emergency Department by ambulance, with a suspected stroke affecting his right arm and leg and his speech.

■ Please make an appropriate and comprehensive assessment of Mr Campbell-Smith, including:

    1   A full neurological assessment
    2   Assessment of his speech and language skills
    3   Assessment of his swallowing.

(If you do not have a model, please read and present the information given on page 381.)

*You will be assessed on the following areas, as well as the content and skills of your examination – take them into account in your presentation.*

### Professionalism

- Professional appearance; maintains infection control standards, including hand cleaning and appropriate use of gloves and aprons
- Maintains patient and personal safety
- Polite introduction; identifies patient and confirms date of birth from name band or other source
- Obtains informal consent; maintains patient privacy and dignity
- Displays empathetic and caring attitudes and behaviours throughout.

### Process

- Appropriate fluency/rhythm/pace to the examination – this may change depending on environment and acute nature of problem
- Organisation and structure of examination; sensitive and empathetic approach
- Uses appropriate clinical techniques throughout
- Maintains privacy and dignity throughout.

### Clinical communication

- Explains proposed examination/procedure: explains examination/procedure as it proceeds
- Offers information in a clear, structured and fluent manner, avoiding jargon
- Listens to patient and responds appropriately
- Demonstrates appropriate body language.

## Station 3

*Data interpretation*        *10-minute station*

The on-call Medical Registrar asks you to review Mr Campbell-Smith's CT head scan with her. This confirms a large right middle cerebral artery infarct. She then uses the hospital radiology server to bring up four other CT head scans from medical patients who she has reviewed over the last few weeks.

■ Please indicate whether each of the statements regarding the scans is TRUE (T) or FALSE (F).

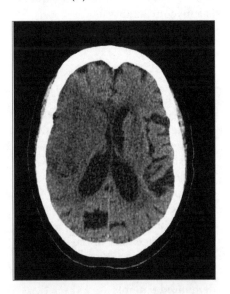

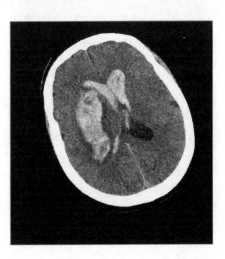

1 This is the CT head scan of a 49-year-old man with a 50 pack year history of cigarette smoking, and a recent diagnosis of type 2 diabetes. He was found by his wife, slumped on the sofa with a dense left hemipareisis.

A There is a large, old posterior infarct on the right

B There is evidence of a left sided subdural haemorrhage

C There is evidence of midline shift

D There is effacement of the lateral ventricle on the right

E The scan is consistent with a large right-sided middle cerebral artery (MCA) infarct

2 This is the CT head scan of a 54-year-old hypertensive woman who was found collapsed in the street.

A This is a contrast enhanced CT head scan

B There is fresh blood extending into the lateral ventricles

C There is mass effect to the left

D There is a large malignant tumour on the right

E The features are typical of a large subarachnoid haemorrhage

SCENARIO 4

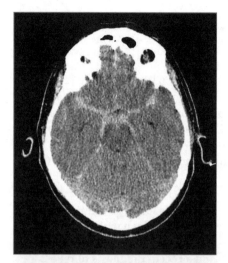

3 This is the CT head scan of a 24-year-old woman who was awoken from sleep with a severe headache. She has vomited twice since arrival in the emergency department and is feeling drowsy and unwell.

1. This is a cerebral angiogram demonstrating the circle of Willis
2. There is blood in the basal cisterns
3. There is an occipital mass
4. A common cause of this appearance is a mycotic aneurysm
5. This patient should be referred for acute thrombolysis

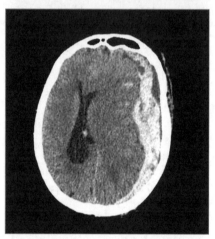

4 This is the CT head scan of a 72-year-old man who presented to the emergency department with a 24-hour history of increasing confusion and right-sided weakness.

A There is a large extradural haemorrhage evident
B There is a large intracererbal haemorrhage evident
C There is effacement of the ventricles
D There is midline shift to the right
E This condition is commonly seen in demented patients

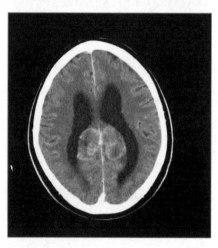

5 This is the CT head scan of a 38-year-old previously fit and well man who presented to his GP with a 2-month history of increasing headaches, blurred vision and nausea

A This is a contrast enhanced scan
B There is evidence of acute intracerebral bleeding
C There is evidence of midline shift
D There are atrophic changes
E The appearances are consistent with a large malignant brain tumour

SCENARIO 4

## Station 4

*Prescribing skills*                    *10-minute station*

Mr Campbell-Smith is admitted to the hyper-acute stroke unit (HASU), where it is agreed he will receive thrombolysis and treatment according to the local HASU protocol.

■ Please write up the patient's thrombolysis regime following the treatment guidelines shown below, along with the regular and as required medications listed.

A Details

o Mr Cameron Campbell-Smith; DOB: 26/08/1960; Hospital no.: 221343; Ward: HASU; Consultant: Dr Jackson

o Height: 1.78m; weight: 88 kg; U&Es: normal; RBG: 11.3 mmol/l; TChol: 9.9 mmol/l

o Observations – HR 130 bpm regular, good volume, BP 198/123 mmHg, RR 22 bpm, $O_2$ sats 94% on air, temperature 38.6 °C, CBG 12.6 mmol/l, GCS 10/15 (E 3, M 4, V 3)

o Regular medications – patient not taking any regular medications prior to admission.

---

**Remember: DRUG DRs D**on't **F**orget **S**igning **O**ff (page 396)

---

## Acute stroke protocol

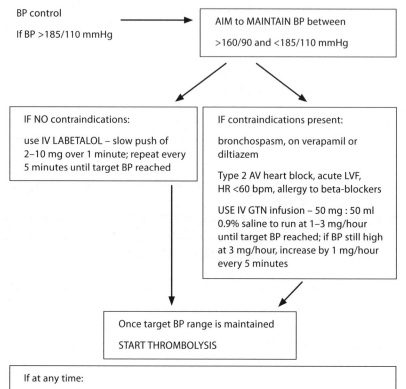

BP control

If BP >185/110 mmHg

→

AIM to MAINTAIN BP between

>160/90 and <185/110 mmHg

---

IF NO contraindications:

use IV LABETALOL – slow push of 2–10 mg over 1 minute; repeat every 5 minutes until target BP reached

---

IF contraindications present:

bronchospasm, on verapamil or diltiazem

Type 2 AV heart block, acute LVF, HR <60 bpm, allergy to beta-blockers

USE IV GTN infusion – 50 mg : 50 ml 0.9% saline to run at 1–3 mg/hour until target BP reached; if BP still high at 3 mg/hour, increase by 1 mg/hour every 5 minutes

---

Once target BP range is maintained

START THROMBOLYSIS

---

If at any time:

BP falls below target range – stop infusions

BP rises again >185/110 mmHg then repeat bolus labetalol or reintroduce GTN infusion; once thrombolysis has been completed – introduce IV GTN infusion if BP rises above target

### B  Thrombolysis
### Calculate rtPA dose
- 0.9 mg/kg to a maximum dose of 90 mg
- First approx 10% given as bolus over 2 minutes, remaining approx 90% over 1 hour; you will need to draw up the dose in 2 × 50 ml syringes and calculate rate in ml/hour (the nurse will draw up the solution to have a concentration of 1 mg/ml).

### C  Routine monitoring to maintain:
- $O_2$ sats at 95–98%: use supplemental $O_2$ if necessary via nasal prongs or mask
- Blood sugar between 4.0 and 11.0 mmol/l; if CBG >11.0 mmol/l, use FRIVII at 0.1 unit of insulin/kg; use IV dextrose to maintain CBG >4.0 mmol/l
- Temperature 36–37.5 °C; if greater than 37.5 °C, bring temperature down using po/pr or IV paracetamol; fanning and cooling devices
- If BP >185/110 mmHg post-thrombolysis, use GTN infusion to reduce BP to between 185/110 and 160/90 mmHg.

D  Regular medications for secondary prophylaxis (unless contraindicated)
o  Simvastatin – 40 mg od
o  Aspirin 300 mg – 2/52; then 75 mg od
o  Clopidogrel 300 mg stat, then 75 mg od for 1 year

By calculation

Total dose = 88 kg × 0.9 mg/kg = 79 mg

Thus there will be:

a  bolus = 8 mg in 8 ml – given as bolus over 1 minute
b  90% infusion as 71 mg; 1 mg/ml thus 71 mg at rate of 71 ml/hour
  i   syringe infusion 1–50 mg in 50 ml at 71 ml/hour
  ii  syringe infusion 2–21 mg in 21 ml at 71 ml/hour.

## Station 5

*Clinical communication skills*                    *10-minute station*

You are the FY1 on the stroke rehabilitation ward that Mr Campbell-Smith has been repatriated to following his admission to the HASU at St. James', the local teaching hospital. The Nursing Sister on the ward is concerned that despite relatively good speech and language reports Mr Campbell-Smith shows little or no understanding of his medications, risk factors and condition. She asks you to explain these issues to him.

■  Please explore how Mr Campbell Smith is getting on with his rehabilitation. He is due for discharge in the next few days and you should re-explain the diagnosis, further management and the medications that have been prescribed.

**Observations today**
o  HR 68 bpm, BP 143/82 mmHg, $O_2$ sats 95% on air, temperature 36.6 °C, CBG 6.0 mmol/l
o  Height 1.78 m, weight 88 kg, BMI $94/(1.78)^2$ = 27.8 kg/m$^2$.

**Present medication**
o  Aspirin 300 mg od
o  Clopidogrel 75mg od
o  Simvastatin 40 mg od
o  Perindopril 10 mg od
o  Indapamide 2.5 mg od
o  Nicotine patches.

# Answers

## Station 1 – History

**Patient script**

You are Mr Cameron Campbell-Smith (DOB 26 August 1960), a black Caribbean man aged 51 years old. You are a right-handed painter and decorator who is fit and well and often works a 6-day week, 0800–1800 h. You have had high blood pressure since just before your 45th birthday but take your medicines 'almost every day'.

This morning you woke feeling fine. You were driving to a new customer's house about 5 miles away when you suddenly started to feel 'really strange'. Your head felt 'as if it wasn't attached to my shoulders', 'all light and floating'. It didn't really feel like dizziness or that you were about to lose consciousness. However, your vision went blurred and you had to stop the van at the side of the road. Then your right arm and leg went numb and weak, and your arm flopped down by your side.

You speed-dialled your wife but then found your speech was very slurred and you couldn't get the right words out. You couldn't really hear what she was saying but think you could understand her. The whole episode lasted about 15–20 minutes and completely resolved after 30 minutes, when you were able to drive home. Your wife was frantic and immediately rang the GP practice and they kindly gave you an emergency appointment. You now feel 100% back to normal and hope this is not going to take too long, as you would like to get back to work!

You had no pre-warning symptoms, headaches or features of seizure. You have never experienced anything like this in the past. Your mother had heart surgery aged 80 years old (you think it was for a heart valve); your father died of lung cancer and was a heavy smoker. You smoke 15–20 roll-up cigarettes/day and have done so for many years. You use about 2 oz of tobacco per week. You drink whisky at the weekends (a large bottle lasts a month or so) but like a 'big drink up from time to time'. You do not know about your cholesterol and have never had symptoms suggestive of a stroke, peripheral vascular disease or IHD. You are otherwise fit and well.

The medications you are on are ramipril 5 mg od and amlodipine 10 mg od. You have no known drug allergies.

You are married and live with your wife in a first-floor flat. You have no children. Your brother and his family live close by. Your wife works as a receptionist in a local dentist practice and is very well.

You think you may have had a mini-stroke. Your neighbour had one last year, and this sounded very similar. You are concerned that you might have another in the near future or indeed a full stroke and hope you can do something about it. You are hoping the doctor can give you some medicines: 'Isn't it an aspirin a day?'

| A | B | C | D | E | | A | B | C | D | E | | A | B | C | D | E |
|---|---|---|---|---|---|---|---|---|---|---|---|---|---|---|---|---|
| PROFESSIONALISM | | | | | | PROCESS | | | | | | COMMUNICATION | | | | |

## CONTENT

| A | B | C | D | E |
|---|---|---|---|---|

**Identifies key information**
- Pre-morbid health: fit and well; woke feeling 'normal' and well
- No similar episodes in the past
- Onset: rapid, acute.

**Includes important negatives, including systemic enquiry**
- Symptoms: asks specifically about headache, visual disturbances, speech and language including comprehension, motor and sensory changes in limbs, duration of symptoms, residual deficit or time to 100% resolution, other features of seizures.

**Identifies key information from rest of the history**
- Cardiovascular risk: family history, IHD, stroke or PVD, diabetes mellitus, hypertension, smoking, alcohol, others
- Relevant facts about employment, housing, social support, life stressors.

**Completing the patient history**
- Drug and allergy history: ramipril and amlodipine; no known drug allergies
- Previous medical history: nil known
- Social and occupational history: as above

**Summarises important areas of the history back to the patient**

**Invites patient to ask questions and deals with them appropriately**

**Establishes patient's ideas, concerns and expectations**

SCENARIO 4

## CLINICAL DIAGNOSTIC REASONING

- **Please present your history**
  - Candidate offers a logical, well-structured account of the history.
- **If I tell you that this man's CBG was 6.2 mmol/l, and his BP 189/121 mmHg on arrival at the surgery today, can you work out his ABCD2 score for me [show candidate the score below]?**

| Risk factor | Category | Score |
|---|---|---|
| Age | Age ≥60 | 1 |
| | Age <60 | 0 |
| Blood pressure | SBP >140 or DBP ≥90 | 1 |
| at assessment | Other | 0 |
| Clinical features | Unilateral weakness | 2 |
| | Speech disturbance (no weakness) | 1 |
| | Other | 0 |
| Duration | ≥60 minutes | 2 |
| | 10–59 minutes | 1 |
| | <10 minutes | 0 |
| Diabetes | Present at assessment | 1 |
| | Not present | 0 |
| | TOTAL (Max) | 7 |

**A score ≥4 puts the patient at HIGH RISK of stroke.**

**SCORE**

**Age <60 years old 0, BP 1, Clinical features 2, Duration 1, Diabetes 0**

**Total = 4 – high risk of further stroke.**

- **What would you recommend for this patient now?**
  - Explain to patient high risk of stroke and that he needs early investigation and further treatment
  - Add aspirin, reinforce need for anti-hypertensives to be taken
  - Needs urgent referral to TIA clinic either today or in the next 24 hours – needs blood tests, CT head scan and carotid Doppler.

**Demonstrates safe, sensible and appropriate management plan**

**Demonstrates clear and logical diagnostic reasoning**

## GLOBAL HISTORY MARK

## Station 2 – Examination

**Patient script (also see page 381)**

You are a middle-aged man who has been brought by ambulance to the Emergency Department. You have mild expressive dysphasia but no receptive problems. You have a grade 3+/5 right hemiparesis but not sensory loss. When assessed you should cough and splutter when attempting to drink the water offered.

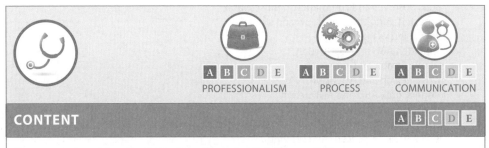

A B **C** D E — PROFESSIONALISM
A B **C** D E — PROCESS
A B **C** D E — COMMUNICATION

### CONTENT
A B **C** D E

**Exposes and positions patient correctly and maintains comfort**

**Comments on wellbeing of patient, ie well or unwell**

**'Feet to face'**
- Observes and comments on patient and surroundings from foot of bed – evidence of obvious neurological deficit, mobility aids.

**Asks for appropriate/relevant clinical observations**
- HR 88 bpm, BP 188/106 mmHg, RR 14 bpm, $O_2$ sats 92% on air, temperature 37.9 °C, CBG 6.1 mmol/l.

**CV and stroke risk assessment**
- Arterial tree, radial pulse, rate and regularity (excludes AF); assesses all peripheral and central pulses; listens for carotid and renal bruits; assesses for AAA
- Assesses heart and praecordium: apex beat, heave and thrills, auscultation
- BP/CBG as above
- Stigmata of hyperlipidaemia
- Tar staining of fingers
- Cranial nerves: observes face, comments on any obvious cranial nerve palsies
- Eyes: V/A using newspaper or similar; both eyes
- Visual fields: EOM, nystagmus
- Pupillary responses: PERL(A)
- Ophthalmoscopy.

- **Why do you wish to do ophthalmoscopy in this patient?**
  - Papilloedema (if there is a large SOL), retinopathy – hypertension
  - Tests: V – motor/sensory; VII – motor; XI and XII.

**Speech tests**
- Comprehension with 1, 2 and 3 stage commands
- Expression - Fluency, appropriate use and content of speech
- Swallowing assessment:

Stages:

Asks patient to
- Sip and hold water in mouth
- Swallow the water: watching and feeling for initiation of swallow
- Comments on presence or absence of cough/spluttering/choking
- Open mouth: looking for pooling in the mouth
- Speak: listening for upper airways pooling (wet quality of voice).

**Upper limb assessment**
- Bulk: observes and comments on muscle bulk
- Tone: left vs right; wrist, elbow and shoulder
- Power: left vs right
- Shoulder: ABD and ADDuction
- Elbow: flexion and extension
- Wrist: flexion and extension
- Fingers: grip, ABD and ADDuction
- Thumb: opposition/abduction
- Coordination: comments that can't assess because of weakness
- Reflexes: biceps, triceps and supinator.

**Lower limb assessment**
- Bulk: observes and comments on muscle bulk
- Tone: left vs right
- Power: left vs right
- Hip: flexion and extension
- Knee: flexion and extension
- Ankle: flexion and extension
- Coordination and gait: comments that can't assess because of weakness
- Reflexes: patella and Achilles.
- Plantar responses.

**Thanks patient, offers assistance, maintains patient's dignity and privacy until they are dressed**

## CLINICAL DIAGNOSTIC REASONING

**Correctly identifies the relevant physical signs, including important negative findings**
- Comments on: cardiovascular risk; neurological deficit, including speech and language, visual problems and limb weakness.

■ **Given the presentations, what immediate and long-term therapeutic interventions would you consider?**
- Acute CT head scan to exclude haemorrhage and other intracranial pathologies
- Anti-platelet treatment; reduction of the blood pressure then thrombolysis with tPA
- Acutely: oxygen via mask or nasal prongs, anti-pyretics
- Secondary prevention lipid-lowering agent (statin), anti-hypertensives and nicotine replacement therapy.

**Demonstrates safe, sensible and appropriate management plan**

**Demonstrates clear and logical diagnostic reasoning**

## GLOBAL EXAMINATION MARK

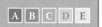

**SCENARIO 4**

## Station 3 – Data interpretation

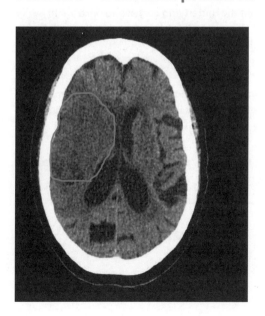

**1. A False, B False, C False, D True, E True**

This unenhanced CT head scan shows a large, acute infarct – there is a wedge of low attenuation (dark grey) within the right MCA territory (circled) with mass effect shown as sulcal and ventricular effacement. If within the time limits of acute stroke protocol and there are no contra-indications, this patient should be referred for urgent thrombolysis in the nearest Hyperacute stroke unit (HASU).

**2. A False, B True, C True, D False, E False**

This non contrast CT head scan shows a large Intracerebral haemorrhage – this is an acute haemorrhage (hence it's white) and is intra-axial, centred on the right basal ganglia which is typical of a hypertensive bleed. The acute haemorrhage has extended into the lateral ventricles and there is mass effect with midline shift to the left.

**3. A False, B True, C False, D False, E False**

This non contrast CT head scan shows a subarachnoid haemorrhage – acute (bright white) haemorrhage in the basal cisterns and surrounding the circle of Willis. Next step should be a CT angiogram (CTA) to look for the aneurysm causing the bleeding.

Mycotic aneurysms are formed by bacterial seeding into the wall of a blood vessel and are relatively rare. They are seen in patients with infective endocarditis.

**4. A False, B False, C True, D True, E True**

This non contrast CT head scan shows an acute left-sided subdural haemorrhage (acute therefore bright white) with mass effect on the ipsilateral left lateral ventricle and midline shift to the right. The key to telling this is a subdural rather than extradural collection is that it is crescentic in shape, and crosses suture lines.

At 7 – 10 days the haemorrhage becomes isodense with the underlying cortex and this may make it difficult to see. Later, it will be darker than the underlying cortex and once again easily visible. Because of the change in density during this period it is important that the radiologist is given as much relevant information as possible.

**5. A True, B False, C False, D False, E True**

This contrast enhanced CT shows a large malignant brain tumour. This is a Glioblastoma multiforme, a brain tumour that is typically a heterogeneous irregular mass which enhances post contrast and often (shown as in this case) crosses the midline.

## GLOBAL DATA INTERPRETATION MARK

SCENARIO 4

# Station 4

## Prescribing skills

| Allergies, sensitivities and adverse drug reactions | | | | | Patient details/addressograph | |
|---|---|---|---|---|---|---|
| No known allergies ✓ | | Initials AF | | Gender (M)/ F | NHS/ Hospital No: 221343 | |
| Not possible to ascertain ☐ | | Date 7/05 | Weight (kg) | Date | | |
| Medicine/substance | Reaction & Severity | Initials & Date | 88kg | 7/05 | Surname: CAMPBELL-SMITH | |
| | | | Height | | First name: CAMERON | |
| | | | 1.78m | | | |
| Alerts | | | Surface area (m²) | | Date of birth: 26.08.60 | |

**IN-PATIENT MEDICATION PRESCRIPTION AND ADMINISTRATION RECORD** — PasTest HOSPITAL

SCENARIO 4

| Consultant JACKSON | Trainee Dr. Name and Bleep no. AF 622 | Date of admission 7.05.12 | Date chart reboarded | Estimated date of discharge |
|---|---|---|---|---|
| This chart is no. ......... of ............. | Transcribing Check by Pharmacy Sign ......... Date ......... | Ward 1. ...HASLL... .. 2. ......... | | |

Supplementary Medication charts in use: Other (please specify): 1 ......... 2 .........

Epidural/PCA ☐  Syringe driver ☐  TPN ☐  Chemotherapy ☐  Insulin sliding scale ☐

Once only medications – loading doses, pre-medication, PGDs or surgical antibiotic propylaxis

| Date | Time to be given | Medicine (approved name) | Dose | Route | Signature and bleep no. | Pharmacy | Time given | Given by | Checked by |
|---|---|---|---|---|---|---|---|---|---|
| 7/05 | Stat | CLOPIDOGREL | 300mg | PO | AF 622 | | | | |
| 7/05 | Stat | ASPIRIN | 300mg | PO | AF 622 | | | | |
| 7/05 | Stat | PARACETAMOL | 1g | PO | AF 622 | | | | |
| 7/05 | Stat | TPA (Bolus) | 8mg/8ml | IV – | To run over 1–2 minutes | | | | |

| Thromboprophylaxis please prescribe treatment regimens in the regular medications section | | | | | | | | | | | | | | | | | | |
|---|---|---|---|---|---|---|---|---|---|---|---|---|---|---|---|---|---|---|
| Choice of mechanical prophylaxis and leg(s) to be applied to | | | | | | Enter Time | Enter details below | | | | | | | | | | | |
| Graduated elastic compression stockings | Intermittent pneumatic compression device (IPC) | Leg | | | | | | | | | | | | | | | | |
| | | Left | Right | Both | | | | | | | | | | | | | | |
| ☑ Start Date: 7/05 | End Date: | Signature and Bleep No. | ☐ | ☐ | ☑ | | | | | | | | | | | | | |
| ☐ Start Date: | End Date: | Signature and Bleep No. AF | ☐ | ☐ | ☐ | | | | | | | | | | | | | |
| Medication NOT FOR HEPARIN | | Dose | | Dose Change | | Enter Time | Enter details below | | | | | | | | | | | |
| Please ensure you have completed the VTE risk assessment form | Date | | | | | | | | | | | | | | | | | |
| | Route | | | | | | | | | | | | | | | | | |
| | Signature | | | | | Instructions | | | | | | | | Pharmacy | | | | ☐ |
| | Bleep no. | | | | | | | | | | | | | | | | | |

| Oxygen | | | | | | | | | | | | | | | | | | |
|---|---|---|---|---|---|---|---|---|---|---|---|---|---|---|---|---|---|---|
| Target Saturation | | 88-92% ☐ | | 94/98% ☑ | | If oxygen saturation falls below target range on prescribed oxygen, patient needs urgent clinical review. If oxygen saturation is above target range on prescribed oxygen, ask for review. | | | | | | | | | | | | |
| Other (specify) | | | | | | *Device: N= nasal cannula, SM = simple face mask, V = venturi, H = humidified, RM = reservoir mask, OTHER = other eg NCPAP/NIPPV | | | | | | | | Pharmacy | | | | ☐ |
| Target Saturation not applicable | | | | | ☐ | | | | | | | | | | | | | |
| | Date Started | Date Changed | | Enter Time | Enter details below | | | | | | | | | | | | | |
| | 7/05 | | | | | | | | | | | | | | | | | |
| Device | Nasal | | | | | | | | | | | | | | | | | |
| % or L/min (specify a range eg 1-21 L/min) | 2L/MIN | | | | | | | | | | | | | | | | | |
| Signature and Bleep no. | | | | | | | | | | | | | | | | | | |

**Regular prescriptions continued**

**Regular medications**

| | Dose | | | Date | 7 | 8 | 9 | 10 | 11 | 12 | | | | | |
|---|---|---|---|---|---|---|---|---|---|---|---|---|---|---|---|
| Date | 7/05/12 | | | Medication | | | | Instructions | | | | Signature and bleep no. | | Pharmacy | |
| Route | PO | | | SIMVASTATIN | | | | | | | | AF 622 | | | |
| Signature | | | | | | | | | | | | | | | |
| 06 | | | | | | | | | | | | | | | |
| 09 | | | | | | | | | | | | | | | |
| 12 | | | | | | | | | | | | | | | |
| 18 | | | | | | | | | | | | | | | |
| (22) | 40mg | | | | | | | | | | | | | | |
| 24 | | | | | | | | | | | | | | | |

**Regular prescriptions continued**

**Regular medications**

| | Dose | | | Date | | | | | | | | | | | |
|---|---|---|---|---|---|---|---|---|---|---|---|---|---|---|---|
| Date | 7/05/12 | | | Medication | | | | Instructions | | | | Signature and bleep no. | | Pharmacy | |
| Route | PO | | | ASPIRIN | | | | 300mg – 2 weeks > | | | | AF 622 | | | |
| Signature | | | | | | | | Reduce 75mg | | | | | | | |
| 06 | | | | | | | | | | | | | | | |
| (09) | 300mg | | | | | | | | | | | | | | |
| 12 | | | | | | | | | | | | | | | |
| 18 | | | | | | | | | | | | | | | |
| 22 | | | | | | | | | | | | | | | |
| 24 | | | | | | | | | | | | | | | |

**Regular prescriptions continued**

**Regular medications**

| | Dose | | | Date | | | | | | | | | | | |
|---|---|---|---|---|---|---|---|---|---|---|---|---|---|---|---|
| Date | 7/05/12 | | | Medication | | | | Instructions | | | | Signature and bleep no. | | Pharmacy | |
| Route | PO | | | CLOPIDOGREL | | | | | | | | AF 622 | | | |
| Signature | | | | | | | | | | | | | | | |
| 06 | | | | | | | | | | | | | | | |
| (09) | 75mg | | | | | | | | | | | | | | |
| 12 | | | | | | | | | | | | | | | |
| 18 | | | | | | | | | | | | | | | |
| 22 | | | | | | | | | | | | | | | |
| 24 | | | | | | | | | | | | | | | |

**Regular prescriptions continued**

**Regular medications**

| | Dose | | | Date | | | | | | | | | | | |
|---|---|---|---|---|---|---|---|---|---|---|---|---|---|---|---|
| Date | 7/05/12 | | | Medication | | | | Instructions | | | | Signature and bleep no. | | Pharmacy | |
| Route | PO | | | PARACETAMOL | | | | To maintain 7° | | | | AF 622 | | | |
| Signature | | | | | | | | below 37.5° | | | | | | | |
| 06 | | | | | | | | | | | | | | | |
| (09) | 1g | | | | | | | | | | | | | | |
| (12) | 1g | | | | | | | | | | | | | | |
| (18) | 1g | | | | | | | | | | | | | | |
| (22) | 1g | | | | | | | | | | | | | | |
| 24 | | | | | | | | | | | | | | | |

## Infusion prescriptions continued

| SC = subcutaneous | IVC = intravenous central |
|---|---|
| | IVP = intravenous peripheral |

| Date & time | Route | Infusion Fluid — Name & strength | Volume | Medication — Approved name with expiry / unit number | Dose | Duration | Rate | Prescriber's signature & bleep no. | Date given | Given by / Added by | Check by | Start time | Finish time | Pharmacy |
|---|---|---|---|---|---|---|---|---|---|---|---|---|---|---|
| 7/05 | IV | 0.9% Saline  Exp:  Batch/unit no: | 50ml | TPA | 50 mg | TO RUN AT 71mg/HOUR | | AF 622 | | | | | | |
| 7/05 | IV | 0.9% Saline  Exp:  Batch/unit no: | 21ml | TPA | 21 mg | TO RUN AT 71mg/HOUR | | | | | | | | |
| | | Exp:  Batch/unit no: | | PATIENT WEIGHS 88.0kg | | | | | | | | | | |
| 7/05 | IV | 0.9% Saline  Exp:  Batch/unit no: | 50ml | ACTRAPID INSULIN | 50 UNITS | TO RUN AT 0.1 UNITS/kg/HOUR  ≡ 8.8 UNITS/HOUR | | | | | | | | |
| | | Exp:  Batch/unit no: | | TO MAINTAIN CAPILLARY BLOOD GLUCOSE BETWEEN >4.0<10 MMOL/L | | | | | | | | | | |
| | | Exp:  Batch/unit no: | | | | | | | | | | | | |
| | | Exp:  Batch/unit no: | | | | | | | | | | | | |
| | | Exp:  Batch/unit no: | | | | | | | | | | | | |
| | | Exp:  Batch/unit no: | | | | | | | | | | | | |
| | | | | | | | | | | | | | | |
| | | | | | | | | | | | | | | |

### As required medications

| Medication | Date | | | | | | | | | | | | | | | | | | |
|---|---|---|---|---|---|---|---|---|---|---|---|---|---|---|---|---|---|---|---|
| CODEINE PHOSPHATE | | | | | | | | | | | | | | | | | | | |
| Indication  PAIN | Time | | | | | | | | | | | | | | | | | | |
| Dose 30 mg | Route PO | Maximum frequency / dose  6 HOURLY | Start date 5/7/12  Stop date | Dose | | | | | | | | | | | | | | | |
| | | | | Route | | | | | | | | | | | | | | | |
| Signature  AF | | | Bleep no. 622 | Given | | | | | | | | | | | | | | | |
| Additional instructions: | | | | | | | | Pharmacy | | | | | | | | | | | |

### As required medications

| Medication | Date | | | | | | | | | | | | | | | | | | |
|---|---|---|---|---|---|---|---|---|---|---|---|---|---|---|---|---|---|---|---|
| METOCLOPRAMIDE | | | | | | | | | | | | | | | | | | | |
| Indication  NAUSEA/VOMITING | Time | | | | | | | | | | | | | | | | | | |
| Dose 10 mg | Route S/Ci IM IV | Maximum frequency / dose  8 HOURLY | Start date 7/05  Stop date | Dose | | | | | | | | | | | | | | | |
| | | | | Route | | | | | | | | | | | | | | | |
| Signature  AF | | | Bleep no. 622 | Given | | | | | | | | | | | | | | | |
| Additional instructions: | | | | | | | | Pharmacy | | | | | | | | | | | |

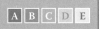

**GLOBAL PRESCRIBING MARK**  A B C D E

## Station 5 – Clinical communication skills

**Patient script**

You are Mr Campbell-Smith (DOB 26 August 1960), 51-years-old. You were originally taken to St. James' Hospital, where you were treated for a 'large stroke' affecting your speech, right arm, right leg and vision. With the treatment and the fantastic therapists, you are now able to walk on your own with just a stick. Your speech is much better and most people can understand you, but you still get the odd word wrong, and this is very frustrating! You get dressed 'pretty much' on your own, go to the toilet without help, although 'I occasionally still make a bit of a mess on the floor when I'm peeing'. You can feed yourself and eating and drinking are fine. You can get in and out of bed, and on and off chairs and the toilet, without help. Overall you're pretty positive (like the therapists) about how you are doing.

You are expecting to go home this week and are really looking forward to being back home, but a little anxious about how your friends and family will treat you. You have seen your brother and his wife almost daily but you've been reluctant to see friends whilst you were unable to speak properly.

'The doctors and nurses have told me I must take all my pills but I'm not convinced that they are doing me any good'. 'My blood pressure and things always seem to be normal whenever someone checks them!'

You have tried to stop smoking but 'still sneak a crafty one here and there when no one is looking'. You are happy to wear the patches and try to stop but you are worried that you will slowly go back to it once home.

You've had a talk with the social worker about financial support but have made no real plans for a pension and 'mainly lived for the day'. You are worried because you don't think you could just stop working and need to be out and about doing something. You have thought about other things you could do and your brother has talked about some things with him in his mini-cab business, but this is not really what you want to do.

You think you will find it all very difficult once home and 'may well end up back here with another stroke'. You know your wife will be very supportive and are hoping you can do it for her.

SCENARIO 4

PROFESSIONALISM      PROCESS

## CONTENT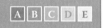

**Confirms reason for discussion**

**Establishes what patient wishes to know; gains agreement/informal consent to participate in the discussion**

**Investigates patient's present level of understanding of scenario**

**Summarises and confirms what has happened so far**
- Went to St. James' after suffering a stroke; given thrombolysis
- Transferred back to local hospital, where he's been receiving therapy
- Present level of functioning: mobility and transfers; speech and language; eating and drinking/feeding; washing and dressing; toileting and continence
- Due to go home this week.

**Establishes patient's ideas, concerns and expectations**

**Explains the key, important information**
- **Medications: actions, frequency, side effects**
    - Aspirin and clopidogrel – anti-platelet; stop blood clots forming in the blood vessels (arteries) of the neck and brain; really important to take these as they stop the strokes occurring; take one each daily; side effects are indigestion, abdominal pain and bruising or bleeding; if excessive or constant need to see a doctor straight away
    - Perindopril – this is a drug that principally reduces blood pressure and is known to reduce further strokes ; take one daily; may cause low blood pressure and dizziness; may also affect kidneys so needs to be monitored by GP
    - Indapamide – lowers blood pressure; works with the perindopril; acts on the kidneys so again needs to be monitored by GP
    - Simvastatin – lowers blood cholesterol; side effects are jaundice and liver problems, muscle aches and pains
    - Nicotine patches – will help give up smoking; this is really important to avoid further strokes and heart attacks.
- **Lifestyle changes**
    - Smoking cessation: really important; can also go to support group if patient thinks this would help
    - Alcohol: down to safe limits (21 units per week); avoid bingeing
    - Weight loss: reinforce healthy eating; low fat; low salt; cut out sweet things – sugar, cakes, biscuits
    - Help with finances and work – to discuss with social workers; think about retraining; think about skills he is able to continue.

**Invites patient to ask questions and is able to deal with them appropriately**

**Summarises important areas of the consultation back to the patient**

**Formally ends the consultation and ensures appropriate follow-up has been discussed**

SCENARIO 4

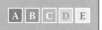

## GLOBAL COMMUNICATION MARK

A B C D E

## Scenario 4:
## Reflection and consolidation

### History

Mr Cameron Campbell-Smith is a right-handed 51-year-old Black Caribbean man who is a previously fit and well painter and decorator. Of note he has had high blood pressure for the past 6 years. This morning he woke feeling fine and was driving to a new job when he suddenly began to feel unwell, with no pre-warning symptoms. His head felt 'as if it wasn't attached to his shoulders', 'light and floating'. He denies dizziness, syncope or pre-syncope but had to stop the van he was driving at the side of the road. He managed to speed-dial his wife but his speech was slurred and he was unable to find the right words.

His right upper and lower limb then became numb and weak and his arm flopped down by his side. The whole episode lasted about 15–20 minutes and completely resolved after 30 minutes, when he was able to drive home. He now feels 100% back to normal with no residual disabilities. He has never experienced a similar episode.

Apart from hypertension, Mr Campbell-Smith's CV risk factors include smoking (he is a lifelong smoker, using about 2 oz of tobacco per week) and alcohol (he drinks a small whisky most nights, but occasionally binges; a large bottle of whisky lasts him about a month); there are no other CV risk factors of note.

Mr Campbell-Smith's current medications are ramipril (5 mg od) and amlodipine (10 mg od). He has no known drug allergies.

Mr Campbell-Smith is married and lives with his wife in a first-floor flat. His wife works as a receptionist in a local dentist practice and is very well. They have no children. His brother and his family live close by.

### Examination

Three weeks after his initial assessment in the GP practice, Mr Campbell-Smith is seen in the Emergency Department of the local teaching hospital, St. James'. Examination of this middle-aged Black Caribbean man revealed him to be overweight with heavy tar staining of the fingers of his right hand. He was hypertensive (BP 187/120 mmHg) with a heart rate of 96 bpm in a regular rhythm. He had a murmur consistent with aortic stenosis but no signs of cardiac failure or peripheral vascular disease.

Neurological assessment revealed Mr Campbell-Smith to have signs consistent with a left hemisphere TACS, as evidenced by a right homonymous hemipanopia, a right hemiparesis (grade 3–4/5) and a mild expressive dysphasia. His swallow was deemed to be unsafe.

### Data interpretation

Patients presenting with TIA or stroke require radiological confirmation of the diagnosis, whilst excluding other pathologies mimicking stroke presentation. Initially all patients should undergo a CT scan of the brain. Where the diagnosis remains inconclusive, a secondary MRI scan may be undertaken.

Other investigations include clinical tests, BP, $O_2$ monitoring, temperature and ECG, all of which impact on the acute management. Blood tests may include FBC, U&Es, glucose, lipids, ESR and clotting screen.

A chest radiograph should be performed to exclude co-morbidities such as cardiovascular disease and primary and secondary lung cancers.

Once the diagnosis has been confirmed, secondary investigations such as Doppler scan of the carotid arterial system, carotid angiogram and potentially carotid endarterectomy should be considered.

## Management

The management of acute stroke in the UK has changed very rapidly over the past five years. In a similar manner to the treatment of patients with ACS and acute STEMI, TIA and stroke patients' risk is now being stratified using objective scoring systems such as the ABCD2 (TIAs) and ROSIER score (stroke). These help identify high-, moderate- and low-risk patients and allow for the planning and delivery of acute intervention. Acute stroke is now treated in a similar manner to acute STEMI, with patients treated with thrombolysis on a hyperacute stroke unit (HASU), located at larger centres of excellence. Once over the initial episode, patients are transferred back to their local hospital, where they are cared for by an expert multidisciplinary team on a dedicated stroke unit. During their rehabilitation, secondary prophylaxis should be started and all cardiovascular and stroke risk assessed and managed.

A third community-based stream is now being successfully introduced allowing early discharge of the patient to their own home, with community-based rehabilitation and follow-up.

## Further reading and web links

*ABCD2 score*:

Johnston SC, Rothwell PM, et al. Validation and refinement of scores to predict very early stroke risk after transient ischaemic attack. *Lancet* 2007;369:283–92.

Nor AM, Davis J, et al. The Recognition of Stroke in the Emergency Room (ROSIER) scale: development and validation of a stroke recognition instrument. *Lancet Neurol* 2005;4:727–34.

*Scottish guidelines on acute stroke management*:

www.sign.ac.uk/pdf/qrg118.pdf

*NICE guidelines on TIA and stroke management*:

www.nice.org.uk/CG68

# Scenario 5: 'Breast lump'

## Station 1

*History*                    *10-minute station*

You are a final year medical student on rotation at a GP practice – the next patient that your GP has arranged for you to see is a 36-year-old lady called Mrs Charlotte North.

■ **Please take a history, which you will then present to your GP, who may ask you some questions.**

*You will be assessed on the following areas, as well as the content and diagnostic reasoning of your history – take them into account in your presentation.*

### Professionalism

- Professional appearance (NHS dress code) – including general appearance, hair and jewellery
- Maintains patient and personal safety
- Polite introduction; identifies patient or interviewee correctly; confirms patient's date of birth from name band or other source
- Obtains informal consent; maintains patient's privacy
- Displays empathetic and caring attitudes and behaviours throughout.

### Process

- Good organisation and structure; appropriate use of open and closed questions
- Appropriate fluency/rhythm/pace to the interview – this may change depending on environment and acute nature of the problem
- Appropriate time for the patient to respond/reply to questions
- Appropriate acknowledgement of difficult or emotional areas of the patient's history.

### Communication skills

- Demonstrates caring and sympathetic attitude
- Asks open questions
- Invites patient to ask questions and answers them appropriately
- Addresses patient's ideas, concerns and expectations.

## Station 2

*Examination*            *10-minute station*

■ Please perform a focussed breast examination while your supervising GP observes you. If required, you may ask for a set of clinical observations, as one of the practice nurses has performed some before the appointment began (if you do not have a model, please read and present the information given on page 381).

*You will be assessed on the following areas, as well as the content and skills of your examination – take them into account in your presentation.*

### Professionalism

- Professional appearance; maintains infection control standards, including hand cleaning and appropriate use of gloves and aprons
- Maintains patient and personal safety
- Polite introduction; identifies patient and confirms date of birth from name band or other source
- Obtains informal consent; maintains patient privacy and dignity
- Displays empathetic and caring attitudes and behaviours throughout.

### Process

- Appropriate fluency/rhythm/pace to the examination – this may change depending on environment and acute nature of the problem
- Organisation and structure of examination; sensitive and empathetic approach
- Uses appropriate clinical techniques throughout
- Maintains privacy and dignity throughout.

### Clinical communication

- Explains proposed examination/procedure: explains examination/procedure as it proceeds
- Offers information in a clear, structured and fluent manner, avoiding jargon
- Listens to patient and responds appropriately
- Demonstrates appropriate body language.

## Station 3

*Data interpretation*            *10-minute station*

■ Please answer the following two questions.
  1 Risk factors for malignancy: for each of the risk factors (a–e) choose the malignancy from the list with which there is the greatest association.
    A   Colorectal carcinoma

SCENARIO 5

B    Squamous cell carcinoma of the bladder
C    Gastric carcinoma
D    Breast carcinoma
E    Cervical carcinoma
F    Hepatocellular carcinoma
G    Prostate carcinoma
H    Ovarian carcinoma
I    Testicular seminoma
J    Malignant melanoma
a.   Type 2 diabetes
b.   Pernicious anaemia
c.   Schistosomiasis
d.   Human papillomavirus
e.   Hormone replacement therapy

2  For each of the malignant diseases listed below indicate whether the statements
   are TRUE (T) or FALSE (F).

A  Colorectal carcinoma:
   a.   Is twice as common in males
   b.   Most commonly metastasises to the spine
   c.   Is often staged using the Dukes' staging system
   d.   Is associated with Crohn's disease
   e.   Is the most common cancer in the UK.

B  Malignant melanoma:
   a.   Is more common in males
   b.   Is never seen in the Afro-Caribbean population
   c.   Cerebral metastases are common
   d.   Breslow thickness >4 mm is associated with a 5-year survival of less than
        10%
   e.   Is most prevalent in the Australasian continent.

C  Lung carcinoma:
   a.   Is the most common cancer in the UK
   b.   Is more common in males
   c.   Non-small cell carcinoma is more common than small cell carcinoma
   d.   Adenocarcinoma is associated with ACTH secretion
   e.   Intestinal metastases are the most common.

SCENARIO 5

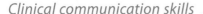

## Station 4

*Clinical communication skills*　　　　　*10-minute station*

Now that you have completed the history and examination, you are asked to explain to
Mrs North what investigations will be arranged for her.

■ Please speak to Mrs North about the investigations and answer any questions she
  may have.

# Answers

## Station 1 – History

**Patient script**

You are Charlotte North (DOB 19 March 1976). You work as a teacher at the local primary school.

You have come to the GP surgery today because about 3 weeks ago you noticed a lump in your left breast. You were examining yourself, as you understand that regular self-examination is advised, and had not noticed anything before this. You initially thought that it would probably be nothing to worry about, but the lump is still there and you now feel you need to have it checked.

The lump is not painful or itchy, nor does it seem to have got bigger or smaller since you noticed it. It does not seem to move position. You have not noticed any discharge from the nipple, and have not noticed any redness or swelling at the skin of the breast. You have never noticed anything like this in the past.

You feel generally well, and have not noticed any other symptoms lately. You have put on a bit of weight since going back to work after taking 3 years off after the birth of your son. Your only medical problem is that you have mild asthma, for which you carry a salbutamol inhaler, and use it approximately once every fortnight. You do not take any other regular medications and are not allergic to any medicines that you know of.

You have been married for 8 years, and have a 4-year-old son. You stopped breastfeeding when your son was 9 months old. You would like to have more children, and you and your husband are trying to have another (ie no contraception at present). You have never had any miscarriages to your knowledge. Your menstrual cycle has always been regular since you started having periods at the age of 14.

You do not smoke, and never have. Most evenings you share a bottle of wine with your husband but rarely drink more than that.

You have a family history of breast cancer – your mother died of breast cancer 11 years ago at the age of 54, and her sister (your aunt) had a scare several years ago and had to undergo some surgery, although you do not know exactly what she had done, as she lives in Australia. You are not aware of any other family history.

A B C D E
PROFESSIONALISM

A B C D E
PROCESS

A B C D E
COMMUNICATION

## CONTENT

A B C D E

### Identifies key information
- Breast lump for last 3 weeks

### Includes important negatives, including systemic enquiry
- No pain or itching
- No nipple discharge
- Does not move position within the breast
- No previous history of breast lumps.

### Identifies key information from rest of history
- Feels generally well, no other symptoms, including weight loss
- Menarche at 14 years, regular menstrual cycles
- One child, breastfed for 9 months; no miscarriages
- Strong family history (see below).

### Completing the patient history
- Drug and allergy history: salbutamol inhaler (prn fortnightly)
- Previous medical history: mild asthma
- Social and occupational history: primary school teacher; married with one child; moderate alcohol; non-smoker
- Family history: mother (died) and maternal aunt (surgery) – breast cancer.

### Summarises important areas of the history back to the patient

### Invites patient to ask questions and deals with them appropriately

### Establishes patient's ideas, concerns and expectations

SCENARIO 5

## CLINICAL DIAGNOSTIC REASONING

■ **Please present your history**
  • Candidate offers a logical, well-structured account of the history.

■ **What are the important differential diagnoses of a breast lump?**
  • Fibroadenoma
  • Breast cancer
  • Fibrocystic disease
  • Duct ectasia
  • Fat necrosis
  • Breast abscess
  • Breast cyst
  • Galactocoele
  • Lipoma
  • Sebaceous cyst.

**Demonstrates clear and logical diagnostic reasoning**

## GLOBAL HISTORY MARK

## Station 2 – Examination

**Patient script (see also page 381)**

You are a generally healthy young woman and should appear comfortable at rest. You have no symptoms of pain and your only concern has been the lump that you have identified in your left breast (upper outer quadrant).

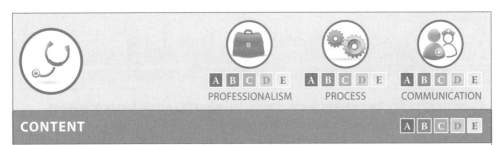

A B C D E
PROFESSIONALISM

A B C D E
PROCESS

A B C D E
COMMUNICATION

## CONTENT

A B C D E

**Exposes and positions patient correctly and maintains comfort**
- Inspection with patient in sitting position followed by palpation with patient lying down.

**Comments on wellbeing of patient, ie well or unwell**

**'Feet to face'**
- Observes and comments on patient and surroundings from foot of bed.

**Asks for appropriate/relevant clinical observations**
- Observations: HR 58 bpm, BP 108/71 mmHG, RR 14 bpm, $O_2$ sats 100% on air.

**Breast examination (must examine normal and abnormal sides)**
- Starts with patient sitting upright with hands resting on thighs (to relax pectoral muscles)
- Inspects breasts for asymmetry, swelling and changes to the skin or the nipples
- Repeats inspection:
  - With patient pushing hands into hips, contracting pectoral muscles
  - With hands raised behind head, to stretch pectoral muscles and skin
  - With patient leaning forward such that the breasts become pendulous.
- Positions patient in lying position (or at 45°) with arm (of side to be examined first) behind head
- Palpation with palm of hand in systematic sequence (clockface or quadrants), compressing tissue of breast against chest wall; includes tissue beneath nipple
- Identifies mass and characterises its nature: size, texture, fixation to underlying structures, tethering to skin
- Observes for signs of pain or discomfort
- Determines fixation by holding lesion between finger and thumb, and asks patient to contract pectoral muscles
- Examines nipple by holding gently and attempts to express discharge
- Examines axillary tail between finger and thumb
- Palpates regional lymph nodes and axilla; examines axilla with arms tensed on hips and with arms relaxed
- Compares findings on each side.

**Thanks patient, offers assistance, maintains patient's dignity and privacy until they are dressed**

SCENARIO 5

## CLINICAL DIAGNOSTIC REASONING

**Correctly identifies the relevant physical signs, including important negative findings**

- **What are the causes of breast swelling in men?**
    - Gynaecomastia may occur normally in pubertal boys due to the high levels of circulating oestradiol, but may be seen in other conditions associated with increased oestrogen production including Cushing's, thyrotoxicosis, acromegaly, prolactinoma and teratoma
    - Breast cancer in men, although rare, must not be disregarded as a potential cause of breast swelling in men (especially if unilateral); it accounts for 1% of all breast cancer cases, but is associated with a worse prognosis compared with women
    - Several drugs can cause gynaecomastia, including:
        - digoxin; spironolactone; cimetidine; oestrogens; vincristine.
    - Other causes of gynaecomastia include cirrhotic liver disease and cannabis use.

- **Is breast cancer hereditary?**
    - There is a strong familial link with breast cancer
    - A positive family history in a first-degree relative is significant, as up to 10% of breast cancers are inherited (autosomal dominant with limited penetrance)
    - Patients that inherit breast cancer tend to present earlier in life, and there may be a family association of other cancers such as bowel and ovarian
    - The *BRCA1*, *BRCA2* and *p53* genes are all implicated in the inheritance of breast cancer.

**Demonstrates clear and logical diagnostic reasoning**

## GLOBAL EXAMINATION MARK

# Station 3 – Data interpretation

**1**

   a.  F
   b.  C
   c.  B
   d.  E
   e.  H

**2**

**A**      **Colorectal carcinoma**

   a.  False
   b.  False
   c.  True
   d.  False
   e.  False

Colorectal carcinoma (adenocarcinoma affecting the colon ± rectum) is the second most common cancer in the UK, with a M : F ratio of 1 : 1. The prinicipal risk factors include fat and cholesterol-rich diet, ulcerative colitis, adenomatous polyps and family history. Right-sided (caecum, ascending and proximal transverse colon) tumours usually present with weight loss and symptoms of anaemia whilst left-sided (distal transverse, descending and sigmoid colon and rectum) tumours more often present with abdominal pain, altered bowel habit and rectal bleeding. They can also present with bowel obstruction or perforation leading to peritonitis. The most common site of metastasis is the liver (via the portal vein) but also lungs, adrenal glands, kidneys and bones. The Dukes' classification is used to stage colorectal cancer. Surgical resection, radiotherapy and chemotherapy are all important in the management of colorectal cancer.

**B**      **Malignant melanoma**

   a.  False
   b.  False
   c.  True
   d.  False
   e.  True

Malignant melanoma is most common in the 20–40 year age group and is more common in females than in males. Melanoma usually derives from a mole or naevus, and the risk factors include asymmetry, border irregularity, colour variation, diameter (>6 mm), evolving (ongoing changes). Two main staging systems are used: Breslow thickness, which measures the tumour from the most superficial to the deepest point (mm), and Clarke's levels, which take into account the anatomical level of skin invaded. Melanoma often metastasises, both to local and regional lymph nodes, remote skin sites, and to the brain, small bowel, lungs, liver, adrenals and heart.

SCENARIO 5

C　　　Lung cancer
  a. True
  b. True
  c. False
  d. False
  e. False

Lung cancer is the most common cancer in the UK, and leads to more than 1 in 5 of all cancer deaths. It is strongly associated with smoking, although can be seen in non-smokers. There is also an association with asbestos exposure. Non-small cell cancers are the most common and include adenocarcinoma, squamous cell carcinoma, and large cell lung cancers. Small cell cancers are less common, but often metastise earlier. There is often an endocrine/paraneoplastic syndrome association, as small cells have a dense concentration of neurosecretory granules, secreting ACTH and ADH (leading to syndrome of inappropriate antidiuretic hormone hypersecretion (SIADH)). Lung cancer most commonly metastasises to the liver, adrenal glands, brain, bones and lymph nodes.

**GLOBAL DATA INTERPRETATION MARK**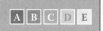

## Station 4 – Clinical communication skills

**Patient script**

You are concerned about the nature of the breast lump that you have discovered. In particular, you are worried that it could be cancer, because your mother and aunt both had breast cancer.

You are anxious to know what tests will be done now and what they involve. Your main concern that is worrying you is that you will have to have a mastectomy, as you don't feel you would manage very well having major surgery like that, and you think you would have to stop your job because you would be worried what people would think or say.

You have the following questions:
  • 'Is this likely to be cancer?'
  • 'What tests do I have to go for now?'
  • 'If all the tests are normal and don't suggest cancer, can I still have the lump removed?'

PROFESSIONALISM    PROCESS

## CONTENT

**Confirms reason for discussion**

**Investigates patient's present level of understanding of scenario**

**Summarises and confirms what has happened so far**
- Recent discovery of a breast lump for which this is her first medical appointment.

**Establishes patient's ideas, concerns and expectations**
- Patient is particularly anxious due to strong family history of breast cancer
- Worried about having major surgery (mastectomy)
- Understands will now need to go for further investigations.

**Explains the key information**
- Explains that breast lumps are very common and can be attributed to a variety of causes, ranging from low to high severity.

**Invites patient to ask questions and is able to deal with them appropriately**
- Reassures that there is high chance that this is not cancer because other causes such as cysts and fibroadenomas are more common; however, given her family history, she is at higher risk than someone without a family history, and so thorough investigation is essential
- Explains that all persistent breast lumps are investigated thoroughly with:
  - Mammography – X-ray (if >35 years)
  - Ultrasound
  - Fine-needle aspiration cytology (FNAC) – needle aspiration of sample of cells from the lump, which can be looked at under microscope for evidence of cancerous (malignant) cells
- Explains that the treatment that she will be offered will depend on the results of the test
- She may have the lump excised if she wishes to, even if all the tests suggest that it is not cancerous
- If the investigations do suggest cancer, she is unlikely to require a mastectomy, as this is only advised if the lesion is large, central, multiple, ill-defined or involves the nipple, or if she chooses mastectomy over wide local excision (WLE).

**Summarises important areas of the consultation back to the patient**

**Formally ends the consultation and ensures appropriate follow-up has been discussed**
- She will be referred to the hospital in the normal way for all patients presenting with breast lumps that require investigation – she will receive appointments for her mammogram, ultrasound and fine-needle aspiration cytology tests.

SCENARIO 5

## GLOBAL COMMUNICATION MARK

## Scenario 5: Reflection and consolidation

### History

Ms North is a 36-year-old primary school teacher who presents with a lump to her left breast. She noticed the lump on routine self-examination three weeks ago, and it has not caused any symptoms of pain. The lump is neither growing nor diminishing, and does not seem to change position. She has not noticed any discharge or other changes to the nipple. She does not report any previous episodes. Of note, she does not report any weight loss. Her menarche was at age 14 years, and she has one child age four years who was breast-fed until 9 months old. She has had no other pregnancies, but is not currently using contraception.
She is generally fit and well, other than mild asthma for which she requires the use of a salbutamol inhaler approximately every fortnight. She does not report any allergies. She does not smoke, but drinks approximately two glasses of wine most evenings (approx. 28 units per week).
She has a strong family history of breast cancer, her mother having died age 54, and a maternal aunt having undergone surgical intervention for a breast-related problem.

### Examination

This lady is generally well in appearance, is of medium build, and her observations are within normal limits. Breast examination reveals no asymmetry. The right breast is normal. Palpation of the left breast demonstrates a 3cm, firm, non-tender mass in the upper outer quadrant. The mass is not fixed to the skin and is not associated with overlying skin changes. The nipple is normal; there is no associated lymphadenopathy, hepatomegaly or bone tenderness.

### Investigations

There is a variety of differential causes of breast lumps, but given that breast cancer remains the most common female cancer in Europe, with a lifetime risk of 1 in 9 women in the UK, all women that present with a breast lump should be investigated with triple assessment:
- History and clinical examination
- Bilateral mammography, usually in combination with ultrasound
- Fine-needle aspiration cytology and/or core biopsy.

### Management

Currently, the UK Breast Screening Programme invites women age 50 to 64 for three-yearly mammograms, after which age women are encouraged to refer for ongoing scans. By 2016, there are plans to extend this age range for invitational scans from 47 to 73 years.
**Carcinoma of the breast:**
These lesions are often characteristically solid, with a firm texture, an irregular outline, but are also often painless. They may be confined to the breast tissue or extend to the surrounding structures: skin, pectoral fascia, pectoral muscle. The TNM (tumour, node, metastasis) system of classification is used, and should be understood. Treatment targets: (1) the breast (wide local excision or mastectomy); (2) the axilla (clearance or radiotherapy); and (3) systemic therapy (including radiotherapy, chemotherapy and hormonal treatment with eg oestrogen-receptor antagonists such as tamoxifen, or aromatase inhibitors such as anastrazole.
**Fibroadenoma:**
These are commonly seen in the 20–35 years age group and represent 20% of all breast lumps. They are often described as 'breast mice' as they appear mobile, and are firm in nature. They arise from overgrowth of terminal duct lobules, and are neither pre-malignant nor associated with higher risk of later breast cancer.

**Breast cysts:**

Breast cysts are more particularly seen in post-menopausal women, but are the most common cause of a breast lump in women between 35 and 50 years. They represent 15% of all breast lumps. The cause is thought to be due to a variation of normal lobular change within the breast tissue, and they sometimes occur in clusters. The intracystic pressure dictates how soft or firm they appear on palpation, and they may be fluctuant and mobile.

**Breast abscesses:**

There are two types of breast abscesses. Lactational abscesses occur in women that are breastfeeding and tend to be sited peripherally. Non-lactational abscesses are most commonly seen in smokers, and occur as a sequela of periductal mastitis and are typically found at the edge of the nipple, and are therefore often associated with nipple inversion.

**Further reading and web links**

*UK Breast Screening Programme:*
www.cancerscreening.nhs.uk/breastscreen
*NICE guidance on breast cancer:*
http://publications.nice.org.uk/early-and-locally-advanced-breast-cancer-cg80
*Cancer staging including TNM classification system:*
www.cancer.gov/cancertopics/factsheet/detection/staging

SCENARIO 5

# Scenario 6:
# 'Terrible legs'

## Station 1

*History*                                           *10-minute station*

You are the FY1 attending the community leg ulcer clinic with the Vascular Nurse Specialist (VNS). He has asked you to see the first patient, Mrs Geraldine Smith (DOB 16/05/1940), a 72-year-old woman who has been sent up by her GP this morning as an emergency. She is happy to talk to you and is very concerned about her legs.

■ Please take a focussed, diagnostic history with a view to presenting it to the VNS.

*You will be assessed on the following areas, as well as the content and diagnostic reasoning of your history – take them into account in your presentation.*

### Professionalism

- Professional appearance (NHS dress code) – including general appearance, hair and jewellery
- Maintains patient and personal safety
- Polite introduction; identifies patient or interviewee correctly; confirms patient's date of birth from name band or other source
- Obtains informal consent; maintains patient's privacy
- Displays empathetic and caring attitudes and behaviours throughout.

### Process

- Good organisation and structure; appropriate use of open and closed questions
- Appropriate fluency/rhythm/pace to the interview – this may change depending on environment and acute nature of the problem
- Appropriate time for the patient to respond/reply to questions
- Appropriate acknowledgement of difficult or emotional areas of the patient's history.

### Communication skills

- Demonstrates caring and sympathetic attitude
- Asks open questions
- Invites patient to ask questions and answers them appropriately
- Addresses patient's ideas, concerns and expectations.

# Station 2

*Examination*                                                    *5-minute station*

- After presenting your history, please perform a focussed clinical assessment of Mrs Smith, to include:
  1. The patient's wellbeing
  2. An assessment of the ulcerated area.

(If you do not have a model, please read and present the information given on page 382.)

*You will be assessed on the following areas, as well as the content and skills of your examination – take them into account in your presentation.*

| Professionalism |  |
| --- | --- |

- Professional appearance; maintains infection control standards, including hand cleaning and appropriate use of gloves and aprons
- Maintains patient and personal safety
- Polite introduction; identifies patient and confirms date of birth from name band or other source
- Obtains informal consent; maintains patient privacy and dignity
- Displays empathetic and caring attitudes and behaviours throughout.

| Process |  |
| --- | --- |

- Appropriate fluency/rhythm/pace to the examination – this may change depending on environment and acute nature of the problem
- Organisation and structure of examination; sensitive and empathetic approach
- Uses appropriate clinical techniques throughout
- Maintains privacy and dignity throughout.

| Clinical communication |  |
| --- | --- |

- Explains proposed examination/procedure: explains examination/procedure as it proceeds
- Offers information in a clear, structured and fluent manner, avoiding jargon
- Listens to patient and responds appropriately
- Demonstrates appropriate body language.

SCENARIO 6

## Station 3

*Examination*                              *10-minute station*

Whilst waiting to refer Mrs Smith to the on-call medical team, the VNS asks you to come to see the next patient, who is nearing the end of her treatment in the clinic.

■ Please perform a formal assessment of the patient's (Mrs Fitzpatrick's) venous system of the lower limbs, including ankle brachial pressure indices (ABPIs). You should use the following equipment:

- Tourniquet
- Appropriate sized cuff and sphygmomanometer
- Doppler machine.

*You will be assessed on the following areas, as well as the content and skills of your examination – take them into account in your presentation.*

### Professionalism

- Professional appearance; maintains infection control standards, including hand cleaning and appropriate use of gloves and aprons
- Maintains patient and personal safety
- Polite introduction; identifies patient and confirms date of birth from name band or other source
- Obtains informal consent; maintains patient privacy and dignity
- Displays empathetic and caring attitudes and behaviours throughout.

### Process

- Appropriate fluency/rhythm/pace to the examination – this may change depending on environment and acute nature of the problem
- Organisation and structure of examination; sensitive and empathetic approach
- Uses appropriate clinical techniques throughout
- Maintains privacy and dignity throughout.

### Clinical communication

- Explains proposed examination/procedure: explains examination/procedure as it proceeds
- Offers information in a clear, structured and fluent manner, avoiding jargon
- Listens to patient and responds appropriately
- Demonstrates appropriate body language.

## Station 4

*Clinical communication skills*          *10-minute station*

Given the patient's presentation, the VNS would you please explain the immediate and long-term management to Mrs Smith and address any concerns she may have.

## Station 5

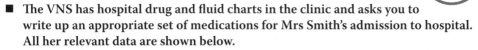

*Prescribing skills*          *10-minute station*

■ The VNS has hospital drug and fluid charts in the clinic and asks you to write up an appropriate set of medications for Mrs Smith's admission to hospital. All her relevant data are shown below.

**Details**

   o Mrs Geraldine Smith, DOB: 16/05/40, Hospital no: 087651, Ward: MAU, Consultant: Dr Hubbard, FY1 bleep number: 201

   o Weight: approx. 90 kg, Height: 1.54 m

   o U&Es: $Na^+$ 139 mmol/l, $K^+$ 3.8 mmol/l, urea 10.8 mmol/l, creatinine 131 µmol/, blood glucose 21.3 mmol/l

   o Allergies: nil known

# Answers

## Station 1 – History

**Patient script**

You are Mrs Geraldine Smith, DOB 16 May 1940 (72 years old). You are now a full-time carer for your husband, but you were previously a factory worker and worked in the local Tate and Lyle sugar factory, in the canning section (no dusts).

You went to see the doctor this morning because 'my terrible legs just got worse... if that's possible'. You have suffered with your legs ever since your children were born. You had three lovely children, but you had a 'really bad thrombosis' in your left leg during your first pregnancy (that was 50 years ago) and your legs, well your veins, just got worse and worse after each pregnancy.

Since then, your left leg, and to a lesser extent your right leg, have been full of varicose veins, really discoloured. Both are swollen below the knees, and 'are just really very ugly'. You hated your legs so much when you were younger, that you wouldn't go out, even on holiday, without a pair of trousers or something to cover them up completely. You were never offered or wore support stockings.

You did think of having 'the operation for the veins' but as time passed by you just learned to accept them, and then as you got to middle age you couldn't be bothered... 'I'd lost all my vanity by then'. You'd had several leg ulcers over the years, mainly on the left, but also on the right. They've always healed up (eventually); some needed 'that really tight bandaging the district nurses used to put on'.

Nearly 3 weeks ago now, you were walking around the local supermarket when a little girl 'crashed' a shopping trolley into the side of your left shin... 'Oh it hurt – little blighter she was, didn't even say sorry'.

Since then it's just got worse and worse – the ulcer has got bigger, increasingly painful, and the edges seem to be 'parting like the Red Sea'. Over the last week or so it's got really mucky, smelly and is leaking everywhere. You've been dressing it yourself but it started to smell, and then you started to feel like you had the flu, so today you thought you had better see the doctor.

Risk factors for leg ulcers:
- ◆ Venous risk – as above
- ◆ Arterial risk – known dietary controlled diabetes, no history of ischaemic heart disease (IHD), stroke, peripheral vascular disease (PVD), hypertension
- ◆ Ex-smoker – gave up 20 years ago; previously smoked 20/day for about 30 years
- ◆ Alcohol – 'I like a glass or two of sherry now and again'; 'If I go out (not very often), I'll have a glass of white wine'
- ◆ Lipids – not known
- ◆ Neuropathic risk – diabetes mellitus (DM); nil else (see drugs below)
- ◆ No other risk.

Previous medical history:
- ◆ 'Suffer with my nerves and depression', but on treatment
- ◆ Seizures (since aged 30 years old) – just came on all of a sudden; last fit 18 months ago; only have one or two a year (if that)
- ◆ Dietary-controlled diabetes – but it hasn't been checked for years!

Medications: amitriptylline 75 mg od, phenobarbitone 120 mg od.

Allergies: ibuprofen – 'makes me feel sick'

You live with your husband (Bill), who is wheelchair-bound since an industrial accident (he was a builder and fell down a broken ladder and broke his lower back; he never walked again). You are his main carer.

You live in a ground-floor flat and have good neighbours who help out, but no formal carers. Your oldest son visits on weekends and buys the shopping; your daughter lives in Vancouver; and your youngest son is in prison for murder ('It wasn't his fault – he's a good boy really').

Ideas – 'I know this is a bad one doc – I'm going to need some bandaging again aren't I?'

Concerns – 'Really need to get this sorted as Bill needs his lunch soon' (you are very reluctant to be admitted to hospital if it's suggested).

Expectations – 'Lets get these legs wrapped and I'll be on my way.'

SCENARIO 6

93

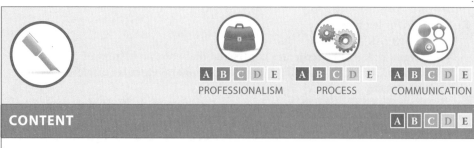

**PROFESSIONALISM**    **PROCESS**    **COMMUNICATION**

## CONTENT

### Identifies key information
- Elicits history of chronic venous diseases of the legs:
  - Suffered extensive left leg deep vein thrombosis (DVT) during first pregnancy
  - Veins progressively worse with each pregnancy
  - Venous disease so extensive wouldn't go out without being covered up – 'terrible legs'
  - No operative intervention; no support stockings
  - Several episodes of venous ulceration, including some requiring compression bandaging
- History of presenting complaint – started 3 weeks ago:
  - Trauma – child crashed shopping trolley into left shin
  - Initially not too bad but then became increasingly diffuse
  - Now affecting most of left shin
  - Increasingly painful, and more recently leaking an offensive odour
  - Dressing the ulcerated area herself – didn't seek help until today
- Risk factors for leg ulceration:
  - Trauma – as above
  - Venous disease – as above
  - Arterial risk – IHD, PVD, stroke, DM, hypertension, lipids, smoking, alcohol excess, family history
  - Neuropathy risk – DM, alcohol, drugs
  - Others – sickle cell disease and drug injection (both highly unlikely in this woman).

### Completing the patient history
- Drug and allergy history: allergies to antibiotics
- Social and occupational history: carer for disabled husband, no formal carers at home; occupation.

### Summarises important areas of the history back to the patient

### Invites patient to ask questions and deals with them appropriately

### Establishes patient's ideas, concerns and expectations

SCENARIO 6

## CLINICAL DIAGNOSTIC REASONING

- **Please present your history**
  - Candidate offers a logical, well-structured account of the history.

- **What is your diagnosis?**
  - Infected traumatic/venous leg ulceration.

- **Could you tell me five different aetiologies of leg ulcers?**
  - Trauma
  - Venous
  - Arterial
  - Neuropathic – primarily at pressure points
  - Other vascular – intravenous drug users, sickle cell disease, Buerger's and other vasculitides
  - Malignant ulceration
  - Other differentials include pyoderma gangrenosum.

- **Could you tell me five investigations you would arrange in this patient?**
  - Bloods – FBC, U&Es, glucose, blood cultures, CRP
  - Venous blood gas – acid base (unwell)
  - Wound swab – MC&S
  - Given her chronic disease and poor use of health services, you may also do a number of chronic disease/'screening' blood tests including LFTs, $B_{12}$/folate, TFTs and HBA-1c.

**Demonstrates safe, sensible and appropriate management plan**

**Demonstrates clear and logical diagnostic reasoning**

## GLOBAL HISTORY MARK

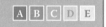

# Station 2 – Examination

> **Patient script (see also page 382)**
>
> You are a 72-year-old woman with features of systemic infection from a 'nasty' venous/traumatic leg ulcer. You are able to participate in the assessment with no real problems but you are feeling 'poorly' and your leg is very painful, which makes it difficult for you to transfer and mobilise.

**SCENARIO 6**

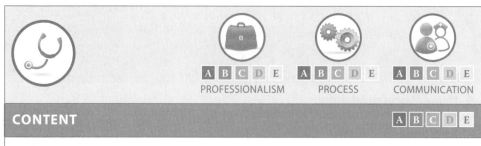

PROFESSIONALISM     PROCESS     COMMUNICATION

## CONTENT

A B C D E

**Exposes and positions patient correctly and maintains comfort**
- Both legs fully exposed to the upper thigh.

**Comments on wellbeing of patient, ie well or unwell**

**'Feet to face'**
- Observes and comments on patient and surroundings from foot of bed.

**Asks for appropriate/relevant clinical observations**
- Observations – HR 104 bpm, BP 156/96 mmHg, RR 22 bpm, $O_2$ sats 95% on air, temperature 38.1 °C, CBG 16.3 mmol/l
- Level of consciousness – Glasgow coma scale (GCS) or APVU (Alert; Pain; Voice; Unresponsive)
- Hydration.

**Assessment of the lower limbs**
- Patient should be standing and legs fully exposed
- Observes/comments on:
  - Varicosities
  - Venous changes – eczema, haemosiderosis, lipodermatosclerosis, loss of leg hair, oedema, swelling, old surgical and non-surgical scars (healed ulcers/venous stripping)
  - Signs of arterial and neuropathic disease
  - Ulceration.
- If candidate attempts assessment of varicosities or other venous assessment refer them back to the instructions.
- Assessment of ulcerated area (BASE):
  - Base
  - Associated features – venous disease, pulses, sensation (light touch, vibration, joint position sense)
  - Site, size, shape
  - Edges.

**Thanks patient, offers assistance, maintains patient's dignity and privacy until they are dressed**

SCENARIO 6

## CLINICAL DIAGNOSTIC REASONING

**Correctly identifies the relevant physical signs, including important negative findings**

- **Can you explain your immediate management of this patient?**
  - Needs admission to hospital for intravenous antibiotics and wound care – including de-sloughing agent
  - Analgesia and compression bandaging (see below)
  - Intravenous sliding scale insulin as hyperglycaemic
  - If 'hospital at home' or equivalent is available then hospital admission may be avoidable but given co-morbidities better to be admitted
  - Husband will also need help/care if she is admitted
  - ABPIs will be required prior to compression bandaging being applied – this may be challenging in this case because of the extensive nature and pain of the ulcerated areas.

**Demonstrates safe, sensible and appropriate management plan**

**Demonstrates clear and logical diagnostic reasoning**

## GLOBAL EXAMINATION MARK

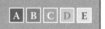

# Station 3 – Examination

**Patient script**

You are Mrs Rosie Fitzpatrick, a 58-year-old woman who is coming to the end of her treatment for a venous leg ulcer on her left shin. You've had 8 weeks of compression bandaging and the ulcer is now almost healed. You are happy to be assessed by the doctor. You have had varicose veins for many years and have 'endured this assessment many times' with the medical students.

SCENARIO 6

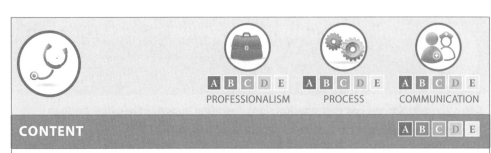

PROFESSIONALISM  PROCESS  COMMUNICATION

## CONTENT

A B C D E

**Exposes and positions patient correctly and maintains comfort**
- Both legs fully exposed to the upper thigh.

**Comments on wellbeing of patient, ie well or unwell**

**'Feet to face'**
- Observes and comments on patient and surroundings from foot of bed.

**Assessment of the lower limbs**
- Patient should be standing and legs fully exposed
- Observes/comments on:
  - Varicosities – defines the course of any varicosities left and right; long and short saphenous veins
  - Venous changes – eczema, haemosiderosis, lipodermatosclerosis, loss of leg hair, oedema, swelling, old surgical and non-surgical scars (healed ulcers/venous stripping)
  - Signs of arterial and neuropathic disease
  - Small area of ulceration.

**Candidate performs the following tests:**
- Cough test – with fingers placed over S-FJ – attempts to elicit a thrill when patient coughs (right and left)
- Tap test – with fingers placed distally over the long saphenous vein, tries to elicit a palpable pressure wave by tapping the SF-J (left and right)
- Trendelenburg's test (left and right) – with patient on the examination couch, elevates patient's leg (ensuring no distress) to 50 degrees and empties the thigh veins (distal to proximal); applies tourniquet approx 5 cm below the SF-J; assists patient to stand; observes and comments on venous filling distal to tourniquet
- Perthe's test – (right and left) asks patient to lie down again on examination couch; applies tourniquet to upper/mid thigh– superficial veins will fill; asks patient to stand up and then asks them to stand up onto the balls of their feet and back down 5–10 times (patient may need support whilst doing this)
- ABPIs – left and right; measures and records systolic blood pressure in brachial artery and corresponding dorsalis pedis artery; correctly calculates ratios expressed as fractions and decimals, eg ankle 120 mmHg : brachial 125 mmHg ($120/125 = 0.96$).

**Thanks patient, offers assistance, maintains patient's dignity and privacy until they are dressed**

## CLINICAL DIAGNOSTIC REASONING

**Correctly identifies the relevant physical signs, including important negative findings**

- **Can you tell me the location of the sapheno-femoral junction?**
  - 4 cm lateral and 4 cm below the pubic tubercle.

- **Can you explain what the likely results of the Trendelenburg's test mean?**
  - If superficial veins refill, incompetence is below the level of the tourniquet
  - If veins don't refill, incompetence is at the SF-J.

- **Can you explain what the likely results of the Perthe's test mean?**
  - If the deep veins are competent, the superficial veins will collapse as blood is pumped proximally by the deep venous system
  - If the deep veins are incompetent, the superficial veins will remain filled.

- **Is there any other clinical test you would perform at this point?**
  - Candidate mentions the need for Doppler assessment of SF-J and popliteal junction.

**Demonstrates safe, sensible and appropriate management plan**

**Demonstrates clear and logical diagnostic reasoning**

## GLOBAL EXAMINATION MARK

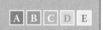

SCENARIO 6

99

## Station 4 – Clinical communication skills

**Patient script**

You are Mrs Geraldine Smith, a 72-year-old woman who has been referred to the community leg ulcer clinic by her GP. You have already met the junior doctor who is explaining the treatment of your leg ulcer to you, and are happy to talk to them.

What you've been told so far – 'I was told by your colleague there (the VNS) that the leg ulcer is really mucky and unpleasant (I think I could have told him that!) and that it needs further treatment but then he went off to phone someone and didn't really explain anything else'.

Ideas – 'I know this is a bad one; its paining me something rotten and smells to high heaven... so it's not good is it?'

Concerns – 'I don't want to take too long over this, 'cause I have to get back to Bill for his lunch'.

Expectations – 'OK... tell me the worst... I need that tight bandaging on again don't I?'

If the doctor says you need to be admitted, challenge them to justify why – 'If it's not life threatening I'd rather take my chances looking after Bill'.

If they don't give you an adequate explanation or are unsympathetic you should refuse to be admitted and ask to be taken home.

PROFESSIONALISM    PROCESS

## CONTENT

**Confirms reason for discussion**
- To talk to Mrs Smith about the management of her leg ulcer.

**Establishes what patient wishes to know; gains agreement/informal consent to participate in the discussion**

**Investigates patient's present level of understanding of scenario**

**Explains the key, important information**
- Immediate management:
  - Leg ulcer is infected and this has now caused systemic/constitutional symptoms – this is making the patient feel like she has flu (the infection has spread)
  - This means the patient needs admission for antibiotics in the vein
  - Won't be as effective if given by mouth as patient is so unwell
  - May be able to arrange 'hospital at home' (if available locally) but given other co-morbidities (hyperglycaemia) may be best to come into hospital
  - Duration of admission – about 5–7 days
  - If admitted will ensure husband Bill is cared for – either at home or with respite admission
  - Once infection improving, will need compression bandaging to left calf
  - Will also need strong painkillers (analgesia) and possibly insulin to control diabetes.
- Long-term management:
  - Compression bandaging until leg ulcer heals
  - Recommend compression hosiery (support stockings) to both legs
  - If similar episode arises, should seek medical help sooner rather than later.

**Establishes patient's ideas, concerns and expectations**

**Invites patient to ask questions and is able to deal with them appropriately**

**Summarises important areas of the consultation back to the patient**

**Formally ends the consultation and ensures appropriate follow-up has been discussed**

## GLOBAL COMMUNICATION MARK

SCENARIO 6

# Station 5 – Prescribing skills

| Allergies, sensitivities and adverse drug reactions | | | | | Patient details/addressograph | |
|---|---|---|---|---|---|---|
| No known allergies ✓ | | Initials | | Gender  M Ⓕ | NHS/ Hospital No:  087651 | |
| Not possible to ascertain ☐ | | Date  9/05 | Weight (kg) | Date | | |
| Medicine/substance | Reaction & Severity | Initials & Date | 90kg | | Surname:  SMITH | |
| | | | Height | | First name:  GERALDINE | |
| Alerts | | | Surface area (m²) | | Date of birth:  16/05/40 | |

## IN-PATIENT MEDICATION PRESCRIPTION AND ADMINISTRATION RECORD

PasTest HOSPITAL

| Consultant  HUBBARD | Trainee Dr. Name and Bleep no.  FEATHER (201) | Date of admission  9/05/12 | Date chart reboarded | Estimated date of discharge |
|---|---|---|---|---|
| This chart is no.  ...1... of ...1... | Transcribing Check by Pharmacy  Sign .......... Date .......... | Ward  1. ....MAU..............  2. .............. | | |

Supplementary Medication charts in use: Other (please specify): 1 .......... 2 ..........

| Epidural/PCA ☐ | Syringe driver ☐ | | TPN ☐ | Chemotherapy ☐ | Insulin sliding scale ☐ |
|---|---|---|---|---|---|

Once only medications – loading doses, pre-medication, PGDs or surgical antibiotic propylaxis

| Date | Time to be given | Medicine (approved name) | Dose | Route | Signature and bleep no. | Pharmacy | Time given | Given by | Checked by |
|---|---|---|---|---|---|---|---|---|---|
| 9/05 | Stat | BENZYLPENICILLIN | 1.2g | IV | AF 201 | | | | |
| 9/05 | Stat | FLUCLOXACILLIN | 1.0g | IV | AF 201 | | | | |
| 9/05 | Stat | METRONIDAZOLE | 500mg | IV | AF 201 | | | | |
| 9/05 | Stat | MORPHINE | 2.5mg | S/C | AF 201 | | | | |
| 9/05 | Stat | CYCLIZINE | 50mg | S/C | AF 201 | | | | |

SCENARIO 6

## Thromboprophylaxis please prescribe treatment regimens in the regular medications section

| Choice of mechanical prophylaxis and leg(s) to be applied to | | | | | | Enter Time | Enter details below | | | | | | | | | | |
|---|---|---|---|---|---|---|---|---|---|---|---|---|---|---|---|---|---|
| Graduated elastic compression stockings | Intermittent pneumatic compression device (IPC) | Leg | | | | | | | | | | | | | | | |
| | | Left | Right | Both | | | | | | | | | | | | | |

NOT FOR STOCKINGS – INFECTED LEG ULCERS

| Graduated elastic compression stockings | Intermittent pneumatic compression device | Signature and Bleep No. | Left ☐ | Right ☐ | Both ☐ |
|---|---|---|---|---|---|
| ☐ Start Date: | ☐ End Date: | | | | |
| ☐ Start Date: | ☐ End Date: | Signature and Bleep No. AF | ☐ | ☐ | ☐ |

| Medication | Dose | Dose Change | Enter Time | Enter details below |
|---|---|---|---|---|
| CLEXANE | 40mg | | | |

| Please ensure you have completed the VTE risk assessment form | Date | 9/05 | | |
| | Route | S/C | | |
| | Signature | AF | | Instructions |
| | Bleep no. | 201 | | |

Pharmacy ☐

---

## Regular prescriptions continued

### Anti-infectives prescription   prescribe long term prophylaxis and anti-tuberculosis medications in regular medications section

| For 7 Days | Dose | | | Date | | | | | | | | | | | | |
|---|---|---|---|---|---|---|---|---|---|---|---|---|---|---|---|---|
| Date 9/05 | | | | Medication BENZYLPENICILLIN | | | Indication INFECTED LEG ULCER | | | Signature and bleep no. AF 201 | | | Pharmacy ☐ | | | |
| Route IV | | | | | | | | | | | | | | | | |
| Signature | | | | | | | | | | | | | | | | |
| 06 | 1.2g | | | | | | | | | | | | | | | |
| 09 | | | | | | | | | | | | | | | | |
| 12 | 1.2g | | | | | | | | | | | | | | | |
| 18 | 1.2g | | | | | | | | | | | | | | | |
| 22 | | | | | | | | | | | | | | | | |
| 24 | 1.2g | | | | | | | | | | | | | | | |

---

## Regular prescriptions continued

| For 7 Days | Dose | | | Date | | | | | | | | | | | | |
|---|---|---|---|---|---|---|---|---|---|---|---|---|---|---|---|---|
| Date 9/05 | | | | Medication FLUCLOXACILLIN | | | Indication LEG ULCERS | | | Signature and bleep no. AF 201 | | | Pharmacy ☐ | | | |
| Route IV | | | | | | | | | | | | | | | | |
| Signature | | | | | | | | | | | | | | | | |
| 06 | 1g | | | | | | | | | | | | | | | |
| 09 | | | | | | | | | | | | | | | | |
| 12 | 1g | | | | | | | | | | | | | | | |
| 18 | 1g | | | | | | | | | | | | | | | |
| 22 | | | | | | | | | | | | | | | | |
| 24 | 1g | | | | | | | | | | | | | | | |

SCENARIO 6

103

## 'TERRIBLE LEGS'

| | Dose | | | Date | | | | | | | | | | | | | |
|---|---|---|---|---|---|---|---|---|---|---|---|---|---|---|---|---|---|
| For 7 Days | | | | | | | | | | | | | | | | | |
| Date 9/05 | | | | Medication | | | | Indication | | | Signature and bleep no. | | | | Pharmacy | | |
| Route IV | | | | METRONIDAZOLE | | | | LEG ULCERS | | | AF 201 | | | | ☐ | | |
| Signature | | | | | | | | | | | | | | | | | |
| (06) | 500mg | | | | | | | | | | | | | | | | |
| 09 | | | | | | | | | | | | | | | | | |
| (12) | 500mg | | | | | | | | | | | | | | | | |
| 18 | | | | | | | | | | | | | | | | | |
| 22 | | | | | | | | | | | | | | | | | |
| (24) | 500mg | | | | | | | | | | | | | | | | |

**Regular prescriptions continued**
**Regular Medications**

| | Dose | | | Date | | | | | | | | | | | | | |
|---|---|---|---|---|---|---|---|---|---|---|---|---|---|---|---|---|---|
| Date 9/05 | | | | Medication | | | | Instructions | | | Signature and bleep no. | | | | Pharmacy | | |
| Route PO | | | | CODEINE PHOSPHATE | | | | | | | AF 201 | | | | ☐ | | |
| Signature | | | | | | | | | | | | | | | | | |
| 06 | | | | | | | | | | | | | | | | | |
| (09) | 60MG | | | | | | | | | | | | | | | | |
| (12) | 60MG | | | | | | | | | | | | | | | | |
| (18) | 60MG | | | | | | | | | | | | | | | | |
| (22) | 60MG | | | | | | | | | | | | | | | | |
| 24 | | | | | | | | | | | | | | | | | |

**Regular prescriptions continued**

| | Dose | | | Date | | | | | | | | | | | | | |
|---|---|---|---|---|---|---|---|---|---|---|---|---|---|---|---|---|---|
| Date 9/05 | | | | Medication | | | | Instructions | | | Signature and bleep no. | | | | Pharmacy | | |
| Route PO | | | | PARACETAMOL | | | | | | | AF 201 | | | | ☐ | | |
| Signature | | | | | | | | | | | | | | | | | |
| 06 | | | | | | | | | | | | | | | | | |
| (09) | 1g | | | | | | | | | | | | | | | | |
| (12) | 1g | | | | | | | | | | | | | | | | |
| (18) | 1g | | | | | | | | | | | | | | | | |
| (22) | 1g | | | | | | | | | | | | | | | | |
| 24 | | | | | | | | | | | | | | | | | |

SCENARIO 6

| Regular prescriptions continued | | | | | | | | | | | | | | | | | | |
|---|---|---|---|---|---|---|---|---|---|---|---|---|---|---|---|---|---|---|
| | Dose | | | Date | | | | | | | | | | | | | | |
| Date 9/05 | | | | Medication | | | Instructions | | | | Signature and bleep no. | | | Pharmacy | | | | |
| Route PO | | | | PHENOBARBITONE | | | | | | | AF 201 | | | | | | | |
| Signature | | | | | | | | | | | | | | | | | | |
| 06 | | | | | | | | | | | | | | | | | | |
| (09) | 120mg | | | | | | | | | | | | | | | | | |
| 12 | | | | | | | | | | | | | | | | | | |
| 18 | | | | | | | | | | | | | | | | | | |
| 22 | | | | | | | | | | | | | | | | | | |
| 24 | | | | | | | | | | | | | | | | | | |

| Regular prescriptions continued | | | | | | | | | | | | | | | | | | |
|---|---|---|---|---|---|---|---|---|---|---|---|---|---|---|---|---|---|---|
| | Dose | | | Date | | | | | | | | | | | | | | |
| Date 9/05 | | | | Medication | | | Instructions | | | | Signature and bleep no. | | | Pharmacy | | | | |
| Route PO | | | | AMITRIPTYLINE | | | | | | | AF 201 | | | | | | | |
| Signature | | | | | | | | | | | | | | | | | | |
| 06 | | | | | | | | | | | | | | | | | | |
| 09 | | | | | | | | | | | | | | | | | | |
| 12 | | | | | | | | | | | | | | | | | | |
| 18 | | | | | | | | | | | | | | | | | | |
| (22) | 75mg | | | | | | | | | | | | | | | | | |
| 24 | | | | | | | | | | | | | | | | | | |

| Regular prescriptions continued | | | | | | | | | | | | | | | | | | |
|---|---|---|---|---|---|---|---|---|---|---|---|---|---|---|---|---|---|---|
| Regular Medications | | | | | | | | | | | | | | | | | | |
| | Dose | | | Date | | | | | | | | | | | | | | |
| Date 9/05 | | | | Medication | | | Instructions | | | | Signature and bleep no. | | | Pharmacy | | | | |
| Route PO | | | | SENNA | | | WITH CODEINE | | | | AF 201 | | | | | | | |
| Signature | | | | | | | | | | | | | | | | | | |
| 06 | | | | | | | | | | | | | | | | | | |
| (09) | ºº TT | | | | | | | | | | | | | | | | | |
| 12 | | | | | | | | | | | | | | | | | | |
| 18 | | | | | | | | | | | | | | | | | | |
| 22 | | | | | | | | | | | | | | | | | | |
| 24 | | | | | | | | | | | | | | | | | | |

SCENARIO 6

105

| Infusion prescriptions continued | | | | | | | | SC = subcutaneous | | IVC = intravenous central IVP = intravenous peripheral | | | |
|---|---|---|---|---|---|---|---|---|---|---|---|---|---|
| Date & time | Route | Infusion Fluid | | Medication | | Duration | Rate | Prescriber's signature & bleep no. | Date given | Given by / Added by | Check by | Start time | Finish time | Pharmacy |
| | | Name & strength | Volume | Approved name with expiry / unit number | Dose | | | | | | | | | |
| 9/05 | IV | 0.9% saline Exp: Batch/unit no: | 1l | | | | 6° | AF 201 | | | | | | |
| 9/05 | IV | 0.9% saline Exp: Batch/unit no: | 1l | + 20mmol KCL | | | 8° | AF 201 | | | | | | |
| 9/05 | IV | 0.9% saline Exp: Batch/unit no: | 1l | + 20mmol KCL | | | 8° | AF 201 | | | | | | |
| 9/05 | IV | 0.9% saline Exp: Batch/unit no: | 1l | | | | 8° | AF 201 | | | | | | |
| 9/05 | IV | 0.9% saline Exp: Batch/unit no: | 1l | + 20mmol KCL | | | 10° | AF 201 | | | | | | |
| | | TITRATE FLUIDS AGAINST U.O; BP > 100mmHg (Systolic); HR < 100 bpm Exp: Batch/unit no: | | | | | | | | | | | | |
| 9/05 | IV | 0.9% saline Exp: Batch/unit no: | 50ml | ACTRAPID INSULIN | 50 UNITS | | TO RUN IV AT 0.1 UNITS/kg/HR ≡ 9 UNITS/HR | | | | | | | |
| | | Exp: Batch/unit no: | PATIENT WEIGHT = 90kg | | | | | AF 201 | | | | | | |
| | | Exp: Batch/unit no: | | | | | | | | | | | | |
| | | | | | | | | | | | | | | |
| | | | | | | | | | | | | | | |

**As required medications**

| Medication | | | | Date | | | | | | | | | | | | | | | | | | | | | | | | | |
|---|---|---|---|---|---|---|---|---|---|---|---|---|---|---|---|---|---|---|---|---|---|---|---|---|---|---|---|---|---|
| CYCLIZINE | | | | | | | | | | | | | | | | | | | | | | | | | | | | | |

| Indication | | | | Time | | | | | | | | | | | | | | | | | | | | | | | | | |
|---|---|---|---|---|---|---|---|---|---|---|---|---|---|---|---|---|---|---|---|---|---|---|---|---|---|---|---|---|---|
| | | | | | | | | | | | | | | | | | | | | | | | | | | | | | |

| Dose | Route | Maximum frequency / dose | Start date | Dose |
|---|---|---|---|---|
| 50 mg | IV/ IM/ SC | 80 | 9/05 | |
| | | | Stop date | Route |
| Signature | | | | |
| AF 201 | | | Bleep no. | Given |

Additional instructions:      Pharmacy

---

**As required medications**

| Medication | | | | Date | | | | | | | | | | | | | | | | | | | | | | | | | |
|---|---|---|---|---|---|---|---|---|---|---|---|---|---|---|---|---|---|---|---|---|---|---|---|---|---|---|---|---|---|
| TRAMADOL | | | | | | | | | | | | | | | | | | | | | | | | | | | | | |

| Indication | | | | Time | | | | | | | | | | | | | | | | | | | | | | | | | |
|---|---|---|---|---|---|---|---|---|---|---|---|---|---|---|---|---|---|---|---|---|---|---|---|---|---|---|---|---|---|
| | | | | | | | | | | | | | | | | | | | | | | | | | | | | | |

| Dose | Route | Maximum frequency / dose | Start date | Dose |
|---|---|---|---|---|
| 50 mg | PO | 8 | 9/05 | |
| | | | Stop date | Route |
| Signature | | | | |
| AF 201 | | | Bleep no. | Given |

Additional instructions:      Pharmacy

---

**As required medications**

| Medication | | | | Date | | | | | | | | | | | | | | | | | | | | | | | | | |
|---|---|---|---|---|---|---|---|---|---|---|---|---|---|---|---|---|---|---|---|---|---|---|---|---|---|---|---|---|---|
| MORPHINE | | | | | | | | | | | | | | | | | | | | | | | | | | | | | |

| Indication | | | | Time | | | | | | | | | | | | | | | | | | | | | | | | | |
|---|---|---|---|---|---|---|---|---|---|---|---|---|---|---|---|---|---|---|---|---|---|---|---|---|---|---|---|---|---|
| | | | | | | | | | | | | | | | | | | | | | | | | | | | | | |

| Dose | Route | Maximum frequency / dose | Start date | Dose |
|---|---|---|---|---|
| 2.5 mg– 5 mg | SC/ IM | As Req. | 9/05 | |
| | | | Stop date | Route |
| Signature | | | | |
| AF 201 | | | Bleep no. | Given |

Additional instructions:      Pharmacy

---

**GLOBAL PRESCRIBING MARK**      A B C D E

SCENARIO 6

# Scenario 6: Reflection and consolidation

## History

Mrs Geraldine Smith is a 72-year-old full-time carer who previously worked in the local Tate and Lyle sugar factory in the canning section.

She has had chronic venous problems of both legs since her first pregnancy. During this pregnancy she suffered an extensive DVT of her left leg. During her subsequent two pregnancies her veins got 'worse and worse', to the point that she was unable to be seen in public without covering her legs.

Over the next few years she suffered several episodes of venous ulcers, some of which required compression bandaging. She has never worn compression hosiery during this period. She thought about having her varicose veins operated on but 'never got round to it'.

Approximately 3 weeks ago she was walking around the local supermarket when a little girl 'crashed' a shopping trolley into the side of her left shin. This has developed into a large ulcerated area affecting most of the left shin.

She poetically describes the edges 'parting like the Red Sea' as the ulceration got worse. It has become offensive, painful and leaking, despite her dressing the area herself. Over the last few days she has become systemically unwell with malaise and fever. Of note her risk factors for ulceration include: venous risk (as above); arterial risk (known dietary-controlled diabetes, no history of IHD, stroke, PVD, hypertension); ex-smoker given up 20 years ago (she previously smoked 20/day for about 30 years); she has occasional glasses of sherry and white wine. Her lipids are not known.

Her neuropathic risk is DM, and nil else (see drugs below). No other risk.

Mrs Smith is being treated for long-term depression and epilepsy; there is nil else of note in her previous medical history. Her current medications are amitriptyline 75 mg od and phenobarbitone 120 mg od. She is allergic to ibuprofen, which makes her feel sick.

She lives with her husband Bill, who is wheelchair-bound since an industrial accident. She is his main carer. They live in a ground-floor flat; they have good neighbours who help out but no formal carers. Her oldest son visits at the weekends and buys the shopping.

## Examination

On examination, this is an unwell-looking older woman who had signs of systemic sepsis. She was tachycardic (HR 104 bpm, pyrexial (temperature 38.1 °C) and hyperglycaemic. Her CBG is 16.3 mmol/l. She is also hypertensive (BP 156/96 mmHg). The general examination was otherwise unremarkable.

On assessment of her lower limbs, Mrs Smith has marked varicosities of the short and long saphenous veins (left and right) and bilateral leg oedema. On the right there is evidence of chronic venous changes and a healed ulcerated area over the medial and anterior shin, approx 4 × 5 cm. On the left there are similar chronic venous changes, but these are mainly lost to a large circumferential, ulcerated area extending over most of the left shin. This is malodorous. Its maximum width is approximately 8–10 cm with a minimum width of approx 4–5 cm. The base is very sloughy and pusy; there are occasional areas of granulation seen. The edges are ragged and uneven.

Sensory and arterial assessments are normal in both feet.

## Investigations

Given her diagnoses of infected leg ulcers, systemic upset and hyperglycaemia, this patient needs investigation to prove the microbiological agent.

As she is a full-time carer for her husband, she has tended to neglect her own health (common amongst carers) and so needs a full set of screening tests as well.

Investigations should include:

- Bloods – FBC, U&Es, RBG, LFTs, $B_{12}$, folate, CRP, TFTs, HbA-1c, blood cultures
- Venous blood gases, including lactate
- Wound swabs.

Other tests may include chest radiograph and ECG (previous heavy smoker and hypertensive).

## Management

Venous disease is often underestimated in younger patients, and they pay the price for this in older age. Young and old patients alike suffering with extensive venous thrombosis and varicosities should be offered compression hosiery to assist with the venous pump in the lower limbs. Extensive venous disease often causes ulceration in later life and this may cause multiple problems, including systemic sepsis.

Infected ulcers may require treatment with intravenous antibiotics, and once improving, compression bandaging. This should always be preceded by measurement and recording of the patient's ABPIs, excluding significant arterial disease.

Supportive treatment including good analgesia, sedatives at night and optimisation of the treatment of co-morbidities (especially heart failure, fluid overload and diabetes mellitus) is essential for adherence to compression, which can prove to be an extremely challenging therapy.

### Further reading and web links

*SIGN guidelines on chronic venous leg ulcer management*:
www.sign.ac.uk/pdf/qrg120.pdf
*RCN guidelines on the treatment of venous leg ulcers*:
www.rcn.org.uk/__data/assets/pdf_file/0003/107940/003020.pdf

SCENARIO 6

# Scenario 7: 'Heart broken'

## Station 1

*History*                                                    *10-minute station*

You are a FY1 doctor on placement in a general practice. Mr Daly has attended with his wife with a history of increasing shortness of breath.

- Please take a history from Mr Daly and then present it to your GP supervisor with your differential diagnosis.

*You will be assessed on the following areas, as well as the content and diagnostic reasoning of your history – take them into account in your presentation.*

### Professionalism

- Professional appearance (NHS dress code) – including general appearance, hair and jewellery
- Maintains patient and personal safety
- Polite introduction; identifies patient or interviewee correctly; confirms patient's date of birth from name band or other source
- Obtains informal consent; maintains patient's privacy
- Displays empathetic and caring attitudes and behaviours throughout.

### Process

- Good organisation and structure; appropriate use of open and closed questions
- Appropriate fluency/rhythm/pace to the interview – this may change depending on environment and acute nature of the problem
- Appropriate time for the patient to respond/reply to questions
- Appropriate acknowledgement of difficult or emotional areas of the patient's history.

### Communication skills

- Demonstrates caring and sympathetic attitude
- Asks open questions
- Invites patient to ask questions and answers them appropriately
- Addresses patient's ideas, concerns and expectations.

## Station 2

*Examination*                    *10-minute station*

After presenting your history, you have been asked to perform a relevant cardiorespiratory examination of Mr Daly.

■ Please present this to your GP supervisor along with your initial management plan. (If you do not have a model, please read and present the information given on page 383.)

*You will be assessed on the following areas, as well as the content and skills of your examination – take them into account in your presentation.*

### Professionalism

- Professional appearance; maintains infection control standards, including hand cleaning and appropriate use of gloves and aprons
- Maintains patient and personal safety
- Polite introduction; identifies patient and confirms date of birth from name band or other source
- Obtains informal consent; maintains patient privacy and dignity
- Displays empathetic and caring attitudes and behaviours throughout.

### Process

- Appropriate fluency/rhythm/pace to the examination – this may change depending on environment and acute nature of the problem
- Organisation and structure of examination; sensitive and empathetic approach
- Uses appropriate clinical techniques throughout
- Maintains privacy and dignity throughout.

### Clinical communication

- Explains proposed examination/procedure: explains examination/procedure as it proceeds
- Offers information in a clear, structured and fluent manner, avoiding jargon
- Listens to patient and responds appropriately
- Demonstrates appropriate body language.

SCENARIO 7

## Station 3

*Data interpretation*                    *10-minute station*

■ Please match each of the clinical pictures below with the most likely underlying diagnosis.

    A   Mitral valve insufficiency
    B   Dilated cardiomyopathy
    C   HIV cardiomyopathy
    D   Ischaemic cardiomyopathy
    E   Myocarditis
    F   Severe aortic stenosis
    G   Hypertensive cardiomyopathy
    H   Takotsubo 'stress-induced' cardiomyopathy
    I   Amyloidosis

1. An 82-year-old man presents with progressive shortness of breath, orthopneoa and an episode of transient loss of consciousness. On examination his apex beat is displaced to the mid axillary line and he has an ejection systolic murmur.

2. A 62-year-old man presents with progressive pitting oedema to the thighs, a displaced apex beat and bibasal crackles on auscultation of the lungs. He has been drinking 40–50 units of whisky a week for the last 4 years.

3. A 65-year-old woman with type 2 diabetes, hypertension and hypercholesterolaemia present with dyspnoea, orthopnea and paroxysmal nocturnal dyspnoea.

4. A 57-year-old man is brought to the Emergency Department having been suffering from crushing central chest pain for 2 hours. Soon after arrival he became acutely short of breath with pulmonary oedema and a loud pan systolic murmur at the apex.

5. A 22-year-old man presents to the Emergency Department with chest pain and shortness of breath. He has been at home with a flu-like illness for the past 10 days. His electrocardiogram (ECG) shows widespread ST elevation in all leads and his chest radiograph (CXR) demonstrates pulmonary oedema.

## Station 4

*Prescribing skills*                    *10-minute station*

Your GP supervisor has received the investigation results shown below.

■ Please prescribe medications to improve the patient's left ventricular function and also to improve his symptoms. Use the FP10 and BNF provided to start the medication.

**Details**

o CXR – shows prominent interstitial shadowing suggestive of pulmonary oedema

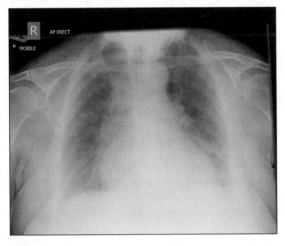

o ECHO – impaired left ventricular function with an estimated ejection fraction of 35–40%.

o FBC × Hb 13.7 g/dl, MCV 89 fl, WCC 8.2 × 10⁹/l, neutrophils 6.2 × 10⁹/l, platelets 345 × 10⁹/l

o U&Es – Na⁺ 137 mmol/l, K⁺ 4.5 mmol/l, urea 8.4 mmol/l, creatinine 92 μmol/l

o RBG – 5.2 mmol/l

o Clotting – INR 1.1.

**Medications to improve prognosis:**

1. ACE inhibitor

2. Beta blocker

3. Aspirin.

**Medications to improve symptoms:**

4. Furosemide.

---

**Remember: DRUG DRs D**on't **F**orget **S**igning **O**ff (page 396)

---

## Station 5

*Clinical communication skills*　　*10-minute station*

Despite Mr Daly's medical treatment he continues to suffer with breathlessness and oedema. In the last 6 months he has been admitted three times to the Cardiology ward for IV diuresis. He is not a candidate for heart transplantation or biventricular pacing and is now taking maximal dose ramipril, beta blockers, spironolactone and a small dose of digoxin. His repeat ECHO now shows an ejection fraction of 15–20%. You are now the FY2 doctor on the Cardiology ward and as you have been involved in his care for some time your Consultant feels it would be appropriate for you to discuss the issues regarding Mr Daly's prognosis and treatment while he observes you in the clinic.

■ Please discuss:
  • Plans for palliation of symptoms as his condition progresses
  • Wishes for end-of-life care
  • Do not attempt resuscitation orders.

SCENARIO 7

# Answers

## Station 1 – History

**Patient script**

You are Mr Michael Daly (DOB 24 November 1935), a 76-year-old man who has come to see your GP with increasing shortness of breath on exertion. You first noticed this about 6 months ago when you started becoming short of breath on climbing your stairs. You are now short of breath after walking 50 m on the flat. Prior to this you had unlimited exercise tolerance.

You have not had any fever, cough, wheeze or sputum production. You have had no weight loss or haemoptysis. You have not felt any chest pain or palpatations.

You have a medical history that includes hypertension, for which you used to take a medication (you are unsure of its name). However, as you did not have any symptoms you stopped taking it and have not been to your GP for over 5 years. You have never had a heart attack, and deny any history of diabetes, high cholesterol or lung disease. You have no allergies.

When asked directly you describe increasing swelling of your ankles, which worsens throughout each day. Your breathlessness is worse on lying down at night and over the last 2 weeks you have been using three pillows to sleep on at night to relieve your breathlessness. You have also woken up gasping for breath on a number of occasions.

You used to work as a train driver but have been retired for 15 years. You have smoked 10 cigarettes per day since you were 15 and drink 10–15 pints of bitter per week. You live with your wife of 50 years, who is in good health. You were very active prior to this illness and enjoyed doing DIY projects. Your mother and father both died in their seventies from a stroke and a heart attack, respectively.

You are concerned that this breathlessness is due to your smoking and would like an inhaler to improve things.

SCENARIO 7

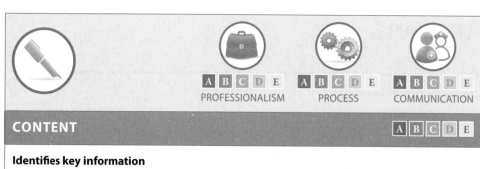

## CONTENT

**Identifies key information**
- Establishes duration of illness
- Establishes shortness of breath, exercised tolerance, orthopnea and paroxysmal nocturnal dyspnoea.

**Includes important negatives, including systemic enquiry**
- Absence of cough, fever, sputum or wheeze
- Absence of weight loss or haemoptysis
- Absence of chest pain or palpitations.

**Completing the patient history**
- Drug and allergy history: nil regular medications and no allergies
- Previous medical history: untreated hypertension; no angina or heart attacks
- Social and occupational history: 30 pack year cigarette history; alcohol intake 10–20 units of alcohol per week
- Family history: no relevant family history.

**Summarises important areas of the history back to the patient**

**Invites patient to ask questions and deals with them appropriately**

**Establishes patient's ideas, concerns and expectations**
- Mr Daly believes that your breathlessness is due to smoking and thinks an inhaler will improve matters.

## CLINICAL DIAGNOSTIC REASONING

- **Please present your history**
  - Candidate offers a logical, well-structured account of the history.

- **What is your differential diagnosis?**
  - Congestive cardiac failure is the most likely diagnosis
  - It is important to exclude severe respiratory disease and associated right heart failure or a large pericardial effusion.

- **What are the most likely underlying causes for this diagnosis?**
  - Untreated hypertension – hypertensive cardiomyopathy
  - Alcoholic cardiomyopathy
  - Occult ischaemia – ischaemic cardiomyopathy
  - Valvular heart disease.

- **How do you categorise the severity of symptoms in heart failure?**
  - The NYHA classification of symptoms in congestive cardiac failure is the most common.

| Class | Patient symptoms |
|---|---|
| Class I (Mild) | No limitation of physical activity |
| Class II (Mild) | Slight limitation of physical activity |
| Class III (Moderate) | Marked limitation of physical activity; comfortable at rest, but less than ordinary exertion leads to symptoms |
| Class IV (Severe) | Unable to carry out any physical activity without discomfort; symptoms of cardiac insufficiency at rest |

- **What category of symptom is Mr Daly suffering from?**
  - Class III symptoms.

## GLOBAL HISTORY MARK

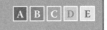

## Station 2 – Examination

**Patient script (see also page 383)**

You are comfortable sitting up at rest. You have swelling of your calves but you are able to breathe comfortably.

SCENARIO 7

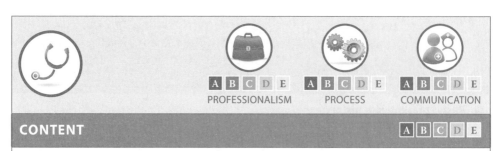

## CONTENT

A B C D E

**Exposes and positions patient correctly and maintains comfort**

**Comments on wellbeing of patient, ie well or unwell**

**'Feet to face'**
- Observes and comments on patient and surrounding from foot of bed.

**Asks for appropriate/relevant clinical observations**
- Observations: HR 94 bpm, BP 182/102 mmHg, RR 16 bpm, O$_2$ sats 95% on air, temperature 36.2 °C, BM 5.2

**General/systemic examination**
- Hands – no cyanosis, nails normal
- Pulse regular in rhythm at the wrist and normal in volume at the carotid
- JVP assessed with patient at 45 degrees, measures to be over 5 cm above the sternum
- Pitting oedema to the knees.

**Focussed examination**
- Inspection – inspects for scars and use of accessory muscles
- Palpation – assesses trachea, assesses chest expansion anteriorly and posteriorly, assesses apex beat
- Auscultation – auscultates in all areas, anteriorly and posteriorly, auscultates lung bases
- Assesses for either tactile vocal fremitus or vocal resonance.

**Completes examination by identifying relevant additional clinical signs**
- Assesses for sacral oedema and hepatomegaly.

**Thanks patient, offers assistance, maintains patient's dignity and privacy until they are dressed**

SCENARIO 7

## CLINICAL DIAGNOSTIC REASONING

A B C D E

Correctly identifies the relevant physical signs, including important negative findings

Does not identify signs that are not present

Demonstrates safe, sensible and appropriate management plan

Demonstrates clear and logical diagnostic reasoning

## GLOBAL EXAMINATION MARK

A B C D E

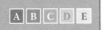

## Station 3 – Data interpretation

**1       F       Severe aortic stenosis**

Severe aortic stenosis leads to left ventricular hypertrophy as the ventricle attempts to expel the small volume of blood through a narrower opening. Eventually, the ventricle is unable to overcome the outflow obstruction, and left ventricular failure occurs. The aim is to replace the valve before this occurs.

**2       B       Dilated cardiomyopathy**

This man has an extremely high alcohol intake, and alcohol itself has a toxic effect on the myocardium. The heart muscle is damaged and dilated cardiomyopathy ensues.

**3       D       Ischaemic cardiomyopathy**

This woman has a number of risk factors for coronary artery disease, and although there is no definite history of myocardial infarction, patients with diabetes often have 'silent myocardial infarction'.

**4       A       Mitral valve insufficiency**

This patient presents with a typical history of a myocardial infarction leading to rupture of a mitral papilla, leading to mitral valve regurgitation. This needs acute cardiothoracic intervention.

**5       E       Myocarditis**

This patient presents with a viral prodrome and then an ischaemic ECG and acute left ventricular dysfunction. This is most likely the result of direct damage to the myocardium by a viral trigger.

SCENARIO 7

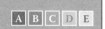

**GLOBAL DATA INTERPRETATION MARK**      A B C D E

## Station 4 – Prescribing skills

1          ACE inhibitor – ramipril 2.5 mg od.

Blood tests will be required in 2–4 weeks to ensure no acute deterioration in renal function, which can occur on initiation of ACE inhibitor therapy, especially in those with risk factors for reno-vascular disease.

2          Beta blocker – bisoprolol 2.5 mg od.

Beta blockers have been shown in many large-scale prospective trials to improve life expectancy in left ventricular dysfunction. Important side effects include bronchospasm in asthmatics, erectile dysfunction and lethargy.

3          Aspirin – 75 mg aspirin od.

4          Furosemide – 40–80 mg od mane.

Furosemide is an important medication in heart failure to aid fluid removal and improve symptoms. This can be titrated to effect. It is important to give in the morning so the diuresis that occurs does not affect the patient's sleep pattern.

SCENARIO 7

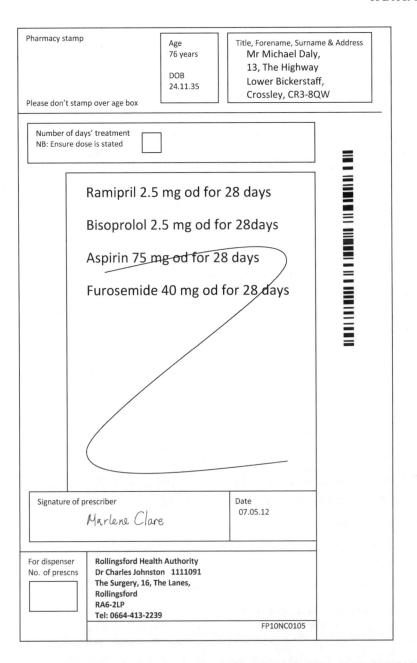

| Pharmacy stamp | Age 76 years<br><br>DOB 24.11.35 | Title, Forename, Surname & Address<br>Mr Michael Daly,<br>13, The Highway<br>Lower Bickerstaff,<br>Crossley, CR3-8QW |
|---|---|---|

Please don't stamp over age box

Number of days' treatment
NB: Ensure dose is stated

Ramipril 2.5 mg od for 28 days

Bisoprolol 2.5 mg od for 28days

Aspirin 75 mg od for 28 days

Furosemide 40 mg od for 28 days

| Signature of prescriber<br>Marlene Clare | Date<br>07.05.12 |
|---|---|

For dispenser
No. of prescns

**Rollingsford Health Authority**
**Dr Charles Johnston  1111091**
**The Surgery, 16, The Lanes,**
**Rollingsford**
**RA6-2LP**
**Tel: 0664-413-2239**

FP10NC0105

**GLOBAL PRESCRIBING MARK**

A B C D E

SCENARIO 7

## Station 5 – Clinical communication skills

### Patient script

You are a 76-year-old man with severe congestive cardiac failure. You are now breathless at rest and have to sleep sitting up downstairs at home. You and your wife are both extremely tired as you have spent much of the last 6 months in the hospital on a drip to improve your oedema.

When the issue is raised you are aware that your heart failure is not curable and the worsening symptoms are your main concern. After discussion with your wife you have decided that you would rather not go back to hospital if your symptoms worsen but are very concerned that you will suffer from pain and shortness of breath if you are not in hospital. You would like to know if there is any support available in the community.

When the issue is raised sensitively, you agree to not attempting resuscitation if your heart stopped.

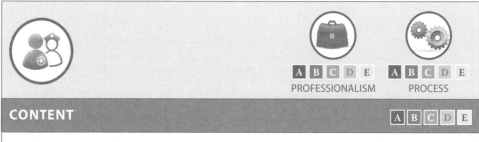

PROFESSIONALISM  A B C D E

PROCESS  A B C D E

### CONTENT   A B C D E

**Confirms reason for discussion**

**Establishes what the patient wishes to know; gains agreement/informal consent to participate in the discussion**

**Investigates patient's present level of understanding of scenario**

**Summarises and confirms what has happened so far**
- Summarises history of congestive cardiac failure on maximal medical therapy
- Establishes current main symptoms of breathlessness, orthopnoea and low mood.

**Establishes patient's ideas, concerns and expectations**
- Identifies that the patient understands that his condition is incurable and that he wishes to now remain at home.
- Establishes concerns regarding symptom control at home.

SCENARIO 7

**Explains the key, important information**

- Explains therapies available for symptom control, including diuresis in the home, antidepressants and oxygen
- Explains that palliative care support is available in the home
- Sensitively raises issue of DNR status.

**Invites patient to ask questions and is able to deal with them appropriately**

**Summarises important areas of the consultation back to the patient**

**Formally ends the consultation and ensures appropriate follow-up has been discussed**

- Ensure discussion of palliative care input and referral to the heart failure community team.

## GLOBAL COMMUNICATION MARK

A B C D E

# Scenario 7: Reflection and consolidation

### History

Mr Daly is a 76-year-old man who presents with a 6-month history of progressive exertional dyspnoea, associated with orthopnea and paroxysmal nocturnal dyspnoea. Exercise tolerance is now 50 m on the flat and was unlimited prior to this. He also has increasing pedal oedema. He has no respiratory symptoms, chest pain or weight loss. His medical history includes untreated hypertension but no known IHD. He takes no regular medication and has no allergies. He is a retired train driver who has a 30 pack year smoking history and drinks 20–30 units of alcohol per week.

### Examination

Mr Daly is comfortable at rest sitting at 45 degrees. He is not tachypnoeic, with a respiratory rate of 16 breaths per minute. On examination he has bilateral pitting oedema to the knees, and elevated jugular venous pressure (JVP) at 5 cm above the sternal notch. He is not cyanosed and his saturations on air are 95%. He has a heart rate of 94 bpm, which is regular in rhythm and normal in volume. His apex beat is displaced laterally to the anterior axillary line but on auscultation there are no murmurs or added sounds. There are bilateral crackles audible at both bases. There is no sacral oedema or hepatomegaly. However, the patient is noticeably hypertensive at 182/102 mmHg.

The most likely diagnosis is of congestive cardiac failure due to uncontrolled hypertension.

The examination of a patient with suspected cardiac failure can give a great deal of information about the aetiology and severity of heart failure and will help to guide ongoing treatment. The signs can be broadly split into those related to left ventricular dysfunction (left-sided signs) and those related to right heart failure (right-sided signs).

SCENARIO 7

123

Left-sided failure:
- Tachypnoea and increased work of breathing
- Bibasal (initially) and then throughout the lung fields, suggesting the development of pulmonary oedema (fluid in the alveoli)
- Cyanosis, which suggests severe hypoxemia
- Lateral displacement of the apex beat (an enlarged heart)
- A gallop rhythm (additional third heart sound), which is a marker of fluid overload.

Right-sided failure:
- Pitting peripheral oedema, ascites and hepatomegaly
- JVP elevation
- If the right ventricular pressure is increased, a parasternal heave may be present.

Biventricular failure:
- Dullness of the lung fields to percussion and reduced breath sounds at the bases of the lung may suggest the development of pleural effusions.

## Investigations

Angiography, cardiac MRI

## Management

The chronic management of heart failure is a challenge in both primary and hospital care. The chronic management has been explored above. However, chronic heart failure can easily decompensate and present with an acute deterioration in symptoms due to pulmonary oedema.

The initial approach to these patients requires an ABC approach with prompt diagnosis and treatment. The mainstays of treatment are:
- Nitrates – GTN infusions and buccal nitrates
- CPAP non-invasive ventilation to improve oxygenation
- Loop diuretics – will help with ongoing fluid overload
- Small dose opiates – more to help with the sensation of extreme dyspnoea that is associated with this presentation.

### Further reading and web links
*British Heart Foundation, patient information resource*:
www.bhf.org.uk/heart-health/conditions/heart-failure.aspx
*NICE guidelines on the management of heart failure*:
http://guidance.nice.org.uk/CG108

SCENARIO 7

# Scenario 8: 'Running on empty'

## Station 1

*History*                                          *10-minute station*

You are the FY1 on the Medical Admissions Unit (MAU). A 45-year-old woman, Karen Revell, has been referred by her GP with anaemia.

- Please take a focussed history and present this along with your differential diagnosis to the Acute Medicine Registrar.

*You will be assessed on the following areas, as well as the content and diagnostic reasoning of your history – take them into account in your presentation.*

### Professionalism

- Professional appearance (NHS dress code) – including general appearance, hair and jewellery
- Maintains patient and personal safety
- Polite introduction; identifies patient or interviewee correctly; confirms patient's date of birth from name band or other source
- Obtains informal consent; maintains patient's privacy
- Displays empathetic and caring attitudes and behaviours throughout.

### Process

- Good organisation and structure; appropriate use of open and closed questions
- Appropriate fluency/rhythm/pace to the interview – this may change depending on environment and acute nature of the problem
- Appropriate time for the patient to respond/reply to questions
- Appropriate acknowledgement of difficult or emotional areas of the patient's history.

### Communication skills

- Demonstrates caring and sympathetic attitude
- Asks open questions
- Invites patient to ask questions and answers them appropriately
- Addresses patient's ideas, concerns and expectations.

## Station 2

*Examination*                                          *10-minute station*

After presenting your history you have been asked to examine Mrs Revell, focussing on possible causes of anaemia.

- Please complete your examination and present your positive findings to your Registrar.

(If you do not have a model, please read and present the information given on page 383.)

*You will be assessed on the following areas, as well as the content and skills of your examination – take them into account in your presentation.*

### Professionalism

- Professional appearance; maintains infection control standards, including hand cleaning and appropriate use of gloves and aprons
- Maintains patient and personal safety
- Polite introduction; identifies patient and confirms date of birth from name band or other source
- Obtains informal consent; maintains patient privacy and dignity
- Displays empathetic and caring attitudes and behaviours throughout.

### Process

- Appropriate fluency/rhythm/pace to the examination – this may change depending on environment and acute nature of the problem
- Organisation and structure of examination; sensitive and empathetic approach
- Uses appropriate clinical techniques throughout
- Maintains privacy and dignity throughout.

### Clinical communication

- Explains proposed examination/procedure: explains examination/procedure as it proceeds
- Offers information in a clear, structured and fluent manner, avoiding jargon
- Listens to patient and responds appropriately
- Demonstrates appropriate body language.

SCENARIO 8

# Station 3

*Procedural skills*                    *10-minute station*

After your initial examination you need to complete your examination of Mrs Revell by completing a digital rectal examination.

**Procedure**
■ Please perform this skill on the model provided and speak to the examiner as if they are the patient.

**Equipment provided**
- Rectal examination model
- Lubricant jelly
- Gauze swabs
- Non-sterile gloves.

# Station 4

*Data interpretation*                    *10-minute station*

Mrs Revell's initial investigation results are below.
■ 1. Please identify three abnormalities.

**Investigation results**
- Blood results – FBC: Hb 5.4 g/dl, MCV 70 fl, WCC 7.9 × 10⁹/l, neutrophils 6.4 × 10⁹/l, platelets 167 × 10⁹/l
- U&Es – Na⁺ 137 mmol/l, K⁺ 4.2 mmol/l, urea 5.8 mmol/l, creatinine 98 μmol/l
- RBG – 6.2 mmol/l
- CCa₂⁺ 2.43 mmol/l, PO₄⁻ 0.98 mmol/l, Mg 0.9 mmol/l
- Clotting screen – INR 1.2
- LFTs – ALT 178 iu/l, ALP 378 iu/l, Alb 21 g/l, bilirubin 48 μmol/l
- Fe 5 μmol/l (9–30.4 μmol/l); ferritin 15 μg/l (20–250 μg/l); TIBC 150 μg/dl (250–370 μg/l)
- CXR – normal
- ECG – sinus tachycardia.
■ 2. Please match the following clinical scenarios to the likely underlying cause of anaemia.
    A  Myelodysplasia
    B  Autoimmune haemolytic anaemia
    C  Multiple myeloma
    D  G6PD deficiency
    E  Aplastic anaemia
    F  B₁₂/folate deficiency
    G  Beta thalassemia
    H  Sickle cell disease

I    Erythropoietin deficiency

a)   A 19-year-old Afro-Caribbean man presents with severe pain in his right hip and leg. His haemoglobin (Hb) is 6.4 and his mean corpuscular volume (MCV) is 65.

b)   A 74-year-old woman presents with weight loss, fatigue and lethargy, and has pain in her back and thighs. Her Hb is 7.8, her MCV is 84 and her erythrocyte sedimentation rate (ESR) is 78.

c)   A 57-year-old man with a history of alcoholism is found to have an Hb of 8.9 and an MCV of 109 on routine bloods with his GP.

d)   A 27-year-old Kenyan man presents to the Emergency Department with an Hb of 6.4, an MCV of 80 and bilrubin of 78. He reports that he was treated for malaria a week ago in Kenya.

e)   A 74-year-old man is seen in the nephrology clinic with diabetes and hypertension and is increasingly lethargic. His Hb is 8.2, MCV is 82, urea is 34 mmol/l and creatinine 654 µmol/l.

## Station 5

*Prescribing skills*                    *10-minute station*

After the post-take ward round with the Acute Medicine Consultant, you have been asked to prescribe a blood transfusion of 3 units.

■  Please prescribe using the BNF and drug chart provided.

**Details**

o  Mrs Karen Revell
o  DOB 16/02/1967
o  Hospital number: 7653451
o  Ward: MAU
o  Consultant: Dr Neves
o  No known drug allergies

# Station 6

*Procedural skills*                    *10-minute station*

Now that you have prescribed the blood transfusion you have been asked to administer the first unit.

**Procedure A**

■ With the nurse caring for Mrs Revell, please check and administer the first unit of blood. Give any further instructions regarding monitoring to the nurse.

**Equipment provided**

- Prescription chart
- Unit of packed red cells with patient's details attached
- Patient arm with cannula in situ
- Blood giving set

**Blood Unit issue sheet**

| Name | DOB | Hosp number | Unit | Exp date |
|------|-----|-------------|------|----------|
| Karen Revell | 16/02/1967 | 7653451 | 456123789GA | Dec 2012 |

**Blood label**

> **UNIT: A positive packed red cells**
>
> **Blood compatible for transfusion for**
>
> **Patient: Karen Revell**
>
> **Sex: female**
>
> **Hospital Number: 7653451**
>
> **DOB: 16/02/1967**
>
> **Unit number: 456123789GA**
>
> **Expires Dec 2012**

# Answers

## Station 1 – History

**Patient script**

You are Mrs Karen Revell (DOB 16 February 1967), a 45-year-old retired shop manager. You have been referred to the hospital after your GP performed a blood test that showed that you are anaemic.

You had presented to your GP earlier in the week with a 3-month history of feeling tired all the time. You have been increasingly short of breath on exertion. However, you are not breathless at rest. You have had no chest pain. You have also recently started to feel lightheaded on standing. You have struggled to get to work due to your tiredness in the last week.

Your only previous medical history is that of asthma, for which you use a salbutamol inhaler as you need it. You have never been admitted to hospital with an exacerbation of your asthma. You take no other medications and have no allergies.

You are a smoker of 10 cigarettes per day for the last 30 years. You drink alcohol – approximately 10 units per week. You have a normal diet, which includes red meat and plenty of vegetables. You live with your partner and stepdaughter. Your father died from bowel cancer at 65 years and your mother is still alive.

On direct questioning:

You have lost weight over the last 3 months, approximately 9 kg. You have not been dieting but were pleased, as you have tried to lose weight unsuccessfully before.

You have had no vomiting or diarrhoea but you have been slightly constipated. You have also noticed a little fresh red blood mixed in with your stool in the last few weeks. You have had no heartburn and have not taken any anti-inflammatories.

You still have periods and have an irregular cycle with no heavy blood loss.

You have started no new medications.

You have had no fevers or night sweats. You have had no bruising or bleeding problems.

You are unsure about what could have caused the anaemia but are very keen to just get a transfusion and get home as soon as possible.

| A | B | C | D | E | | A | B | C | D | E | | A | B | C | D | E |
PROFESSIONALISM    PROCESS    COMMUNICATION

## CONTENT

A B C D E

### Identifies key information
- Establishes duration of illness – 3 months of lethargy and weight loss
- Establishes presence of symptoms of anaemia – shortness of breath on exertion, postural lightheadedness but no chest pain
- Establishes history of altered bowel habit with blood in stool
- Assesses history of risk factors for anaemia, to include: no history of menorrhagia; no dyspepsia or malaena; no symptoms of bone marrow failure – spontaneous bruising and infections; normal diet, including red meat and vegetables.

### Completing the patient history
- Drug and allergy history: PRN salbutamol, no allergies
- Previous medical history: asthma – controlled on PRN salbutamol
- Social and occupational history: working as a shop manager; smokes – 15 pack year history; alcohol intake – 10 units per week
- Family history: paternal colon cancer aged 69.

### Summarises important areas of the history back to the patient

### Invites patient to ask questions and deals with them appropriately

### Establishes patient's ideas, concerns and expectations
- Patient is keen to just have a transfusion and get home.

## CLINICAL DIAGNOSTIC REASONING

A B C D E

- ■ **Please present your history**
  - Candidate offers a logical, well-structured account of the history.
- ■ **Your Registrar agrees with you that the history is in keeping with a possible colonic malignancy. What risk factors do you know for colo-rectal cancer?**
  - Family history including familial adenomatous polyposis and hereditary non-polyposis colo-rectal cancer (HNPCC)
  - Diet heavy in red meat and low in fibre-containing vegetables – 'Western diet'
  - Obesity.

## GLOBAL HISTORY MARK

A B C D E

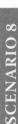
SCENARIO 8

131

## Station 2 – Examination

Patient script (see also page 383)

You are a 45-year-old woman who is comfortable at rest. Your abdomen is soft and non-tender.

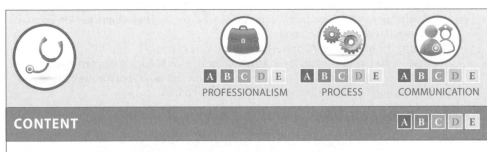

PROFESSIONALISM    PROCESS    COMMUNICATION

### CONTENT    A B C D E

**Exposes and positions patient correctly and maintains comfort**

**Comments on wellbeing of patient, ie well or unwell**
- Patient appears slim but not cachextic
- Obvious pallor of skin.

**Asks for appropriate/relevant clinical observations**
- Observations: HR 102 bpm, BP 110/65 mmHg, RR 12 bpm, $O_2$ sats 96% on air, temperature 37.0 °C

**General examination**
- Hands – assesses for nail signs; leuconychia and koilonychia, assess for palmar erythema
- Face – no cyanosis, assesses eyes for jaundice and pallor, examines mouth for angular stomatitis, glossitis and oral ulceration
- Assesses for lymphadenopathy, to include supra-clavicular nodes (Virchow's node).

**Focussed examination**
- Inspection – comments on absence of distension or scars
- Palpation – palpates all nine quadrants to light touch and deep palpation, palpates for organomegaly (liver, spleen) starting from the right iliac fossa; ballots the kidneys
- Percussion – assesses in all nine quadrants and percusses liver to assess hepatomegaly
- Auscultation – auscultates bowel sounds for at least 30 seconds.

**Completes examination by identifying relevant additional clinical signs**
- Asks to perform a digital rectal examination.

**Thanks patient, offers assistance, maintains patient's dignity and privacy until they are dressed**

## CLINICAL DIAGNOSTIC REASONING

**Correctly identifies the relevant physical signs, including important negative findings**

- **How would you like to complete this examination?**
  - The important final part of the examination of any patient with anaemia is a digital rectal examination in order to assess for any masses or malaena.

- **What is your differential diagnosis?**
  - The differential for this patient must include: lower gastrointestinal malignancy; upper gastrointestinal malignancy; peptic ulcer disease.

- **What diagnostic investigations would you now request?**
  - Bloods tests – FBC to assess Hb and MCV; haematinics, including iron studies, $B_{12}$ and folate; cross-match sample in order to transfuse as required
  - Oesophagogastroduodenoscopy (OGD) and colonsoscopy – to assess for any malignant lesion
  - CT of chest, abdomen and pelvis – as malignancy is likely, this can be performed to assess for any distant metastases.

## GLOBAL EXAMINATION MARK

SCENARIO 8

## Station 3 – Procedural skills

**Procedure: Digital rectal examination**

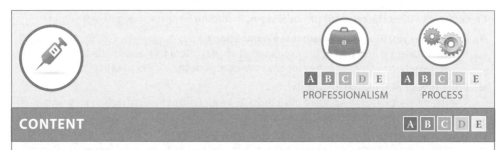

PROFESSIONALISM    A B C D E

PROCESS    A B C D E

### CONTENT    A B C D E

**Explains that they would ask for a chaperone and position the patient correctly on left lateral**

**Identifies and sets out equipment correctly; maintains aseptic technique throughout**

**Correctly performs the procedure**
- Wears gloves
- Inspects the perianal area.
- Lubricates index finger
- Tells the patient that they are now going to insert their finger
- Inserts index finger and comments on the sphincter tone of the anus
- Notes any tenderness, induration, irregularities or nodules
- Inserts index finger further into the rectum and systematically examines the right lateral, posterior, and left lateral surfaces
- Turns the hand so that the finger can examine the anterior surface (and prostate in male patients)
- Withdraws finger and examines finger for faeces, blood and mucus
- Provides the patient with tissue to wipe the anus
- Disposes of the gloves and wipes in the clinical waste bin.

**Ensures patient receives correct advice about what to do next and follow-up**

**Ensures nursing staff or other healthcare professionals receive correct information about the consequences/outcome of the procedure/task**

**Thanks patient, offers assistance, maintains patient's dignity and privacy until they are dressed**

### GLOBAL PROCEDURE MARK

A B C D E

SCENARIO 8

## Station 4 – Data interpretation

**1. Abnormalities (three from):**
- **Microcytic anaemia**
- **Low ferritin and total iron-binding capacity (TIBC), suggesting iron deficiency**
- **Raised alanine amino-transferase (ALT) and alkaline phosphatase (ALP) with elevated bilirubin – may suggest hepatic metastasis**
- **Low albumin – impaired liver synthetic function.**

**2.**

**a) H**

This man is likely to have sickle cell disease and a painful vaso-occlusive sickle crisis. People with sickle cell disease have a chronic anaemia that is profoundly microcytic due to the haemoglobinopathy.

**b) C**

This patient presents with non-specific symptoms including lethargy and weight loss. The presence of a normocytic anaemia and raised ESR with bone pain suggests multiple myeloma as the likely diagnosis.

**c) F**

This man has asymptomatic macrocytic anaemia in the context of chronic alcohol abuse. The poor diet associated with alcoholism often leads to dietary deficiency of vitamin $B_{12}$ and folate, which leads to impaired haemopoietic function. It is often asymptomatic.

**d) D**

This patient was treated for malaria a week ago and now has a normocytic anaemia with a raised bilirubin. It is likely that he was treated with a medication such as primaquine, which can precipitate haemolysis in patients with G6PD deficiency. G6PD levels should be checked prior to a prescription of primaquine.

**e) I**

This patient has renal failure and a normocytic anaemia. Chronic renal failure is associated with anaemia related to a reduced production of erythropoietin by the kidneys, which leads to reduced red cell production by the bone marrow. Erythropoietin can be supplemented with subcutaneous injections.

**GLOBAL DATA INTERPRETATION MARK**

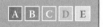

SCENARIO 8

## Station 5 – Prescribing skills

Each unit of blood should be prescribed separately. A non-urgent blood transfusion should be prescribed over 4 hours. Blood is prescribed as packed red cells in order to differentiate from other blood products available.

| Allergies, sensitivities and adverse drug reactions | | | | | | Patient details/addressograph | |
|---|---|---|---|---|---|---|---|
| No known allergies ✓ | | | Initials AF | Gender M (F) | | NHS/ Hospital No: 7653451 | |
| Not possible to ascertain ☐ | | | Date 07/5 | Weight (kg) | Date | | |
| Medicine/substance | Reaction & Severity | Initials & Date | | | | Surname: REVELL | |
| | | | | Height | | First name: KAREN | |
| | | | | | | | |
| Alerts | | | | Surface area (m²) | | Date of birth: 16.02.67 | |

| Infusion prescriptions continued | | | | | | | | | SC = subcutaneous | | IVC = intravenous central IVP = intravenous peripheral | | | | |
|---|---|---|---|---|---|---|---|---|---|---|---|---|---|---|---|
| Date & time | Route | Infusion Fluid | | Medication | | Duration | Rate | Prescriber's signature & bleep no. | Date given | Given by / Added by | Check by | Start time | Finish time | Pharmacy |
| | | Name & strength | Volume | Approved name with expiry / unit number | Dose | | | | | | | | | |
| 7/05 | IV | Blood Exp: Batch/unit no: | 1 unit | | | | 2 HOURS | AF 622 | | | | | | |
| 7/05 | IV | Blood Exp: Batch/unit no: | 1 unit | | | | 2 HOURS | AF 622 | | | | | | |
| 7/05 | IV | Blood Exp: Batch/unit no: | 1 unit | | | | 2 HOURS | AF 622 | | | | | | |
| 7/05 | IV | 0.9% saline Exp: Batch/unit no: | 100ml | | | | 10 mins | AF 622 | | | | | | |
| | | Exp: Batch/unit no: | | | | | | | | | | | | |
| | | Exp: Batch/unit no: | | | | | | | | | | | | |
| | | Exp: Batch/unit no: | | | | | | | | | | | | |
| | | Exp: Batch/unit no: | | | | | | | | | | | | |
| | | Exp: Batch/unit no: | | | | | | | | | | | | |
| | | | | | | | | | | | | | | |
| | | | | | | | | | | | | | | |

## GLOBAL PRESCRIBING MARK

A B C D E

## Station 6 – Procedural skills

**Procedure: Blood transfusion**

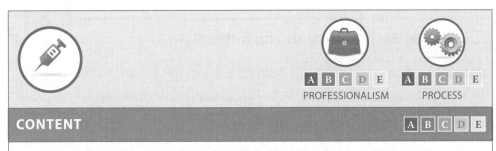

PROFESSIONALISM     PROCESS

### CONTENT

**Exposes and positions patient correctly and maintains comfort**

**Identifies and sets out equipment correctly; maintains aseptic technique throughout**
- Prescription chart
- Unit of blood
- Blood giving set
- Gloves.

**Washes hands**

**Ensures patient consent obtained and documented**

**Ensures baseline observations have been taken and documented**

**Correctly performs the procedure**
- Identifies patient from patient label
- Verbally confirms patient's name, DOB and location with patient
- Confirms patient's details and unit details with nurse
- Puts on gloves
- Removes sterile cap from unit of blood
- Closes valve on giving set and inserts into unit of blood
- Squeezes chamber until filled with blood
- Runs blood through giving set
- Attaches to cannula and adjusts drip rate.

**Obtains an acceptable/appropriate result**

**Disposes of all sharps and other items correctly**

**Ensures nursing staff or other healthcare professionals receive correct information about the procedure/task**
- Explains to nurse that patient needs observations at the start of transfusion, at 15 min and hourly throughout the transfusion; and report all abnormalities immediately to the designated doctor
- Documents on the prescription chart the unit number for each unit administered
- Returns unit label to transfusion department to ensure each unit is traceable to the patient who has received it.

**SCENARIO 8**

137

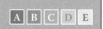

# Scenario 8: Reflection and consolidation

## History

Mrs Revell is a 45-year-old woman who presents with symptomatic anaemia. She was referred by her GP after an outpatient blood test. She has been increasingly lethargic over the last 3 months with exertional shortness of breath and postural lightheadedness. She denies chest pain.

She has a 3-month history of weight loss of 9 kg with altered bowel habit. She has been constipated and noted fresh red blood mixed in with her stool. She has no malaena or dyspepsia. She has an irregular menstrual cycle with no menorrhagia. She has started no new medications. She has had no recurrent infections or spontaneous bruising. She eats a varied diet, which includes red meat and vegetables.

She has a past medical history of asthma, well controlled on PRN salbutamol, with no other new medications. She is a smoker with a 15 pack year history with a moderate alcohol intake. Her father died from bowel cancer at age 69.

The likely diagnosis is that of an iron-deficiency anaemia related to a probable colonic malignancy.

## Examination

On examination, Mrs Revell is pale but comfortable. She is slim in build but not cachextic. She is tachycardic at rest at 102 bpm, her BP is normal at 100/65 mmHg, with a RR of 12 bpm and oxygen saturations of 96% on room air.

Examination of the hands shows no palmar erythema, koilonychia or leuconchyia. Her conjunctiva are pale and there is no evidence of jaundice. She has angular stomatitis but oral examination is otherwise normal. She has no palpable lymphadenopathy.

On examination of the abdomen there are no scars or distension. There is a palpable nodular liver edge at 2 cm below the costal margin with no associated splenomegaly. She has fullness of the right iliac fossa but no palpable discrete mass. Bowel sounds are present and normal in character. I would like to complete the examination with a digital rectal examination.

## Investigations

The decision to transfuse blood is based on a combination of the investigation results and clinical picture as to whether a patient is symptomatic. If an urgent transfusion is not required, iron-deficiency anaemia can be treated with iron supplements.

Each trust has clear guidelines to help in this decision making with a usual guideline of only transfusing asymptomatic individuals when the haemoglobin is less than 7.0 g/dl. In those with symptoms related to their anaemia or significant co-morbidities such as ischaemic heart disease transfusion may be appropriate at a higher haemoglobin level. It is important to realise that transfusions are not without risk.

## Management

Transfusion reactions are a common complication of blood transfusions and most are mild self-limiting reactions related to minor antigen incompatibility. However, it is important to understand the pathophysiology behind these reactions and how to recognise and manage them.

Acute haemolytic transfusion reaction:

- Incompatible transfused red cells react with the patient's own anti-A or anti-B antibodies, which can lead to gross intravascular haemolysis and disseminated intravascular coagulopathy with subsequent cardiovascular collapse
- Infusion of ABO incompatible blood usually arises from errors in labelling sample tubes/request forms or from inadequate checks at the time of transfusion.

Infective shock:

- A unit of blood contaminated with bacteria is transfused, with subsequent onset of hypertension or hypotension and rigours, and collapse rapidly follows the transfusion.

Transfusion-related acute lung injury (TRALI):

- TRALI is a form of acute respiratory distress due to donor plasma containing antibodies against the patient's white cells. This occurs within 6 hours and presents with cough, breathlessness and bilateral pulmonary infiltrates.

Fluid overload

- This occurs when too much fluid is transfused or fluid is transfused too quickly, especially in those who are not hypovolaemic. Furosemide is prescribed with packed red cells in those at risk, such as those with congestive cardiac failure.

Non-haemolytic febrile reactions:

- Fevers (>1 °C above baseline) and rigours may develop during red cell or platelet transfusion due to patient antibodies to transfused white cells
- Most febrile reactions can be managed by slowing or stopping the transfusion and giving paracetamol.

Severe allergic reaction or anaphylaxis:

- Allergic reactions occur when patients have antibodies that react with proteins in transfused blood components. This can range from urticaria to anaphylactic shock.

### Further reading and web links

*UK blood transfusion and tissue transplantation services website:*
www.transfusionguidelines.org.uk/

# Scenario 9:
# 'Frequent and profuse'

## Station 1

*History*                                        *10-minute station*

You are the FY1 on a Gastroenterology firm. You've been called down to Outpatients by your Consultant, Dr Alsted, to admit a patient, Mr Joel Barnet (DOB 07/08/1977 – aged 34 years) who has presented today with worsening symptoms of his inflammatory bowel disease. Unfortunately his old notes are unavailable and Dr Alsted has requested that you take a complete history of his condition, including this present exacerbation.

■ Please take a comprehensive history with a view to presenting it to Dr Alsted.

*You will be assessed on the following areas, as well as the content and diagnostic reasoning of your history – take them into account in your presentation.*

### Professionalism

- Professional appearance (NHS dress code) – including general appearance, hair and jewellery
- Maintains patient and personal safety
- Polite introduction; identifies patient or interviewee correctly; confirms patient's date of birth from name band or other source
- Obtains informal consent; maintains patient's privacy
- Displays empathetic and caring attitudes and behaviours throughout.

### Process

- Good organisation and structure; appropriate use of open and closed questions
- Appropriate fluency/rhythm/pace to the interview – this may change depending on environment and acute nature of the problem
- Appropriate time for the patient to respond/reply to questions
- Appropriate acknowledgement of difficult or emotional areas of the patient's history.

### Communication skills

- Demonstrates caring and sympathetic attitude
- Asks open questions
- Invites patient to ask questions and answers them appropriately
- Addresses patient's ideas, concerns and expectations.

# Station 2

*Examination*                    *10-minute station*

■ **After presenting your history to Dr Alsted, she asks you to perform a focussed clinical assessment of Mr Barnet, to include:**

1. **His acute clinical status**
2. **Signs/complications of his chronic condition.**

**(If you do not have a model, please read and present the information given on page 384.)**

*You will be assessed on the following areas, as well as the content and skills of your examination – take them into account in your presentation.*

## Professionalism

- Professional appearance; maintains infection control standards, including hand cleaning and appropriate use of gloves and aprons
- Maintains patient and personal safety
- Polite introduction; identifies patient and confirms date of birth from name band or other source
- Obtains informal consent; maintains patient privacy and dignity
- Displays empathetic and caring attitudes and behaviours throughout.

## Process

- Appropriate fluency/rhythm/pace to the examination – this may change depending on environment and acute nature of the problem
- Organisation and structure of examination; sensitive and empathetic approach
- Uses appropriate clinical techniques throughout
- Maintains privacy and dignity throughout.

## Clinical communication

- Explains proposed examination/procedure: explains examination/procedure as it proceeds
- Offers information in a clear, structured and fluent manner, avoiding jargon
- Listens to patient and responds appropriately
- Demonstrates appropriate body language.

## Station 3

*Procedural skills*                    *10-minute station*

Dr Alsted – spotting a training opportunity (she tells you this could be written up as a DOPS) – asks you to perform a digital rectal examination (DRE) on Mr Barnet, before she performs a rigid sigmoidoscopy and biopsy.

**Procedure**
■ Please perform a DRE using the manikin provided, explaining your actions to a colleague as if he/she were Mr Barnet.

**Equipment provided**
- DRE manikin
- Gloves
- Lubricant gel
- Tissue paper or similar, to wipe patient.

## Station 4

*Data interpretation*                    *10-minute station*

1. Mr Barnet had routine bloods taken on arrival in the outpatient clinic and Dr Alsted has asked you to review the results and record them in the patient's notes.
■ Please indicate whether each of these statements is TRUE (T) or FALSE (F) regarding Mr Barnet's results (below).

**Details**
- ○ FBC: Hb 7.9 g/dl, MCV 84 fl, WCC 16.6 × $10^9$/l, neutrophils 12.7 × $10^9$/l, platelets 431 × $10^9$/l
- ○ U&Es: Na$^+$ 146 mmol/l, K$^+$ 2.6 mmol/l, urea 15.8 mmol/l, creatinine 114 μmol/l
- ○ RBG: 5.1 mmol/l
- ○ LFTs: TBil 4.7mmol/l, ALT 14 iu/l, AST 18 iu/l, Alk phos 133 iu/l, Alb 27 g/l
- ○ Clotting: INR 1.1; APTT 32 s
- ○ ESR 56 mm/hour
- ○ CRP 364 mg/l

    A   The Hb and MCV are most likely explained by his renal impairment.
    B   The Hb and MCV indicate he has an occult colonic malignancy.
    C   The white cell and differential are in keeping with the acute exacerbation of his Crohn's disease.
    D   The white cell and differential suggest he has a cryptosporidium infection.
    E   The urea : creatinine ratio is suggestive of pre-renal impairment.
    F   The serum potassium is in keeping with a diarrhoeal illness.
    G   Given the serum sodium, he should receive 0.45% saline solution.
    H   Given the serum potassium, he should initially receive 40 mmol potassium supplementation per litre of fluid.

I   The LFTs are highly suggestive of fatty infiltration of the liver.
J   The hypoalbuminaemia is consistent with severe, chronic IBD.
K   The coagulation screen and platelet count are suggestive of early disseminated intravascular coagulopathy (DIC).
L   The inflammatory markers are suggestive of a severe exacerbation of his IBD.

2. Dr Alsted shows you Mr Barnet's plain abdominal X-ray image, which shows a non-specific gas pattern in the small and large bowel, with no other pathological features. She then shows you several other images from gastroenterology patients admitted over the last few months.

■ Please indicate whether each of these statements is TRUE (T) or FALSE (F) regarding the abdominal X-ray images shown below.

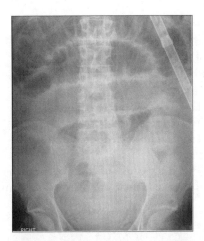

a. This is the plain abdominal image taken of a 28-year-old man with Crohn's disease who presented in the Emergency Department with severe abdominal pain and vomiting.
   A   There are multiple dilated loops of small bowel.
   B   There is an intra-abdominal drain in situ.
   C   Another common cause of this appearance is colonic carcinoma.

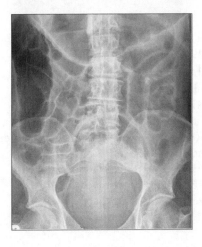

b. This is the plain abdominal image taken of a 46-year-old man with ulcerative colitis who presented in the Emergency Department with severe abdominal pain, diarrhoea and now absolute constipation.
   A   There are features consistent with toxic megacolon.
   B   There is evidence of extra-gastrointestinal complications of his IBD.
   C   This appearance is more commonly seen in pseudomembranous colitis.

SCENARIO 9

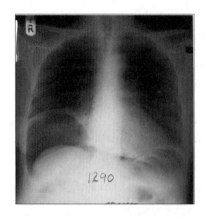

c. This is the image taken of a 33-year old man with a long history of peptic ulcer disease who presented n the Emergency Department with a 12-hour history of severe upper abdominal pain and vomiting.
   A There is evidence of dilated loops of large bowel.
   B There is a large hiatus hernia.
   C The management should be 'drip and suck', and observation for 24–48 hours.

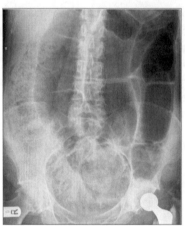

d. This is the plain abdominal image taken of a 76-year-old woman with a 3-month history of weight loss, intermittent constipation and a new microcytic anaemia.
   A There is evidence of dilated small bowel loops.
   B The caecum is loaded with faecal residue.
   C The likely cause of this appearance in this case is post-operative adhesions.

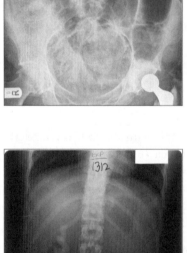

e. This is the plain abdominal image taken of a 39-year-old man with severe right-sided abdominal and back pain, now associated with fever and vomiting.
   A There is evidence of pancreatic calcification.
   B There is evidence of a recent barium study.
   C This appearance is associated with recurrent infection by urease-producing bacteria.

## Station 5

*Clinical communication skills*     *10-minute station*

Dr Alsted is not only concerned about Mr Barnet's acute presentation but also his poor nutritional status. She thinks he might be a candidate for additional nutritional support, and may even require total parenteral nutrition (TPN) if his acute exacerbation fails to settle.

■ Please take a focussed nutritional history, and using the information to date, and the MUST© screening tool below, make a nutritional assessment of Mr Barnet, explaining the results and his likely management to him.

| MUST© screening tool – five-step screening and management plan | | | | |
|---|---|---|---|---|
| **STEP 1 – BMI score** | | **STEP 2 – Weight loss score** | | **STEP 3 – Acute disease effect score** |
| **BMI** | | **Unplanned weight loss in last 6 months** | | **If patient is acutely ill and there has been, or is unlikely to be, no nutritional intake for more than 5 days** |
| **BMI (kg/m²)** | **SCORE** | **% weight loss** | **SCORE** | **SCORE = 2** |
| >20 | 0 | <5.0 | 0 | |
| 18.5–19.9 | 1 | 5.0–10 | 1 | |
| <18.5 | 2 | >10 | 2 | |

**STEP 4 – Calculate risk: Score 0 = low risk; 1 = medium risk; 2 or more = high risk**

| Step 5 – Management guidelines | | |
|---|---|---|
| Low risk – routine clinical care | Medium risk – observe | High risk – treat* |
| Repeat screening | Document dietary intake for 3 days | Refer to dietitian, Nutritional Support Team or implement local policy |
| Hospital – weekly | | |
| Care homes – monthly | If adequate – little concern and repeat screening | Set goals, improve and increase overall nutritional intake |
| Community – annually for special groups, eg those >75 years | Hospital – weekly | Monitor and review care plan |
| | Care home – at least monthly | Hospital – weekly |
| | Community – at least every 2–3 months | Care home – monthly |
| | | Community – monthly |
| | If inadequate – clinical concern – follow local policy, set goals, improve and increase overall nutritional intake, monitor and review care plan regularly | * Unless detrimental or no benefit is expected from nutritional support, eg imminent death. |

## Station 6

*Prescribing skills*                    *10-minute station*

Given the history, examination and data findings, Dr Alsted asks you to write up an appropriate set of medications and fluids for Mr Barnet.

■ Using the drug and fluid charts provided please write up the medications and fluids as if Mr Barnet were being admitted acutely from the clinic.

### Details

- ○ Mr Joel Barnet, DOB 07/08/1977, Hospital no. 757543, Ward: Elm, Consultant: Dr Alsted, FY1, AF: bleep number 622
- ○ Height 1.78 m, weight 62.3 kg, U&Es: $Na^+$ 146 mmol/l, $K^+$ 2.6 mmol/l, urea 15.8 mmol/l, creatinine 114 μmol/l
- ○ Allergies: Infliximab

> **Remember: DRUG DRs D**on't **F**orget **S**igning **O**ff (page 396)

# Answers

## Station 1 – History

**Patient script**

You are Mr Joel Barnet (DOB 07 August 1977 – 34 years old), and work as the Senior Physiotherapist here on the orthopaedic wards. You were seen as an emergency by Dr Alsted this morning as she knows you well and allows you to self-refer when you become acutely unwell. (You have read extensively about your condition and can talk very competently with the medical staff about your disease.)

History of IBD:

Diagnosis – originally you were diagnosed in 1997, aged 20 years old. You had recently returned from a gap year in The Gambia and when the symptoms started everyone thought you had picked up a tropical infection. Despite two courses of antibiotics from your GP you just got 'worse and worse'.

Initially you had several symptoms:

(1) Diarrhoea – loose, brown motions, mixed with blood and mucus. The frequency increased over several days from four to five motions per 24 hours to a maximum of about once every 2 or 3 hours. It was so bad you were getting little or no sleep, and were unable to eat or drink very much. You were referred to Dr Shine (the gastroenterologist before Dr Alsted) and he diagnosed the problem after taking a colonic biopsy. It soon settled down with steroids and the 5-ASA medicines.

(2) Joints – lots of aches and pains in the joints of your hands, feet and back

(3) Eyes – severe red, painful eyes – this was later confirmed as uveitis

(4) Skin – large red blotchy rash on shins – you were told later this was erythema nodosum.

Progression – since then you've had multiple flare-ups (maybe one or two a year for the last 10 years or so). You often manage them yourself with some guidance by Dr Alsted. During these exacerbations you take a course of steroids and 5-ASA and it usually settles down. In between times you are usually OK with a bit of codeine from time to time.

During this period, you've been hospitalised several times and ended up having a small bowel resection about 5 years ago after a particularly nasty episode, and then a further resection 3 years ago. Your last admission was 8 months ago, but that wasn't too bad. You had a trial of infliximab at that time but you weren't able to tolerate it (you had an allergic reaction to the injection, where you became very red, itchy and breathless, and they (the doctors) had to give you adrenaline and steroids, as they were really worried about you).

This episode started slowly about 2 weeks ago and has predictably got worse and worse! Initially, your bowels opened three or four times per day; your motions were loose and brown with associated fresh blood and mucus. Now you are opening your bowels every 3 hours, with lots of fresh blood and mucus. You have had increasing generalised abdominal pain with associated nausea but no vomiting. The pain was originally a dull ache but overnight has become almost unbearable, severe and all over the abdomen.

During the last 4 or 5 days you've been taking increasing doses of painkillers (paracetamol and codeine phosphate) and steroids, but to no avail. You've been eating and drinking poorly, and have had hardly any sleep in the last few days.

As well as the abdominal problems, the joints in your hands and your lumbar spine have been really painful and sore.

Of note – your maternal grandmother and your aunt (mother's sister) both had inflammatory bowel disease; you are a lifelong non-smoker; you have 'occasional binges' of alcohol when your bowels are OK but generally very little; you take no illicit drugs. Your occupation is Senior Physiotherapist in the hospital Orthopaedic Department.

Previous medical history – appendicectomy at 14 years old; fractured left fibula and tibia requiring plating of tibia (motorbike accident aged 23 years old).

Regular medications and allergies – was previously on azathioprine but was changed to methotrexate after last admission. Methotrexate 20 mg once a week. Presently also taking prednisolone 30 mg per day, and olsalazine 1 g bd. Allergic to infliximab (as above).

You are married, and your wife (Julia) is a physiotherapist at the private hospital 'down the road'. You have one daughter (Jessica), aged two and a half. You live in a two-bedroom garden flat, near the hospital.

Ideas – 'This is the worst I've been in a very long time, as bad as when I had to have my operations'. Concerns – 'I'm really worried and just hope it's not too late – I don't want another operation.'

Expectations – 'Just hope the medications can get me better without the intervention of a surgeon.'

| A B C D E | A B C D E | A B C D E |
|---|---|---|
| PROFESSIONALISM | PROCESS | COMMUNICATION |

## CONTENT

A B C D E

**Identifies key information**

**Includes important negatives, including systemic enquiry**
- History of IBD
    - Diagnosis – presenting symptoms; when, where and how
    - Progression
    - Normal control – medications, reviews by healthcare professionals
    - Worst its been – hospital admissions, operations, abdominal and systemic complications
    - Risk factors for IBD – family history, cigarette smoking, appendicectomy (aged 14 years old).
- Present episode
    - Duration and progression
    - Symptoms – gastrointestinal (GI) and extra GI
    - Medications
    - Impact – sleep, oral intake.

**Completing the patient history**
- Drug and allergy history: previously on azathioprine but was changed to methotrexate after last admission; now methotrexate 20 mg once a week; also taking prednisolone 30 mg per day, and olsalazine 1 g bd for last 5 days
- Previous medical history: appendicectomy (14 years old), fractured left fibula and tibia requiring ORIF of tibia (motorbike accident aged 23 years old)
- Social and occupational history: married with one young daughter; accommodation; alcohol rarely but occasional binge.

**Summarises important areas of the history back to the patient**

**Invites patient to ask questions and deals with them appropriately**

**Establishes patient's ideas, concerns and expectations**

## CLINICAL DIAGNOSTIC REASONING

- **Please present your history**
  - Candidate offers a logical, well-structured account of the history.

- **What is your diagnosis?**
  - Acute exacerbation of patient's Crohn's disease – mainly distal colonic symptoms (diarrhoea, mucus and fresh blood) but also has acute arthritis.

- **Could you tell me the investigations you would request for this patient, with a reason for each**
  - Bloods
    - FBC – HB/MCV: anaemia, WCC and differential – acute flare-up; platelets – ensure no thrombocytopenia (DIC and giving 5-ASA)
    - U&Es – renal impairment
    - LFTs – chronic complications of IBD, eg fatty liver; albumin: chronic, poor nutrition and flare-ups lead to hypoalbuminaemia
    - CRP/ESR – markers of acute inflammation
    - Clotting screen – ensure no DIC or coagulopathy (acute bleeding)
    - Blood (and stool cultures) – in case infective element to flare up (especially if pyrexial)
    - Venous blood gases – pH, bicarbonate and lactate.
  - Radiology
    - Plain abdominal X-ray - exclude sinister pathology, eg toxic megacolon or bowel obstruction
    - May require CT abdomen if symptoms not settling.

**Demonstrates safe, sensible and appropriate management plan**

**Demonstrates clear and logical diagnostic reasoning**

## GLOBAL HISTORY MARK

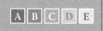

## Station 2 – Examination

**Patient script (see also page 384)**

You are a 34-year-old man with long-standing Crohn's disease. You are in obvious distress with abdominal pain. You are able to cooperate with the doctor's examination. You have diffuse, moderate tenderness throughout the abdomen. You have guarding but no rigidity.

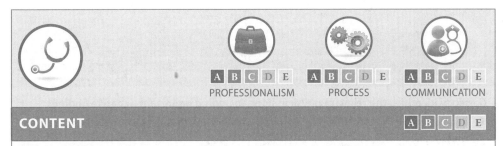

SCENARIO 9

PROFESSIONALISM | PROCESS | COMMUNICATION

## CONTENT

A B C D E

**Exposes and positions patient correctly and maintains comfort**

**Comments on wellbeing of patient, ie well or unwell**
- Suggests giving the patient some appropriate analgesia before continuing.

**'Feet to face'**
- Observes and comments on patient and surroundings from foot of bed – including laparotomy scar.

**Asks for appropriate/relevant clinical observations**
- Observations – HR 110 bpm, BP 105/66 mmHg, RR 20 bpm, $O_2$ sats 97% on air, temperature 38.2 °C, CBG 4.9 mmol/l, height 1.78 m, weight 62.3 kg, BMI 19.7 kg/m$^2$.

**General/systemic examination**
- Specifically comments on associated features of:
- Crohn's/abdominal disease, including: anaemia, clubbing, signs of chronic liver disease; ulceration in the mouth and signs of anaemia and hydration.

**RS and CVS examinations**
- Abdomen – appropriate technique throughout
- Inspection – scars, masses, organomegaly
- Palpation – systematic assessment; superficial and deep palpation; comments on tenderness and signs of peritonism
- Assesses for masses
- Examines for hepatomegaly, splenomegaly and enlarged kidneys
- Assesses hernial orifices
- Auscultation – comments on bowel sounds
- DRE – examiner stops candidate (see next station).

**Assesses for the stigmata of acute/chronic disease**
- Abdomen – as above
- Eyes – uveitis/conjunctivitis
- Joints – assesses small joints of hands and feet; sacro-iliac and lumbar spine (inappropriate in this case due to clinical status of patient)
- Skin – comments on rashes on upper and lower limbs.

**Thanks patient, offers assistance, maintains patient's dignity and privacy until they are dressed**

## CLINICAL DIAGNOSTIC REASONING

A B C D E

**Correctly identifies the relevant physical signs, including important negative findings**

- **Can you name the skin lesions associated with Crohn's disease and one other cause of these rashes?**
  - Pyoderma gangrenosum – associated with rheumatoid arthritis, haematological malignancy and primary biliary cirrhosis
  - Erythema nodosum – tuberculous, sarcoid, oral contraceptive pill
  - Both are commonly idiopathic, with no cause found; this, as always, is a diagnosis of exclusion.

- **Can you tell me five immediate therapeutic interventions you would instigate for this patient?**
  - Analgesia – consider IV opiates and an anti-emetic
  - Intravenous fluids – he may need 5 or 6 litres of fluid in the next 24 hours; he may well be hypokalaemic given the amount of watery diarrhoea he has suffered and will require supplemental potassium added to each bag of fluid
  - Steroids – he may require both intravenous hydrocortisone and steroid enemas
  - 5-ASA compounds, eg mesalazine or olsalazine (if tolerated)
  - Nutritional support –he should be reviewed urgently by a dietician as he may require TPN.

**Demonstrates safe, sensible and appropriate management plan**

**Demonstrates clear and logical diagnostic reasoning**

## GLOBAL EXAMINATION MARK

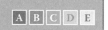
A B C D E

## Station 3 – Procedural skills

**Procedure: Digital rectal examination**

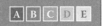

PROFESSIONALISM    PROCESS

## CONTENT

A B C D E

### Identifies and sets out equipment correctly; maintains aseptic technique throughout

- Gloves
- Lubricant gel
- Tissue paper or similar.

### Confirms/introduces presence of chaperone to patient

### Ensures patient privacy prior to starting procedure – checks surroundings, eg curtains are closed

### Fully explains procedure; gains informal consent to proceed

### Exposes and positions patient correctly and maintains comfort

- Left lateral position, underwear removed and knees tucked up into chest (or as best as patient can manage).

### Correctly performs the procedure

- Puts on gloves and prepares gel on tissue or gauze
- Observation – looks for and comments on the presence/absence of perinanal disease, eg skin tags, fistulae (healed and active), abscesses, visible fissures or externalised haemorrhoids
- Wipes gloved index finger into gel and liberally applies to patient's anus
- Confirms to patient imminent insertion of finger
- Inserts finger gently from 6 o'clock position (of anus), arcing finger from perineum into anus (ie not directly into anus)
- Palpates and comments on anterior, posterior and lateral rectal walls: masses, ulceration; in male patient: comments on prostate size and consistency
- Comments on presence/consistency, or absence of faeces
- Withdraws finger and inspects/comments on presence/absence of faeces/blood/melaena
- Cleans/wipes patient's anus with clean tissue paper
- Disposes of gloves and tissue paper into appropriate clinical waste bin
- Washes hands with soap and water.

### Ensures patient receives correct advice about what to do next and follow-up

### Ensures nursing staff or other healthcare professionals receive correct information about the consequences/outcome of the procedure/task

### Thanks patient, offers assistance, maintains patient's dignity and privacy until they are dressed

## CLINICAL DIAGNOSTIC REASONING

■ **What might you find on DRE in a young Crohn's patient presenting like this?**
  • Peri-anal disease – healed and active fistulae; skin tags and abscesses
  • Probably empty rectum
  • May be tender due to peri-anal or rectal abscess, or inflamed loops of bowel
  • Gloved finger – residue of diarrhoeal stool, blood and mucus.

■ **Can you tell me three indications to perform a DRE in any given patient (ie not just this one)?**
  • Suspected local disease – anal or rectal carcinoma; fistulae, haemorrhoids, fissures
  • Constipation/faecal impaction
  • Exclude blood and/or melaena PR.

**Demonstrates appropriate level of knowledge and skills**

**Demonstrates clear and logical diagnostic reasoning**

## GLOBAL PROCEDURE MARK

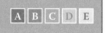

## Station 4 – Data interpretation

**1.**

A **False** – he has a normocytic anaemia that is most likely due to his chronic, relapsing remitting inflammatory bowel disease. Given his poor nutritional state, previous small bowel resections (and his acute PR bleeding) he may well have a mixed iron, $B_{12}$ and folate deficiency, and these should all be excluded by laboratory testing.

B **False** – given this patient's history and presentation he may have had a microcytic anaemia (consistent with an occult GI malignancy) but this would be due to his overt PR blood loss from his colitis rather than a malignancy. Patients with ulcerative colitis for greater than 10 years have a lifetime risk of about 10% of developing colonic carcinoma, it is far lower (but still increased compared to the general population) for Crohn's patients.

C **True** – there is a neutrophilic leucocytosis in keeping with an acute inflammatory process.

D **False** – This patient is very unlikely to have a cryptosporidium infection, a protozoan infection, most commonly found in HIV positive patients. The neutrophilia is more in keeping with a bacterial infection.

E True – the urea 15.8 (approx × 4) : creatinine 114 (approx × 1.3), ie 4 : 1.3 is highly suggestive of pre-renal impairment.

F True – given the severe, profuse watery diarrhoea that he has suffered it would be important to document a laboratory potassium result from this patient.

G False – this patient should receive a mixture of either 0.9% saline or Hartmann's solution, and 5% dextrose. These should be supplemented with 40 mmol/l of potassium. Such fluids are not routinely stocked on wards and it would be advisable to discuss this patient's requirements with the ward pharmacist as early as possible, to ensure adequate supplies of appropriate fluids can be ordered.

H True – see above.

I False – chronic fatty liver (common in patients with IBD) will commonly cause a rise in the transaminases (ALT and AST), as well as mild derangement of the alkaline phosphatise, giving a mixed derangement of the liver function tests (LFTs). However, some patients may have normal LFTs.

J True – this man has several reasons to be hypoalbuminaemic. Hypoalbuminaemia is commonly found in malnutrition, chronic liver disease and chronic protein loss, eg nephrotic syndrome and enteropathies. It is also a sign of severe, acute illness such as overwhelming sepsis or inflammation.

K False – DIC may occur in severe, acute exacerbations of IBD, but this is not the case here.

L True – His erythocyte sedimentation rate (ESR) and C-reactive protein (CRP) are highly suggestive of a serious, acute exacerbation.

2a.
   A True
   B False
   C False

This is a plain abdominal X-ray image showing the typical features of small bowel obstruction. There are multiple dilated loops (>3.5 cm) of small bowel, differentiated from the large bowel by the valvulae conniventes. The tubing shown is extra-abdominal and is probably part of a suction system (drip and suck). Small bowel obstruction is most commonly caused by post-operative adhesions. Other causes include Crohn's disease of the small bowel, malignancy and herniae.

b.
   A True
   B True
   C False

This is a plain abdominal X-ray image showing features of dilated large bowel and toxic megacolon, defined radiologically by large bowel loops >6 cm. There is also evidence of sacro-ilitis with sclerosis and loss of the normal sacro-iliac joint spaces. This is consistent with the patient's presentation of severe ulcerative colitis. Most causes of colitis can cause toxic megacolon, but IBD (UC) remains the most common. Other causes include pseudomembranous colitis (C. difficile), ischaemic colitis, infectious enteritis and radiation-induced colitis.

c.

> A False
> B False
> C False

This is an erect chest image showing gross gas under both hemidiaphragms (right > left). This is consistent with an acute perforation of the bowel. Unless there are contraindications, he requires urgent surgical intervention, intravenous fluids, analgesia and antibiotics.

d.

> A False
> B True
> C False

This is a supine abdominal film showing large bowel obstruction. As indicated in question a, small bowel loops are defined by the valvulae connivente (plicae ciculares) that extend across the width of the loops. Large bowel loops are defined by the haustral pattern. The ground glass appearance in the ascending colon is consistent with faecal loading. There is an incidental left total hip replacement.

Large bowel obstruction is commonly caused by colonic carcinoma, diverticular disease, abscesses, volvulus and extrinisic compression by pelvic and other malignant tumours.

e.

> A False
> B False
> C True

This is a pre-contrast plain abdominal image that shows a large, calcified 'staghorn' calculus in the right renal area. These large stones are associated with recurrent infection with urease producing Gram-negative bacteria such as *Proteus*, *Klebsiella*, *Pseudomonas* and *Enterobacter*. Pancreatic calcification is more centrally located, and is usually 'speckled', rather than solid in appearance.

**GLOBAL DATA INTERPRETATION MARK**

## Station 5 – Clinical communication skills

**Patient script**

You haven't discussed nutritional support with anyone as yet on this admission (you have had this discussion several times on previous admissions) and are happy to talk to the FY1.

After your last admission about 8 months ago you gained quite a lot of weight and had been feeling really well on your new treatment. You weighed yourself on the departmental scales when you returned to work and you were 68.4 kg. Your weight today was 62.3 kg (you are 1.78 m tall).

You and your family eat a 'healthy diet' with lots of fresh vegetables and fruit. On the advice of the dieticians here in the hospital you also supplement your diet with multivitamins and some essential elements, which you buy online.

Over the past 10 days or so you have been eating and drinking very little and haven't managed anything substantial for the best part of the week.

Ideas – you know you've lost lots of weight.

Concerns – when you've been this ill in the past you have needed TPN, including both admissions where you ended up having bowel resection.

Expectations – you are just hoping that TPN can be avoided this time, but 'I'm not going to hold my breath.'

SCENARIO 9

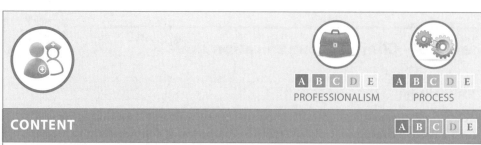

PROFESSIONALISM · A B C D E

PROCESS · A B C D E

## CONTENT · A B C D E

**Confirms reason for discussion**
- To talk to patient about his diet and plans for possible nutritional support.

**Establishes what patient wishes to know; gains agreement/informal consent to participate in the discussion**

**Investigates patient's present level of understanding of scenario**

**Summarises and confirms what has happened so far**

**Establishes patient's ideas, concerns and expectations**

**Explains the key, important information**
- 'Fighting weight' – what is Joel's 'normal'/best weight; when did he last weigh this amount?
- Present weight confirmed at 62.3 kg; present height confirmed at 1.78 m
- Calculates BMI = 19.7 kg/m²
- Calculates percentage weight loss $\frac{(68.4 - 62.3)}{68.4} \times 100 = 8.9\%$
- Calculates MUST© score = 4 (BMI = 1, % weight loss = 1, acute illness with poor intake = 2)
- Discusses normal diet when well
- Discusses diet and oral intake since becoming unwell.

**Establishes further management**
- MUST© score suggests high risk for malnutrition
- Urgent review by dietitian and hospital nutrition team
- Possible need for enteral or parenteral feeding
- Explores patient's understanding of TPN.

**Invites patient to ask questions and is able to deal with them appropriately**

**Summarises important areas of the consultation back to the patient**

**Formally ends the consultation and ensures appropriate follow-up has been discussed**

## GLOBAL COMMUNICATION MARK

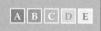

# Station 6 – Prescribing skills

| Allergies, sensitivities and adverse drug reactions | | | | | Patient details/addressograph | |
|---|---|---|---|---|---|---|
| No known allergies ☐ | | Initials  AF | | | NHS/ Hospital No:  757543 | |
| Not possible to ascertain ☐ | | Date | | | | |
| Medicine/substance | Reaction & Severity | Initials & Date | Weight (kg) | Date | Surname:  BARNET | |
| INFLIXIMAB | SEVERE ALLERGIC REACTION | | 62.3kg | | | |
| | | | Height | | First name:  JOEL | |
| | | | 1.78m | | | |
| Alerts | | | Surface area (m²) | | Date of birth:  07.08.77 | |

**IN-PATIENT MEDICATION PRESCRIPTION AND ADMINISTRATION RECORD**

PasTest HOSPITAL

| Consultant | Trainee Dr. Name and Bleep no. | Date of admission | Date chart reboarded | Estimated date of discharge |
|---|---|---|---|---|
| ALSTED | FEATHER 622 | 7/05/12 | | |
| This chart is no. | Transcribing Check by Pharmacy | Ward | | |
| .................... of .................... | Sign ............. Date ............. | 1. ....................  2. .................... | | |

| Supplementary Medication charts in use:  Other (please specify): 1 ....................  2 .................... |
|---|

| Epidural/PCA ☐ | Syringe driver ☐ | | TPN ☐ | Chemotherapy ☐ | Insulin sliding scale ☐ |
|---|---|---|---|---|---|

**Once only medications – loading doses, pre-medication, PGDs  or surgical antibiotic propylaxis**

| Date | Time to be given | Medicine (approved name) | Dose | Route | Signature and bleep no. | Pharmacy | Time given | Given by | Checked by |
|---|---|---|---|---|---|---|---|---|---|
| 7/05 | Stat | HYDROCORTISONE | 100mg | IV | AF 622 | | | | |
| 7/05 | Stat | OLSALAZINE | 1g | PO | AF 622 | | | | |
| 7/05 | Stat | PREDSOL ENEMA | x1 | PR | AF 622 | | | | |
| 7/05 | Stat | MORPHINE | 5mg | IV | AF 622 | | | | |
| 7/05 | Stat | CYCLIZINE | 50mg | IV | AF 622 | | | | |
| 7/05 | Stat | SANDO-K+ | TT | PO | AF 622 | | | | |

SCENARIO 9

| Thromboprophylaxis please prescribe treatment regimens in the regular medications section | | | | | | | |
|---|---|---|---|---|---|---|---|
| **Choice of mechanical prophylaxis and leg(s) to be applied to** | | | | | | Enter Time | **Enter details below** |
| Graduated elastic compression stockings | Intermittent pneumatic compression device (IPC) | Leg | | | | | |
| | | Left | Right | Both | | | |
| ✓ | ☐ | Signature and Bleep No. | ☐ | ☐ | ✓ | | |
| Start Date: 7/05 | End Date: | | | | | | |
| ☐ | ☐ | Signature and Bleep No. AF | ☐ | ☐ | ☐ | | |
| Start Date: | End Date: | | | | | | |

| Medication | Dose | Dose Change | Enter Time | Enter details below | Pharmacy |
|---|---|---|---|---|---|
| NOT FOR HEPARIN PR BLEEDING | Date | | | | |
| Please ensure you have completed the VTE risk assessment form | Route | | | | ☐ |
| | Signature | | Instructions | | |
| | Bleep no. | | | | |

| Regular prescriptions continued | | | | | | | | | |
|---|---|---|---|---|---|---|---|---|---|
| **Regular medications** | | | | | | | | | |
| | Dose | | | Date | 7 | 8 | 9 | 10 | 11 | 12 |

| Date 7-5-12 | | | Medication | Instructions | Signature and bleep no. | Pharmacy |
|---|---|---|---|---|---|---|
| Route PO | | | METHOTREXATE | 20mg ONCE WEEKLY | AF 622 | ☐ |
| Signature | | | | | | |

| Time | | | | 7 | 8 | 9 | 10 | 11 | 12 | | | | |
|---|---|---|---|---|---|---|---|---|---|---|---|---|---|
| 06 | | | | | | | | | | | | | |
| (09) | 20mg | | | ✕ | ✕ | | ✕ | ✕ | ✕ | ✕ | ✕ | | ✕ | ✕ | ✕ | ✕ |
| 12 | | | | | | | | | | | | | |
| 18 | | | | | | | | | | | | | |
| 22 | | | | | | | | | | | | | |
| 24 | | | | | | | | | | | | | |

| Regular prescriptions continued | | | | | | |
|---|---|---|---|---|---|---|
| **Regular medications** | | | | | | |
| | Dose | | | Date | | |

| Date 7-5-12 | | | Medication | Instructions | Signature and bleep no. | Pharmacy |
|---|---|---|---|---|---|---|
| Route PO | | | OLSALAZINE | | AF 622 | ☐ |
| Signature | | | | | | |

| Time | | | | | | | | | | | | | |
|---|---|---|---|---|---|---|---|---|---|---|---|---|---|
| 06 | | | | | | | | | | | | | |
| (09) | 1g | | | | | | | | | | | | |
| 12 | | | | | | | | | | | | | |
| 18 | | | | | | | | | | | | | |
| (22) | 1g | | | | | | | | | | | | |
| 24 | | | | | | | | | | | | | |

SCENARIO 9

### Prescription 1

| | Dose | | | Date | | | | | | | | | | | | | |
|---|---|---|---|---|---|---|---|---|---|---|---|---|---|---|---|---|---|
| **Regular prescriptions continued** | | | | | | | | | | | | | | | | | |
| **Regular medications** | | | | | | | | | | | | | | | | | |
| Date 7/8/12 | | | | **Medication** PREDSOL ENEMA | | | **Instructions** 20 mg/100ml | | | **Signature and bleep no.** AF 622 | | | **Pharmacy** | | | | |
| Route PR | | | | | | | | | | | | | | | | | |
| Signature | | | | | | | | | | | | | | | | | |
| 06 | | | | | | | | | | | | | | | | | |
| 09 | | | | | | | | | | | | | | | | | |
| 12 | | | | | | | | | | | | | | | | | |
| 18 | | | | | | | | | | | | | | | | | |
| (22) | X1 | | | | | | | | | | | | | | | | |
| 24 | | | | | | | | | | | | | | | | | |

### Prescription 2

| | Dose | | | Date | | | | | | | | | | | | | |
|---|---|---|---|---|---|---|---|---|---|---|---|---|---|---|---|---|---|
| **Regular prescriptions continued** | | | | | | | | | | | | | | | | | |
| **Regular medications** | | | | | | | | | | | | | | | | | |
| Date 7/8/12 | | | | **Medication** HYDROCORTISONE | | | **Instructions** | | | **Signature and bleep no.** AF 622 | | | **Pharmacy** | | | | |
| Route IV | | | | | | | | | | | | | | | | | |
| Signature | | | | | | | | | | | | | | | | | |
| 06 | | | | | | | | | | | | | | | | | |
| (09) | 100mg | | | | | | | | | | | | | | | | |
| (12) | 100mg | | | | | | | | | | | | | | | | |
| (18) | 100mg | | | | | | | | | | | | | | | | |
| (22) | 100mg | | | | | | | | | | | | | | | | |
| 24 | | | | | | | | | | | | | | | | | |

### Prescription 3

| | Dose | | | Date | | | | | | | | | | | | | |
|---|---|---|---|---|---|---|---|---|---|---|---|---|---|---|---|---|---|
| **Regular prescriptions continued** | | | | | | | | | | | | | | | | | |
| **Regular medications** | | | | | | | | | | | | | | | | | |
| Date 7/8/12 | | | | **Medication** CODEINE PHOSPHATE | | | **Instructions** (PAIN) | | | **Signature and bleep no.** AF 622 | | | **Pharmacy** | | | | |
| Route PO | | | | | | | | | | | | | | | | | |
| Signature | | | | | | | | | | | | | | | | | |
| 06 | | | | | | | | | | | | | | | | | |
| (09) | 60mg | | | | | | | | | | | | | | | | |
| (12) | 60mg | | | | | | | | | | | | | | | | |
| (18) | 60mg | | | | | | | | | | | | | | | | |
| (22) | 60mg | | | | | | | | | | | | | | | | |
| 24 | | | | | | | | | | | | | | | | | |

### Prescription 4

| | Dose | | | Date | | | | | | | | | | | | | |
|---|---|---|---|---|---|---|---|---|---|---|---|---|---|---|---|---|---|
| **Regular prescriptions continued** | | | | | | | | | | | | | | | | | |
| **Regular medications** | | | | | | | | | | | | | | | | | |
| Date 7/8/12 | | | | **Medication** PARACETAMOL | | | **Instructions** | | | **Signature and bleep no.** AF 622 | | | **Pharmacy** | | | | |
| Route PO | | | | | | | | | | | | | | | | | |
| Signature | | | | | | | | | | | | | | | | | |
| 06 | | | | | | | | | | | | | | | | | |
| (09) | 1g | | | | | | | | | | | | | | | | |
| (12) | 1g | | | | | | | | | | | | | | | | |
| (18) | 1g | | | | | | | | | | | | | | | | |
| (22) | 1g | | | | | | | | | | | | | | | | |
| 24 | | | | | | | | | | | | | | | | | |

161

| Regular prescriptions continued | | | | | | | | | | | | | | | | |
|---|---|---|---|---|---|---|---|---|---|---|---|---|---|---|---|---|
| **Regular medications** | | | | | | | | | | | | | | | | |
| | Dose | | | Date | | | | | | | | | | | | |
| Date 7/5/12 | | | | Medication | | | | Instructions | | | Signature and bleep no. | | | Pharmacy | | |
| Route PO | | | | SANDO-K+ | | | | MONITOR K+ | | | AF 622 | | | ☐ | | |
| Signature | | | | | | | | UNTIL > 3.5mmol/L | | | | | | | | |
| 06 | | | | | | | | | | | | | | | | |
| (09) | ♀♀ ⊤⊤ | | | | | | | | | | | | | | | |
| 12 | | | | | | | | | | | | | | | | |
| (18) | ♀♀ ⊤⊤ | | | | | | | | | | | | | | | |
| 22 | | | | | | | | | | | | | | | | |
| 24 | | | | | | | | | | | | | | | | |

| Infusion prescriptions continued | | | | | | | | | SC = subcutaneous | | IVC = intravenous central IVP = intravenous peripheral | | | |
|---|---|---|---|---|---|---|---|---|---|---|---|---|---|---|
| Date & time | Route | Infusion Fluid | | Medication | | Duration | Rate | Prescriber's signature & bleep no. | Date given | Given by / Added by | Check by | Start time | Finish time | Pharmacy |
| | | Name & strength | Volume | Approved name with expiry / unit number | Dose | | | | | | | | | |
| 7/05 | | 0.9% Saline Exp: Batch/unit no: | 1 L | | | | 30 MINS | AF 622 | | | | | | |
| 7/05 | | 0.9% Saline Exp: Batch/unit no: | 1 L | +40mmol KCL | | | 2 HOURS | | | | | | | |
| 7/05 | | 0.9% Saline Exp: Batch/unit no: | 1 L | +40mmol KCL | | | 4 HOURS | | | | | | | |
| 7/05 | | 0.9% Saline Exp: Batch/unit no: | 1 L | +40mmol KCL | | | 4 HOURS | | | | | | | |
| 7/05 | | 0.9% Saline Exp: Batch/unit no: | 1 L | +40mmol KCL | | | 4 HOURS | | | | | | | |
| 7/05 | | 0.9% Saline Exp: Batch/unit no: | 1 L | +40mmol KCL | | | 6 HOURS | | | | | | | |
| TITRATE FLUIDS AGAINST U.O. > 35ml/HR; BP > 100 systolic; HR < 100 bpm | | Exp: Batch/unit no: | | | | | | | | | | | | |
| | | Exp: Batch/unit no: | | | | | | | | | | | | |
| | | Exp: Batch/unit no: | | | | | | | | | | | | |
| | | | | | | | | | | | | | | |

| As required medications | | | | Date | | | | | | | | | | | | | | | | | | | | | | | | |
|---|---|---|---|---|---|---|---|---|---|---|---|---|---|---|---|---|---|---|---|---|---|---|---|---|---|---|---|---|---|
| Medication MORPHINE | | | | Date | | | | | | | | | | | | | | | | | | | | | | | | |
| Indication PAIN | | | | Time | | | | | | | | | | | | | | | | | | | | | | | | |
| Dose 2.5-5mg | Route IV/IM | Maximum frequency / dose As Reqd | Start date 7/05 | Dose | | | | | | | | | | | | | | | | | | | | | | | | |
| | | | Stop date | Route | | | | | | | | | | | | | | | | | | | | | | | | |
| Signature AF | | | | | | | | | | | | | | | | | | | | | | | | | | | | |
| | | Bleep no. 622 | | Given | | | | | | | | | | | | | | | | | | | | | | | | |
| Additional instructions: | | | | | | | | | | | | | | | Pharmacy | | | | | | | | | | | | | |

| As required medications | | | | Date | | | | | | | | | | | | | | | | | | | | | | | | |
|---|---|---|---|---|---|---|---|---|---|---|---|---|---|---|---|---|---|---|---|---|---|---|---|---|---|---|---|---|
| Medication CYCLIZINE | | | | Date | | | | | | | | | | | | | | | | | | | | | | | | |
| Indication NAUSEA | | | | Time | | | | | | | | | | | | | | | | | | | | | | | | |
| Dose 50 mg | Route IV/IM | Maximum frequency / dose TDS | Start date 7/05 | Dose | | | | | | | | | | | | | | | | | | | | | | | | |
| | | | Stop date | Route | | | | | | | | | | | | | | | | | | | | | | | | |
| Signature AF | | | | | | | | | | | | | | | | | | | | | | | | | | | | |
| | | Bleep no. 622 | | Given | | | | | | | | | | | | | | | | | | | | | | | | |
| Additional instructions: | | | | | | | | | | | | | | | Pharmacy | | | | | | | | | | | | | |

## GLOBAL PRESCRIBING MARK

A B C D E

## Scenario 9: Reflection and consolidation

### History

This is Mr Joel Barnet, a 34-year-old man with long-standing Crohn's disease. He works as the Senior Physiotherapist on the orthopaedic wards here in the hospital. He self-referred to the clinic this morning with an acute flare-up of his Crohn's.

His IBD was originally diagnosed in 1997, and has been relapsing and remitting in nature since then. He originally presented to his GP after returning from The Gambia. His main symptoms were frequent, loose brown, bloody stools and mucus PR. He also had symptoms suggestive of uveitis, arthritis of his hands and lower spine, and erythema nodosum of the shins. The diagnosis was confirmed on colonic biopsy by Dr Shine, Gastroenterologist (here).

Since then he's had multiple flare-ups (at least one or two a year for the last 10 years). He often manages them himself with some guidance by Dr Alsted. During these exacerbations he takes a course of steroids and 5-ASA and it usually settles down. However he's been hospitalised several times and ended up having a small bowel resection about 5 years ago after a particularly nasty episode, and then a further resection 3 years ago. His last admission was 8 months ago, but according to him 'this wasn't too bad'. During that admission he had a trial of infliximab but had an acute allergic reaction to the injection, requiring adrenaline and steroids. He was taking azathioprine until his last admission, but it was then agreed he should be tried on a weekly dose of methotrexate. He is presently on methotrexate 20 mg once weekly.

His present exacerbation started slowly about 2 weeks ago. Initially his bowels were open three or four times per day; he describes the motions as loose, brown with associated fresh blood and mucus. This has worsened and he is now opening his bowels every 3 hours, with lots of fresh blood and mucus. He has had increasing, generalised abdominal pain with associated nausea but no vomiting. The pain was originally a dull ache but overnight has become almost unbearable, severe and all over the abdomen.

During the last 4 or 5 days, he has been taking increasing doses of painkillers and steroids but with little effect. He has been eating and drinking poorly, and has had hardly any sleep in the last few days. As well as the abdominal problems, the joints in his hands and his lumbar spine have been really painful and sore.

Of note: both his maternal grandmother and his mother's sister both had inflammatory bowel disease. He is a lifelong non-smoker and drinks alcohol occasionally. No illicit drug taking.

As well as his weekly methotrexate, he is presently taking prednisolone 30 mg per day, and olsalazine 1 g bd. He is allergic to infliximab, as described above.

He is married and has a daughter who is two and a half years old. His wife is also a physiotherapist. They live in a two-bedroom garden flat near the hospital.

### Examination

On examination, this is a thin-looking, clinically anaemic and dehydrated man. He was in obvious distress lying on the examination couch. He was alert and orientated in time, place and person. He has signs consistent with an acute exacerbation of his Crohn's disease. He is clinically dehydrated, pyrexial (temperature 38.2 °C), tachycardic (HR 110 bpm) but his BP (105/66 mmHg) is just acceptable. He has marked ulceration of his buccal mucosa and of note his BMI is 19.7 kg/m². He had no signs of acute or chronic liver disease.

Examination of his abdomen revealed him to be thin with signs of a previous laparotomy and appendicectomy. He has generalised, moderate tenderness and some guarding, but no signs of peritonism. There is no palpable organomegaly or masses. DRE was deferred at the request of the consultant.

Examination of his eyes and skin were unremarkable but there is evidence of an acute flare-up of the arthritis in his hands and I would like to assess his spine and sacro-iliac joints more thoroughly once he is clinically improved.

## Investigations

A severe acute flare-up of colitis is defined by:
- Stool frequency >6 stools with blood PR, per 24 hours
- Pyrexia – temperature >37.5 °C
- Tachycardia – HR >90 bpm
- Hb <10 g/dl
- Albumin <30 g/l
- ESR >30 mm/hour.

In the case of a patient presenting with an acute, severe exacerbation of their IBD it is essential to also record:
- Bloods – U&Es, LFTs, CRP, glucose and blood cultures
- Venous blood gases – to ascertain acid–base balance; serum lactate (ischaemia, perforation)
- Radiology – plain abdominal X-ray; CT abdomen is now performed routinely in severe episodes of IBD.

## Management

As with all potentially complex and serious conditions, patients with IBD should be cared for by an expert multidisciplinary team.

Acute episode: many mild to moderate exacerbations of Crohn's disease are self-managed by the patient using oral steroids, 5-ASA compounds and loperamide or codeine to reduce the frequency of the diarrhoea. However, more serious episodes often require in-patient care. This will include:
- Symptomatic relief with appropriate analgesia and anti-emetics (avoid pro-peristaltic agents such as metoclopramide in small bowel disease)
- IV fluids with potassium supplementation
- Steroids – consider intravenous hydrocortisone or methylprednisolone; oral budesonide (ileo-caecal disease), and for distal disease (sigmoid and proctitis) steroid foam enemas
- 5-ASA compounds for colitis
- Nutritional assessment and support by hospital nutrition team
- Joint care with a specialist surgical team is common in many centres.

Maintenance of remission – unlike ulcerative colitis, in which 5-ASA compounds are so important in maintenance therapy, Crohn's patients benefit little from long-term 5-ASA (unless they principally have colitis). They are generally maintained either on no drugs at all, and treat themselves symptomatically (as above) or require immunosuppressive treatments such as azathioprine, 6-mercaptopurine (6MP) or mycophenolate mofetil. Methotrexate and ciclosporin are both used when steroids and these other immunosuppressive agents are ineffective.

### Further reading and web links
*British Society of Gastroenterology's latest guidelines on the management of IBD*:
www.bsg.org.uk/clinical-guidelines/ibd/guidelines-for-the-management-of-inflammatory-bowel-disease.html
*MUST screening tool*:
www.bapen.org.uk/pdfs/must/must_full.pdf

# Scenario 10: 'All very confusing'

## Station 1

*History*                                     *10-minute station*

You are the FY1 on a Care of the Elderly firm. You have been asked by the Consultant to attend the Diagnostic Memory Clinic (DMC) to gain experience of assessing patients with memory problems. The next patient is Mrs Jill Michelson, who has been referred by her GP for assessment. She is accompanied by her husband, George, who is to corroborate Jill's history. They are both happy to talk to you.

■ Please take a focussed history from the patient and then her husband, with a view to presenting the history and likely diagnosis to the Consultant. You do not need to do a formal mental state assessment.

*You will be assessed on the following areas, as well as the content and diagnostic reasoning of your history – take them into account in your presentation.*

### Professionalism

- Professional appearance (NHS dress code) – including general appearance, hair and jewellery
- Maintains patient and personal safety
- Polite introduction; identifies patient or interviewee correctly; confirms patient's date of birth from name band or other source
- Obtains informal consent; maintains patient's privacy
- Displays empathetic and caring attitudes and behaviours throughout.

### Process

- Good organisation and structure; appropriate use of open and closed questions
- Appropriate fluency/rhythm/pace to the interview – this may change depending on environment and acute nature of the problem
- Appropriate time for the patient to respond/reply to questions
- Appropriate acknowledgement of difficult or emotional areas of the patient's history.

### Communication skills

- Demonstrates caring and sympathetic attitude
- Asks open questions
- Invites patient to ask questions and answers them appropriately
- Addresses patient's ideas, concerns and expectations.

## Station 2

*Examination*                              *10-minute station*

Mrs Michelson is diagnosed as having mixed Alzheimer's and vascular dementia and is started on appropriate treatment. Three months later she is brought to the Emergency Department by ambulance, having been found on the floor by her husband, who had just popped out to the local shops to get some milk. He reports that she has become increasingly confused and agitated over the last 48 hours but denies any obvious, systemic problems. You are the FY1 working on the Medical Admissions Unit (MAU).

■ Please make an appropriate, diagnostic assessment of Mrs Michelson with a view to presenting your findings to the MAU Consultant on the mid-take ward round.

(If you do not have a model, please read and present the information given on page 384.)

*You will be assessed on the following areas, as well as the content and skills of your examination – take them into account in your presentation.*

### Professionalism

- Professional appearance; maintains infection control standards, including hand cleaning and appropriate use of gloves and aprons
- Maintains patient and personal safety
- Polite introduction; identifies patient and confirms date of birth from name band or other source
- Obtains informal consent; maintains patient privacy and dignity
- Displays empathetic and caring attitudes and behaviours throughout.

### Process

- Appropriate fluency/rhythm/pace to the examination – this may change depending on environment and acute nature of the problem
- Organisation and structure of examination; sensitive and empathetic approach
- Uses appropriate clinical techniques throughout
- Maintains privacy and dignity throughout.

### Clinical communication

- Explains proposed examination/procedure: explains examination/procedure as it proceeds
- Offers information in a clear, structured and fluent manner, avoiding jargon
- Listens to patient and responds appropriately
- Demonstrates appropriate body language.

## Station 3

*Data interpretation*                    *10-minute station*

1 The MAU Registrar asks you to look up Mrs Michelson's data on the computer and record them in her notes.

- Please refer to these data and indicate whether the statements below are TRUE (T) or FALSE (F).
  - FBC × Hb 9.3 g/dl, MCV 104 fl, WCC 19.6 × $10^9$/l (neutrophils 15.9 × $10^9$/l), platelets 91 × $10^9$/l
  - U&Es – $Na^+$ 159 mmol/l, $K^+$ 6.3 mmol/l, urea 35.6mmol/l, creatinine 254 µmol/l
  - RBG – 3.1mmol/l
  - LFTs – TBil 4.5 mmol/l, ALT 32 iu/l, AST 23iu/l, Alk phos 181 iu/l, ALb 28 g/l
  - Clotting – INR 1.3, APTT 35 s
  - $CCa^{2+}$ 2.01 mmol/l, $PO_4^{2-}$ 0.78 mmol/l
  - CRP 364 mg/l
  - ABGs – pH 7.22, $PaO_2$ 10.3 KPa, $PaCO_2$ 3.3 KPa, $HCO_3^-$ 14.9 mmol/l, BXS 7.9 mmol/l, lactate 3.9 mmol/l
  - Blood cultures sent

  A   The Hb and MCV are consistent with folate deficiency.
  B   The white cell and differential are suggestive of an atypical pneumonia.
  C   The thrombocytopenia may be a sign of early disseminated intravascular coagulopathy (DIC).
  D   The urea : creatinine ratio confirms pre-renal impairment.
  E   The calculated serum osmolality is 359.3 mOsmo/kg.
  F   Given this patient's serum sodium, she should receive 0.45% saline solution.
  G   Given this patient's serum potassium, she should not receive potassium supplementation.
  H   The hypoalbuminaemia is consistent with chronic cognitive impairment.
  I   The coagulation screen confirms the DIC.
  J   Given these results, this patient should be given venous thrombo-embolic (VTE) prophylaxis with low molecular weight heparin (LMWH).
  K   The arterial blood gases (ABGs) suggest a severe mixed respiratory/ metabolic acidosis.
  L   The elevated C-reactive protein (CRP) is commonly seen in disorders such as systemic lupus erythematosus (SLE).
  M   This set of data is supportive of an acute bacterial sepsis.

2 The Care of the Elderly ST4 shows you the CT brain scans from three dementia patients presently on her ward.

- Please indicate whether each of the statements regarding the scans is TRUE (T) or FALSE (F).

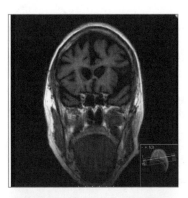

A This is the MRI brain scan of a 66-year-old man with severe dementia.
1 There is evidence of raised intracranial pressure
2 The cortices look normal
3 The ventricles are normal
4 The periventricular white matter shows areas of low attenuation
5 These appearances are commonly seen in patients with alcohol related dementia

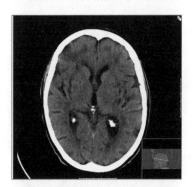

B This is the CT brain scan of an 81-year-old man with a 1-year history of increasing memory problems. Although he is still living at home alone, he is unable to recognise his children or brothers.
1 The sulci are widened
2 There are several subcortical infarcts
3 The ventricles are normal
4 There is evidence of white matter low attenuation
5 These appearances are consistent with hypertensive related disease

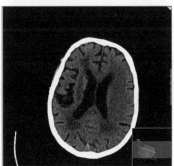

C This is the scan of a 79-year-old woman who presented with fronto-temporal signs and increasing cognitive impairment.
1 There is evidence of an ischaemic stroke
2 There is evidence of small vessel disease
3 The ventricles are dilated
4 There is evidence of a right subdural haemorrhage
5 This patient should be placed on anti-platelet treatment

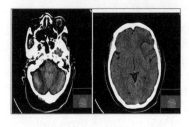

D These are two sections from a CT head scan of a 74-year-old man with a 3-year history of increasing confusion. Of note he has untreated atrial fibrillation.
1 There is evidence of an ischaemic stroke in the right cerebellar lobe
2 There is evidence of small vessel disease
3 The ventricles are dilated
4 There is evidence of a left fronto-temporal lesion
5 This patient should be placed on anti-coagulation therapy

SCENARIO 10

169

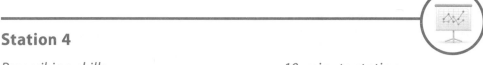

## Station 4

*Prescribing skills*                    *10-minute station*

Mrs Michelson is admitted under the care of the MAU team with a diagnosis of delirium secondary to urinary tract infection (UTI), and acute kidney injury (AKI) secondary to dehydration.

■ Please write up the following:
- An appropriate fluid regime and FRIVII
- An appropriate stat dose of intravenous gentamicin and augmentin
- Regular dosing of augmentin for 3 days
- Loading doses of digoxin
- Oxygen
- Regular medications where appropriate
- VTE prophylaxis.

Details
- o Mrs Jill Michelson; DOB: 06/051938; Hospital no. 987453; Ward: MAU; Consultant: Dr Lightowlers
- o Weight approx. 45 kg; U&Es: $Na^+$ 159 mmol/l, $K^+$ 6.3 mmol/l, urea 35.6mmol/l, creatinine 254 μmol/l
- o Observations – HR 123 bpm, BP 93/65 mmHg, RR 26 bpm, $O_2$ sats 92% on air, temperature 39.1 °C, CBG 16.1 mmol/l
- o Regular medications – donepezil 10 mg od, bendroflumethiazide 2.5 mg od, aspirin 75 mg od.

---

**Remember: DRUG DRs Don't Forget Signing Off** (page 396)

---

## Station 5

*Clinical communication skills*                *10-minute station*

You are the FY1 on the Care of the Elderly rehabilitation ward where Mrs Michelson is recovering/rehabilitating after her acute admission with severe Gram-negative sepsis. At the multidisciplinary meeting this morning the multidisciplinary team (MDT) discussed possible discharge for Mrs Michelson, and in view of this your Consultant has asked you to assess Mrs Michelson's cognition and her capacity, and document these in her notes.

■ Using the 30-point Mini-Mental State Examination (MMSE) Folstein form and the guide to capacity assessment shown below, please assess Mrs Michelson's cognition and capacity.

| Folstein – Mini-Mental State Examination (MMSE) | | Correct | Incorrect |
|---|---|---|---|
| Orientation Score (Max 10) | | | |
| What is today's date? | | | |
| What is the year? | | | |
| What is the month? | | | |
| What day is today? | | | |
| What season is it? | | | |
| What building are we in? | | | |
| What floor are we on? | | | |
| What town are we in? | | | |
| What province are we in? | | | |
| What country are we in? | | | |
| Registration Score (max 3) | | | |
| 'ball', 'flag', 'tree'; ask to repeat. First repetition is score. Repeat until get it right or 6 times | | | |
| Attention & calculation Score (max 5) | | | |
| 100 -7's for 5 subtractions, OR spell 'world' backwards with 1 point for each letter in exactly the right place | | | |
| Recall Score (max 3) | | | |
| 3 previous words (from Registration) | | | |
| Language Score(max 9) | | | |
| Name a watch and a pencil (2 points) | | | |
| Repeat the following 'no ifs, ands or buts' (1 point) | | | |
| Follow a three-stage command: 'take the paper in your right hand, fold it in half and put it on the floor' (3 points) | | | |
| Repeat and obey the following: CLOSE YOUR EYES (1 point) | | | |
| 'Write a sentence'; must have noun, verb and be sensible (1 point) | | | |
| Draw 2 intersecting pentagons each side 1". Must have 10 angles and intersect (1 point) | | | |
| TOTAL | | / 30 | |

There are four criteria set out in the Mental Capacity Act as to why a person may not be able to make a decision. The criteria relates to whether the person is able to:

o   Comprehend the information relevant to the decision (which requires the information to have been presented to that person in a way appropriate to their circumstances)

o   Retain this information for long enough to make the decision (with the fact that the period of retention may be short irrelevant to this consideration)

o   **Use and weigh the information to arrive at a choice (which requires an understanding of the consequences of making a decision one way or the other, or of failing to make a decision)**

o   **Communicate the decision.**

■ **Given the four criteria and the multidisciplinary team reports shown below, please make an assessment of Mrs Michelson's capacity regarding her wishes to go home and make a decision regarding her discharge.**

---

**Physio report**

Jill (Michelson) is unsteady and requires supervision and assistance of one with transfers and mobilising short distances; she has been unable to successfully/safely complete a set of seven stairs with or without assistance.

---

**Occupational therapist report**

Jill requires prompting to get washed and dressed but she can do these with minimal assistance; she can feed herself but often gets distracted and ends up eating very little. She was unable to make toast or a cup of tea safely; she required prompting and supervision throughout her visit to the kitchen. On her home visit she didn't really recognise her home and was slightly perplexed when Ralph and I tried to assure her she was home. She required supervision and support in all aspects of her visit.

---

**Nursing staff report**

Jill is pleasant and easy to care for. She requires minimal assistance and prompting for meals, washing and dressing. She needs prompting about toileting and is occasionally incontinent of urine. She is continent of faeces. She sleeps well and does not wander on the ward.

# Answers

## Station 1 – History

**Patient script**

**Jill's script:**

You are Mrs Jill Michelson. You are able to give your DOB – 6 May 1938 – but if asked how old you are, you should reply 'Oh you shouldn't ask a lady her age.' You are not really sure why you have come to the doctors today (you didn't realise you were at the hospital) but if challenged 'it's some nonsense about my memory.... I wish everyone would stop interfering and leave me alone.'

Concerns – you are not worried about your memory and don't see that it's been a problem.

Expectations – 'I assume you all think I'm mad, but I'm really not!' 'Shall we just get on with it and get it over and done with?'

If asked/challenged on the following points, you should answer:
- Speech and language – 'I sometimes get my words muddled up but that's just normal for people of my age.'
- Mobility – 'I haven't been out much recently.' 'I don't remember any falls.'

Regarding your recall and recognition, you deny any problems with recalling events or recognising people or places. You have no problems getting around 'but always have my Ralph with me just in case'.

If asked, you deny any hallucinations – auditory or visual – self-harm or suicidal ideation and any other problems.

If asked about CV risk factors, you should answer:
- FHx – mother and father are both dead but you deny any illness in the family; your brother and sister are fine
- Smoking – 'I used to smoke as a young woman but not since my children were born.'
- Alcohol – 'Oh yes, I enjoy a glass of wine or three.'

You can't answer the rest – just dismiss them out of hand – 'Oh I've no use remembering things like that.'

At this point you get agitated with the doctor and tell him/her 'Oh that's quite enough for one day.' 'Ask Ralphy – he'll tell you what's been going on.'

The doctor should check that it's OK to talk to your husband Ralph before continuing; if the doctor doesn't ask, you should make a fuss about 'being treated like the family dog' ... 'I would like to be asked if it's OK to talk about me!'

**Husband's script:**

You are Ralph Michelson, Jill's husband of 47 years. You have noticed problems with Jill's memory since the beginning of last summer, and actually if you really think hard, you perhaps can see there were problems for about 4 or 5 months before that. Initially you didn't think much about the odd incident but it's become unavoidable over the past 3–4 months.

During the last few months:

- Speech and language – Jill was always keen on quizzes and word games, and did the crossword in the paper every day; over the past few months this has all stopped. She is often getting her words muddled and can't find the right ones, which really sends her into a rage.
- Mobility – Jill had several falls last summer and has been unsteady on her feet for a good few months; she was a keen ballroom dancer up until last year but this all stopped over last summer. You don't remember her ever hitting her head or complaining of headaches. Jill hasn't wandered outside, but recently you have found her sobbing in the kitchen and I think it's because she hasn't been able to find her way around the house.
- Recall and recognition – Jill can't be left on her own as she gets lost in previously familiar places, like the local shops, the park or the supermarket. She gets your two daughters mixed up and sometimes fails to recognise the grandchildren. She has often mistaken photos of various close family and friends for the wrong people.
- Other mental health issues – no hallucinations; Jill has been low recently but there are no features of depressive illness. There has been no systemic upset of note; she is on no regular medications and has no known drug allergies.

If asked about CV risk factors, you should answer:

- FHx – Jill's mother died of cancer aged about 70 years old; her father died after World War II through alcohol-related problems. Jill's oldest sister (Mary) died last year aged 81 – she had Alzheimer's disease; her sister Sarah (aged 77) is well, with no problems; her younger sister (Violet – 71) has severe heart problems (lifelong smoker).
- Smoking – Jill is an ex-smoker. She gave up after the children were born (about 41 years ago).
- Alcohol – Jill has always enjoyed a glass or two of wine (mostly Chardonnay or Sauvignon blanc) with meals; never excessive but probably drinks 8–10 glasses most weeks.
- No known hypertension, ischaemic heart disease, stroke, peripheral vascular disease or diabetes mellitus. Lipids – not known.
- SHx – Jill is a retired nursing sister; she worked in the operating theatre throughout her career.

You and Jill have been happily married for 47 years; you have two sons – Mark (would have been 45 years old but died in a motorbike accident aged 21 'she never really got over it') and David (42 years old and a bank manager in Stevenage – has three beautiful daughters) – as well as your two daughters.

Ideas – 'She's got the same thing as her sister Mary, hasn't she doc?'

Concerns – 'How long before I have to put her in a home?'

Expectations – 'Aren't there any new treatments you can give her?'

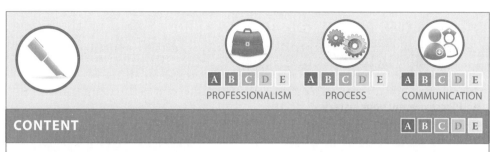

PROFESSIONALISM · PROCESS · COMMUNICATION

SCENARIO 10

## CONTENT

### Identifies key information from patient
- Insight into memory problems
- Specifically asks about speech and language, mobility, recall and recognition, hallucinations, depressive symptoms; tries to get patient to give examples of memory problems.

### Includes important negatives, including systemic enquiry
- Systemic illness.

### Identifies key information from rest of history
- Cardiovascular risk
- Family history.

### Asks permission of patient to talk to her husband

### Identifies key information from husband
- Onset and progression of memory problems
- Specifically asks about speech and language, mobility, recall and recognition, hallucinations, depressive symptoms.

### Includes important negatives, including systemic enquiry
- Systemic illness.

### Identifies key information from rest of history
- Cardiovascular risk
- Family history
- Social history/educational level.

### Completing the patient history
- Drug and allergy history: no regular medication or allergies
- Previous medical history: nil known.

### Summarises important areas of the history back to the patient and husband

### Invites patient and husband to ask questions and is able to deal with them appropriately

### Establishes patient's and husband's ideas, concerns and expectations

SCENARIO 10

## CLINICAL DIAGNOSTIC REASONING

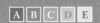

- **Please present your history**
  - Candidate offers a logical, well-structured account of the history.

- **Please tell me five initial investigations you would organise with a reason for each**
  - **Bloods:**
    - FBC: Hb/MCV ($B_{12}$ and folate); WCC and differential (haematological malignancy; platelets (possible intervention with aspirin)
    - U&Es: abnormalities of renal function may exacerbate confusional states; normal renal function is important in terms of drug therapy
    - RBG: vascular risk
    - LFTs: malignancy
    - Calcium: malignancy and exacerbation of confusion
    - ESR: vasculitis
    - $B_{12}$/folate/TFTs/VDRL: so-called 'reversible causes of dementia'.
  - **Radiology:**
    - CXR: exclude associated vascular disease and primary and secondary lung tumours
    - CT head scan: exclude associated vascular disease; raised intracranial pressure; primary and secondary brain tumours.

- **What classes of medications are available to treat this patient's underlying condition(s)?**
  - **For her dementia, possible interventions would include:**
    - Acetylcholinesterase inhibitors, eg donepezil
    - NMDA antagonists, eg memantine.
  - **All vascular risk should be assessed – may require anti-platelet therapy (aspirin or clopidogrel)**

**Demonstrates safe, sensible and appropriate management plan**

**Demonstrates clear and logical diagnostic reasoning**

## GLOBAL HISTORY MARK

## Station 2 – Examination

### Patient script (see page 384)

You are a 73-year-old woman who has been brought by ambulance to the Emergency Department. You have known dementia and are very agitated and confused; you are not aggressive but are not really able to help the doctor with his/her examination. You are unable to consistently follow commands.

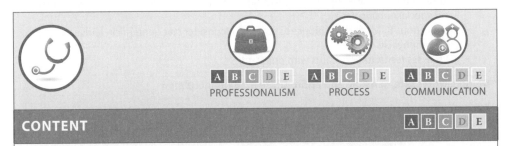

A B **C** D E
PROFESSIONALISM

A B **C** D E
PROCESS

A B **C** D E
COMMUNICATION

## CONTENT

A B **C** D E

**Acknowledges patient is confused and agitated – tries to reassure patient**

**Exposes and positions patient correctly and maintains comfort**

**Comments on wellbeing of patient, ie well or unwell**

**'Feet to face'**
- Observes and comments on patient and surroundings from foot of bed
- Evidence of obvious neurological deficit; mobility aids.

**Asks for appropriate/relevant clinical observations**
- HR 118 bpm, irregular; BP 87/56 mmHg; RR 24 bpm, $O_2$ sats 92% on air; temperature 39.9 °C; CBG 19.4 mmol/l
- Urinalysis: no urine available as yet
- Comments on GCS or AVPU
- AMTS                          /10
- Name                         Recognition of 2xpeople
- Time of day                  DOB
- Address for recall           WWII
- Year                         Monarch
- Place                        20-1

**General examination – J/A/CL/CY/O/LNS**
- Sepsis – excludes signs of meningitis, chest sepsis, intra-abdominal sepsis – including palpating for obstructed bladder – skin and join sepsis, including leg ulcers
- Raised intracranial pressure and focal neurological deficit – full assessment of cranial nerves and peripheral neurology
- Signs of malignancy – pleural effusions, hepatomegaly, intra-abdominal masses, lymphadenopathy.

**Thanks patient, offers assistance, maintains patient's dignity and privacy until they are dressed**

## CLINICAL DIAGNOSTIC REASONING

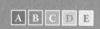

**Correctly identifies the relevant physical signs, including important negative findings**

■ **What is your diagnosis?**
  • Probably a delirium secondary to uro-sepsis, complicating chronic dementia.

■ **Given the presentation, what immediate therapeutic interventions would you consider?**
  • Admission to hospital, ensuring patient safety at all times – may need low-level mattress and special nursing care
  • Intravenous fluids and antibiotics to cover UTI (consider stat gentamicin and augmentin)
  • VTE prophylaxis
  • Discusses resuscitation status with husband.

**Demonstrates safe, sensible and appropriate management plan**

**Demonstrates clear and logical diagnostic reasoning**

## GLOBAL EXAMINATION MARK

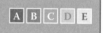

## Station 3 – Data interpretation

**1**

**A      True**

Hb 9.3 g/dl, MCV 104 fl: a macrocytic anaemia, consistent with a folate deficiency.

**B      False**

White cell count (WCC) 19.6 × 10⁹/l (neutrophils 15.9 × 10⁹/l): this is a marked neutrophilic leucocytosis consistent with a typical bacterial infection, such as streptococcus or staphylococcus. This may also occur in trauma or severe inflammation.

**C      True**

Platelets 91 × 10⁹/l: thrombocytopenia may be consistent with early DIC or secondary to drug therapy, alcohol excess or haematological malignancy.

**D      True**

Urea 35.6 mmol/l, creatinine 254 µmol/l: the urea : creatinine ratio of this patient is approximately 9 : 5–6. Thus the urea has risen proportionally more than the creatinine, thus confirming pre-renal impairment.

E      False

The calculated serum osmolality = 2(Na$^+$ + K$^+$) + urea + glucose = 2(159 + 6.3) + 35.6 + 13.1 = 379.3 mOsmo/kg.

F      False

Despite the hypernatraemia (Na$^+$ 159 mmol/l) present, there is no indication to prescribe hypotonic saline (0.45% saline = 'half normal saline'). Hartmann's contains 135 mmol/l sodium, whereas 0.9% saline contains 150 mol/l. Either solution would be appropriate in this patient. Rapid and/or large changes in serum sodium, and thus osmolality, may lead to central pontine myelinolysis, as well as cerebral oedema.

G      True

K+ 6.3 mmol/l: the potassium should be monitored and once back in the normal range should be supplemented at 20 mmol/l.

H      True

Alb 28 g/l: hypoalbuminaemia is common in patients with severe cognitive impairment, as they rarely eat adequate amounts of food. However, if this is not corroborated by carers, other causes should be sought.

I      False

The clotting profile (international ratio (INR) and activated partial thromboplastin time (APTT)) is within normal limits.

J      True

All hospitalised patients should be treated with thrombo-embolic (TED) stockings and LMWH if there are no contraindications.

K      False

This patient has a metabolic acidosis, as evidenced by the low bicarbonate, negative base excess and raised lactate. The low bicarbonate (PaCO$_2$ 3.3 KPa) suggests some attempted respiratory compensation.

L      False

The SLE and other vasculitides commonly cause a markedly elevated erythrocyte sedimentation rate (ESR) with a normal CRP.

M      True

This set of data is consistent with a patient suffering an episode of serious sepsis. There is evidence of multi-organ failure, including AKI, respiratory failure, hypoalbuminaemia and thrombocytopenia. Together, these carry a poor prognosis, especially in frail patients.

**2**

**A**

1 False, 2 False, 3 False,4 True, 5 True

This MRI scan shows gross cerebral atrophy with hugely enlarged sulci and ventricles. This is so gross that there is little normal brain matter left! The periventricualr white matter demonstrates low attenuation consistent with small vessel disease. Such gross cerebral atrophy may occur with Alzheimer's disease but is most commonly seen in alcohol related dementia.

**B**

1 True, 2 False, 3 False, 4 True, 5 True

This CT head scan shows cerebral atrophy with enlarged sulci and ventricles. The periventricular white matter, particularly around the posterior horns, shows the low attenuation of small vessel disease. White matter low attenuation is the pathognomonic change of hypertensive small vessel disease.

**C**

1 True, 2 True, 3 False, 4 False, 5 True

This CT head scan shows a large ischaemic stroke in the right frontal lobe, with mild cerebral atrophy. The ventricular system at this level is not particularly dilated. There is no evidence of a subdural haemorrhage, although this is a common incidental finding in confused patients presenting to hospital. In view of the large frontal infarct this patient should be placed on anti-platelet treatment.

**D**

1 True, 2 False, 3 False, 4 True, 5 False

This CT head scan shows a large wedged infarct in the right cerebellar lobe. There is no evidence of small vessel disease and the ventricles are not dilated at this level. There is a large ill defined lesion in the left fronto-temporal area that on further investigation was shown to be a large infarct with haemorrhagic transformation. In view of his multiple infarcts and atrial fibrillation the patient should theoretically be placed on anticoagulation therapy. However his poor cognition and possible severe disabilities following these strokes may make this impractical in real life.

**GLOBAL DATA INTERPRETATION MARK**

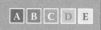

## Station 4

*Prescribing skills*

| Allergies, sensitivities and adverse drug reactions | | | | | | Patient details/addressograph | |
|---|---|---|---|---|---|---|---|
| No known allergies ✓ | | Initials JN | | Gender M /(F) | | NHS/ Hospital No: 987453 | |
| Not possible to ascertain ☐ | | Date | | Weight (kg) | Date | | |
| Medicine/substance | Reaction & Severity | Initials & Date | | 45kg | | Surname: MICHELSON | |
| | | | | Height | | First name: JILL | |
| Alerts | | | | Surface area (m²) | | Date of birth: 06.05.38 | |

### IN-PATIENT MEDICATION PRESCRIPTION AND ADMINISTRATION RECORD

PasTest HOSPITAL

| Consultant LIGHTOWLERS | Trainee Dr. Name and Bleep no. NELSON 061 | Date of admission 13/05/12 | Date chart reboarded | Estimated date of discharge |
|---|---|---|---|---|
| This chart is no. .................... of .................... | Transcribing Check by Pharmacy Sign .................... Date .................... | Ward 1. ......MAU.................... 2. .................... | | |

| Supplementary Medication charts in use:  Other (please specify): 1 .................... 2 .................... | | | | | | | | |
|---|---|---|---|---|---|---|---|---|
| Epidural/PCA ☐ | Syringe driver ☐ | | | TPN ☐ | Chemotherapy ☐ | | Insulin sliding scale ✓ | |

Once only medications – loading doses, pre-medication, PGDs  or surgical antibiotic propylaxis

| Date | Time to be given | Medicine (approved name) | Dose | Route | Signature and bleep no. | Pharmacy | Time given | Given by | Checked by |
|---|---|---|---|---|---|---|---|---|---|
| 13/05 | Stat (11.00) | GENTAMICIN | 80mg | IV | JN 061 | | | | |
| 13/05 | Stat (11.00) | CO-AMOXICLAV | 1.2g | IV | JN 061 | | | | |
| 13/05 | Stat (11.00) | DIGOXIN | 500 micrograms | IV | JN 061 | | | | |
| | 18.00 | DIGOXIN | 250 micrograms | IV | JN 061 | | | | |

**SCENARIO 10**

| Thromboprophylaxis please prescribe treatment regimens in the regular medications section | | | | | | | | |
|---|---|---|---|---|---|---|---|---|
| Choice of mechanical prophylaxis and leg(s) to be applied to | | | | | | Enter Time | Enter details below | |
| Graduated elastic compression stockings | Intermittent pneumatic compression device (IPC) | Leg | | | | | | |
| | | Left | Right | Both | | | | |
| ☑ Start Date: 7/05 End Date: | ☐ | Signature and Bleep No. | ☐ | ☐ | ☑ | | | |
| ☐ Start Date: End Date: | ☐ | Signature and Bleep No. AF | ☐ | ☐ | ☐ | | | |

| Medication CLEXANE | | Dose 20mg | Dose Change | Enter Time | Enter details below | | |
|---|---|---|---|---|---|---|---|
| Please ensure you have completed the VTE risk assessment form | Date | 13/05 | | | | | |
| | Route | SC | | | | | |
| | Signature | JN | | Instructions | | Pharmacy ☐ | |
| | Bleep no. | 061 | | | | | |

| Oxygen | | | | | |
|---|---|---|---|---|---|
| Target Saturation | 88-92% ☐ | 94/98% ☑ | If oxygen saturation falls below target range on prescribed oxygen, patient needs urgent clinical review. If oxygen saturation is above target range on prescribed oxygen, ask for review. | | |
| Other (specify) | | | *Device: N= nasal cannula, SM = simple face mask, V = venturi, H = humidified, RM = reservoir mask, OTHER = other eg. NCPAP/NIPPV | Pharmacy ☐ | |
| Target Saturation not applicable | | ☐ | | | |

| | Date Changed | Date Changed | Enter Time | Enter details below |
|---|---|---|---|---|
| | 13/05 | | | |
| Device | NASAL | | | |
| % or L/min (specify a range eg 1-21 L/min) | 2L/MIN | | | |
| Signature and Bleep no. | JN 061 | | | |

| Regular prescriptions continued | | | | | | | | |
|---|---|---|---|---|---|---|---|---|
| Anti-infectives prescription   *prescribe long term prophylaxis and anti-tuberculosis medications in regular medications section* | | | | | | | | |
| For 3 days | Dose | | | Date | 7 | 8 | 9 | 10 |
| Date 13/05 | | | | Medication CO-AMOXICLAV | | Instructions UTI | Signature and bleep no. JN 061 | Pharmacy ☐ |
| Route | IV | | | | | | | |
| Signature | | | | | | | | |
| (06) | 600mg | | | | | | | |
| 09 | | | | | | | | |
| 12 | | | | | | | | |
| 18 | | | | | | | | |
| (22) | 600mg | | | | | | | |
| 24 | | | | | | | | |

**Regular prescriptions continued**

| | Dose | | | Date | 7 | 8 | 9 | 10 | 11 | 12 | | | | | | | |
|---|---|---|---|---|---|---|---|---|---|---|---|---|---|---|---|---|---|
| Date 13/05 | | | | Medication | | | Instructions | | | Signature and bleep no. | | | Pharmacy | | | | |
| Route | PO | | | BENDROFLUMETHI-AZIDE | | | NOT WHILST AKI/BP | | | JN 061 | | | ☐ | | | | |
| Signature | | | | | | | | | | | | | | | | | |
| 06 | | | | | | | | | | | | | | | | | |
| (09) | 2.5mg | | | ✕ ✕ ✕ ✕ ✕ | | | | | | | | | | | | | |
| 12 | | | | | | | | | | | | | | | | | |
| 18 | | | | | | | | | | | | | | | | | |
| 22 | | | | | | | | | | | | | | | | | |
| 24 | | | | | | | | | | | | | | | | | |

**Regular prescriptions continued**

| | Dose | | | Date | | | | | | | | | | | | | |
|---|---|---|---|---|---|---|---|---|---|---|---|---|---|---|---|---|---|
| Date 13/05 | | | | Medication | | | Instructions | | | Signature and bleep no. | | | Pharmacy | | | | |
| Route | PO | | | DONEPEZIL | | | | | | JN 061 | | | ☐ | | | | |
| Signature | | | | | | | | | | | | | | | | | |
| 06 | | | | | | | | | | | | | | | | | |
| 09 | | | | | | | | | | | | | | | | | |
| 12 | | | | | | | | | | | | | | | | | |
| 18 | | | | | | | | | | | | | | | | | |
| (22) | 5mg | | | ✕ ✕ ✕ ✕ | | | | | | | | | | | | | |
| 24 | | | | | | | | | | | | | | | | | |

**Regular prescriptions continued**

| | Dose | | | Date | | | | | | | | | | | | | |
|---|---|---|---|---|---|---|---|---|---|---|---|---|---|---|---|---|---|
| Date 13/05 | | | | Medication | | | Instructions | | | Signature and bleep no. | | | Pharmacy | | | | |
| Route | PO | | | DIGOXIN | | | | | | JN 061 | | | ☐ | | | | |
| Signature | | | | | | | | | | | | | | | | | |
| 06 | | | | | | | | | | | | | | | | | |
| (09) | 125 micro-grams | | | | | | | | | | | | | | | | |
| 12 | | | | | | | | | | | | | | | | | |
| 18 | | | | | | | | | | | | | | | | | |
| 22 | | | | | | | | | | | | | | | | | |
| 24 | | | | | | | | | | | | | | | | | |

SCENARIO 10

183

# 'ALL VERY CONFUSING'

## Regular prescriptions continued

### Anti-infectives prescription  *prescribe long term prophylaxis and anti-tuberculosis medications in regular medications section*

| | Dose | | | Date | | | | | | | | | |
|---|---|---|---|---|---|---|---|---|---|---|---|---|---|
| **Date** 13/05 | | | | **Medication** ASPIRIN | | | **Instructions** | | | **Signature and bleep no.** JN 061 | | **Pharmacy** ☐ | |
| **Route** | PO | | | | | | | | | | | | |
| **Signature** | | | | | | | | | | | | | |
| 06 | | | | | | | | | | | | | |
| (09) | 75mg | | | | | | | | | | | | |
| 12 | | | | | | | | | | | | | |
| 18 | | | | | | | | | | | | | |
| 22 | | | | | | | | | | | | | |
| 24 | | | | | | | | | | | | | |

## Infusion prescriptions continued

*\* NO ADDED K+ – K+ = 6.3 mmol/L*

SC = subcutaneous  
IVC = intravenous central  
IVP = intravenous peripheral

| Date & time | Route | Infusion Fluid | | Medication | | Duration | Rate | Prescriber's signature & bleep no. | Date given | Given by / Added by | Check by | Start time | Finish time | Pharmacy |
|---|---|---|---|---|---|---|---|---|---|---|---|---|---|---|
| | | Name & strength | Volume | Approved name with expiry / unit number | Dose | | | | | | | | | |
| 13/05 | IV | 0.9 % Saline Exp: Batch/unit no: | 1l | | | | 4° | JN 061 | | | | | | |
| 13/05 | IV | 0.9 % Saline Exp: Batch/unit no: | 1l | | | | 4° | JN 061 | | | | | | |
| 13/05 | IV | 0.9 % Saline Exp: Batch/unit no: | 1l | | | | 6° | JN 061 | | | | | | |
| 13/05 | IV | 0.9 % Saline Exp: Batch/unit no: | 1l | | | | 8° | JN 061 | | | | | | |
| 13/05 | IV | 0.9 % Saline Exp: Batch/unit no: | 1l | | | | 10° | JN 061 | | | | | | |
| | | TITRATE FLUIDS TO U.O. > HR, BP > 100 Systolic; HR < 100 BPM Exp: Batch/unit no: | | | | | | | | | | | | |
| 13/05 | IV | 0.9 % Saline Exp: Batch/unit no: | 50ml | ACTRAPID INSULIN | 50 UNITS | TO RUN AT 0.1 U/Kg/HR 1.5 UNITS/HOUR | | JN 061 | | | | | | |
| | | Exp: Batch/unit no: | | | | | | | | | | | | |
| | | Exp: Batch/unit no: | | | | | | | | | | | | |

## As required medications

| Medication PARACETAMOL | | | | Date | | | | | | | | | | |
|---|---|---|---|---|---|---|---|---|---|---|---|---|---|---|
| Indication | | | | Time | | | | | | | | | | |
| **Dose** 1g | **Route** IV/ IM | **Maximum frequency / dose** 4g/ 24° | **Start date** 13/05 | **Dose** | | | | | | | | | | |
| | | | **Stop date** | **Route** | | | | | | | | | | |
| **Signature** JN 061 | | | | | | | | | | | | | | |
| | | | **Bleep no.** | **Given** | | | | | | | | | | |
| **Additional instructions:** | | | | | | | | **Pharmacy** | | | | | ☐ | |

| As required medications | | | | | | | | | | | | | | | | | | | | | |
|---|---|---|---|---|---|---|---|---|---|---|---|---|---|---|---|---|---|---|---|---|---|
| **Medication**<br>METOCLOPRAMIDE | | | **Date** | | | | | | | | | | | | | | | | | | |
| **Indication** | | | **Time** | | | | | | | | | | | | | | | | | | |
| **Dose**<br>10 mg | **Route**<br>IV/ IM | **Maximum frequency / dose**<br>/8° | **Start date**<br>13/05 | **Dose** | | | | | | | | | | | | | | | | | | |
| | | | **Stop date** | **Route** | | | | | | | | | | | | | | | | | | |
| **Signature**<br>JN 061 | | | **Bleep no.** | **Given** | | | | | | | | | | | | | | | | | | |
| **Additional instructions:** | | | | | | | | | | | | | | **Pharmacy** | | | | | | | |

## GLOBAL PRESCRIBING MARK

A B C D E

## Station 5 – Clinical communication skills

**Patient script**

You should try to be consistent with your answers to the 30-point MMSE (Folstein) and the capacity assessment (ie getting similar areas of questions incorrect, rather than scattering your incorrect answers throughout the various themes). You should aim to get a score of around 15–20 on the Folstein but when assessed for capacity should give answers that suggest you don't retain capacity.

You don't remember anyone else discussing these issues with you, and are horrified that the doctor is implying that you can't go home, and may end up in a 'home'; however when asked you deny having been on a home visit and don't remember any of the events at home that led to your original admission. You have no insight into your own safety issues and can't understand why anyone would be concerned about you. However, if asked again about going into a care home you should act ambivalent 'I wouldn't mind that really', but then should be indignant about 'going to be with Ralph'.

If asked to repeat the discussions around discharge, you should be vague and confabulate about home but should not be able to give any evidence that you have retained the important parts of the discussion, and are therefore not competent to make decisions about discharge.

A B C D E
PROFESSIONALISM

A B C D E
PROCESS

## CONTENT

A B C D E

**Confirms reason for assessments**

**A memory test and a test to 'see if you are able to decide about going home'.**

**Gains agreement/informal consent to participate in the assessments**

**MMSE**
- Allows patient appropriate time; gives clear and understandable instruction, avoids complex descriptions and jargon.

**Capacity assessment**

**Investigates patient's present level of understanding of discharge plans**
- Asks if anyone else has discussed them with her and what they have told her
- Recall around events leading up to original admission and progress since then; asks about recall of home visit and how it went

**Establishes patient's ideas, concerns and expectations**
- Ideas and concerns about going home or into a care home
- Understanding and insight into safety issues, eg 'Do you understand why people might be worried and concerned about you?'

**Explains the key, important information**
- Presents facts to patient around MDT concerns and risks of discharge
- Asks patient to repeat major discussion points
- Asks patient to communicate their final decision about going home.

**Invites patient to ask questions and is able to deal with them appropriately**

**Summarises important areas of the consultation back to the patient**

**Formally ends the consultation and ensures appropriate follow-up has been discussed**

## CLINICAL DIAGNOSTIC REASONING

■ **Given your discussions with the patient, what do you think about her capacity to make decisions about her discharge?**
  - The patient does not fulfil all the criteria of capacity and was inconsistent and vague at times
  - Given these facts she does not have capacity to make a competent decision about discharge.

■ **What would you suggest should happen next? If Mrs Michelson didn't have any family or close friend to advocate for her what would you do?**
  - There should be a care planning meeting involving Jill, her husband Ralph and members of the MDT, co-ordinated by a social worker. The team and Mr Michelson should work together to produce a safe and effective discharge plan.
  - If Mr Michelson feels he can look after Jill at home, then adaptations to the home must be made, and formal care and support should be put in place. If he is unable to care for her at home, then extra care, sheltered accommodation or residential care may be required if there is no-one to advocate on the patient's behalf an Independent Mental Capacity Advocate (IMCA) should be appointed.

**Demonstrates safe, sensible and appropriate management plan**

**Demonstrates clear and logical diagnostic reasoning**

## GLOBAL COMMUNICATION MARK

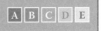

# Scenario 10: Reflection and consolidation

## History

Mrs Jill Michelson has been suffering with memory problems for about 8–10 months, although she herself does not seem to think she has any problems. She does admit to word-finding problems, but this she just dismisses as part of getting old. She is easily distracted and seems rather agitated when questioned. She rapidly loses patience with the doctor and asks him /her to speak to her husband, Ralph. Despite this instruction, it is always appropriate to gain the patient's permission before talking about them to second parties.

Jill's husband Ralph confirms that his wife's memory problems started about 6–8 months ago but have been much worse in the last few months. He admits to the following issues:

- Word-finding and language problems (suggesting Alzheimer's disease)
- Problems of recognition and recall; getting lost in familiar places
- Reduced mobility and falls
- No hallucinations; low mood but no overt features of depression.

## Examination

Three months later Mrs Michelson is brought to the Emergency Department after having been found on the floor by her husband after he popped out to get some milk from the local shops.

Examination of this elderly woman with known dementia revealed her to be acutely unwell and overtly septic, with a temperature of 39.1 °C. She was agitated and confused and had an abridged mental test score of 1/10. Her urinalysis was positive for blood, protein, leucocytes and nitrites.

She was tachycardic, clinically in fast atrial fibrillation with a blood pressure of 93/65, a CBG of 16.1 and hypoxic and tachypnoeic. Cardiovascular examination showed her to have a loud systolic murmur consistent with mitral regurgitation, but there were no signs of heart failure, and her chest was clear. Abdominal examination revealed she was constipated with hard pellet-like stools on digital rectal examination, but was otherwise unremarkable; neurological assessment was likewise unremarkable.

She is very confused, and this suggests she is suffering from a delirium, or acute on chronic confusion. There are multiple causes of delirium; these need to be excluded through systematic examination and investigation. Common causes include:

- Sepsis – thus one should record general features suggesting sepsis – pyrexia, hot and vasodilated pripheries, flushed, tachycardia, hypotension (severe sepsis), and specific features of meningism, ENT infections, chest, intra-abdominal, urinary, skin and joint infection, including leg ulcers (you must take down any dressings or bandaging present)
- Metabolic disturbance – hyper- or hypoglycaemia and hypoxia are easily defined through clinical testing; others such as electrolyte disturbances, hypercapnia, hyper- and hypocalcaemia, uraemia and deranged liver function tests should be sought with appropriate blood tests.
- Intracranial events – infarction, haemorrhage, space-occupying lesions, signs of raised intracranial pressure – these may be excluded through examination and appropriate investigations, including a CT scan of the brain
- Drug toxicity – this may deliberate, or accidental. Toxicology is often a forgotten test in the acutely delirious. Medications may often exacerbate or contribute to the delirium even when not the principle cause, especially sedatives and drugs that act on the central nervous system.

Your history and examination should be targeted at defining/excluding these common causes. In this case, the patient had signs consistent with a severe uro-sepsis, including:

- BP 93/65 mmHg, HR 123 bpm; temperature 39.1 °C = septic shock
- CBG 16.1 mmol/l = hyperglycaemia; new onset diabetes mellitus or stress-related hyperglycaemia
- RR 26 bpm, $O_2$ sats 92% on air – tachypnoea and mild hypoxia
- Urinalysis: blood ++, protein ++, leuc ++, nitrite + – consistent with a UTI
- General examination – hot and vasodilated peripheries.

Other causes, eg subdural haemorrhage, must be considered given the degree of bruising, suggesting multiple falls.

## Data interpretation

Patients presenting with delirium need a comprehensive examination before ordering targeted blood and other investigations. However, even when this is achievable (which it isn't always because of the patient's agitation and confusion), investigations should also be comprehensive, as there may be several contributing factors, including multi-organ failure (as in this case).

Common investigations that should be considered include:

- Bloods – FBC, U&Es, RBG, LFTs, calcium, CRP, blood cultures
- Urinalysis and MSU
- ECG, CXR, ABGs, CT head scan
- If intra-abdominal pathology is suspected – consider serum amylase, abdominal ultrasound or CT scan.

## Management

The initial management of such a confused, agitated patient should include specialist nursing care, preferably on a Care of the Elderly ward. If sedation is required (it should be avoided if at all possible) small aliquots of IV or IM haloperidol should be administered; the patient may require a low-level bed to keep them safe.

Generic management will include appropriate IV antibiotics, IV fluids and in view of the hyperglycaemia, a FRIVII or sliding scale. Her diuretic and donepezil should be stopped in the acute phase.

Once in the recovery/rehabilitation phase a full MDT assessment should be made and, in conjunction with the patient and her husband, discharge planning should be set in motion. For safe discharge patients with cognitive impairment should have formal documentation of their cognitive state, and their capacity and reports from all members of the MDT. If disagreement and conflict arise among family, patient and the MDT, a care planning meeting should be organised, in which areas of disagreement and safe discharge should be negotiated.

When patients have no advocates, an independent person may be formally appointed to advocate for them. This person is called an Independent Mental Capacity Advocate (IMCA). Other agencies that may be required include the Court of Protection.

## Further reading and web links

Folstein MF, Folstein SE, McHugh PR. 'Mini-mental state'. A practical method for grading the cognitive state of patients for the clinician. *Journal of Psychiatry Research* 1975; 12: 189–98.
*Great article about teaching decision-making capacity*:
http://chestjournal.chestpubs.org/content/137/2/248.full.pdf+html
*Further article on assessing decision-making capacity*:
http://chestjournal.chestpubs.org/content/137/2/421.full.pdf+html
*BGS guidelines on the diagnosis and management of patients with dementia*:
www.sign.ac.uk/pdf/sign86.pdf
*NICE guidelines for care of patients with dementia*:
www.nice.org.uk/CG042
*Summary of Mental Capacity Act (2005)*:
www.dh.gov.uk/en/Publicationsandstatistics/Bulletins/theweek/Chiefexecutivebulletin/DH_4108436
*BGS guidelines on capacity*:
www.bgs.org.uk/index.php?option=com_content&view=article&id=40:gpgtestamentarycapacity&catid=12:goodpractice&Itemid=106

# Scenario 11: 'Hyper, hyper'

SCENARIO 11

## Station 1

*History*                                        *10-minute station*

You are the FY1 on a GP placement. This morning you are seeing patients on your own before presenting them to the senior partner, Dr Shah. You are keen to make a good impression, as you are thinking about a career in general practice. The next patient is Mr Adam Bellows (DOB 13/09/58), who is attending the surgery this morning for his annual diabetes review.

■ Please take a full history of this patient's condition, with a view to presenting it to Dr Shah, as a 'history of a long-term condition'.

*You will be assessed on the following areas, as well as the content and diagnostic reasoning of your history – take them into account in your presentation.*

### Professionalism

- Professional appearance (NHS dress code) – including general appearance, hair and jewellery
- Maintains patient and personal safety
- Polite introduction; identifies patient or interviewee correctly; confirms patient's date of birth from name band or other source
- Obtains informal consent; maintains patient's privacy
- Displays empathetic and caring attitudes and behaviours throughout.

### Process

- Good organisation and structure; appropriate use of open and closed questions
- Appropriate fluency/rhythm/pace to the interview – this may change depending on environment and acute nature of the problem
- Appropriate time for the patient to respond/reply to questions
- Appropriate acknowledgement of difficult or emotional areas of the patient's history.

### Communication skills

- Demonstrates caring and sympathetic attitude
- Asks open questions
- Invites patient to ask questions and answers them appropriately
- Addresses patient's ideas, concerns and expectations.

## Station 2

*Examination*                                    *10-minute station*

Having presented the history, Dr Shah asks you to perform a 'holistic' assessment of Mr Bellows, appropriate to a diabetes annual review. He has provided the following equipment:

- Ophthalmoscope
- Urine dipsticks
- Neurology assessment kit
- Stethoscope
- Sphygmomanometer
- Snellen chart

■ Please perform the examination and present the relevant findings (given within the station) to Dr Shah in an appropriate manner for a busy GP.

(If you do not have a model, please read and present the information given on page 385.)

*You will be assessed on the following areas, as well as the content and skills of your examination – take them into account in your presentation.*

### Professionalism

- Professional appearance; maintains infection control standards, including hand cleaning and appropriate use of gloves and aprons
- Maintains patient and personal safety
- Polite introduction; identifies patient and confirms date of birth from name band or other source
- Obtains informal consent; maintains patient privacy and dignity
- Displays empathetic and caring attitudes and behaviours throughout.

### Process

- Appropriate fluency/rhythm/pace to the examination – this may change depending on environment and acute nature of problem
- Organisation and structure of examination; sensitive and empathetic approach
- Uses appropriate clinical techniques throughout
- Maintains privacy and dignity throughout.

### Clinical communication

- Explains proposed examination/procedure: explains examination/procedure as it proceeds
- Offers information in a clear, structured and fluent manner, avoiding jargon
- Listens to patient and responds appropriately
- Demonstrates appropriate body language.

## Station 3

*Procedural skills*                    *10-minute station*

**Procedure**

It is very important to assess a diabetic patient's eyes.

■ Please show Dr Shah how you would perform a full eye assessment on Mr Bellows, including ophthalmoscopy.

**Equipment provided**

- Volunteer for eye assessment – if willing they may also be used for ophthalmoscopy, otherwise an ophthalmoscopy manikin should be used
- Snellen chart
- Pen torch
- Ophthalmoscope
- 'Red' pin.

## Station 4

*Data interpretation*                    *10-minute station*

Seven months later Mr Bellows is admitted to his local hospital after having been unwell for several days with a 'real nasty' chest infection. You are the FY1 on the diabetes and endocrine firm and you have been asked to review and record Mr Bellows' blood test results from his admission the previous morning.

■ Please review Mr Bellows' data shown below and indicate whether the statements are TRUE (T) or FALSE (F).

- ○ FBC: Hb 8.3 g/dl, MCV 104 fl, Hct 0.56, WCC 6.6 × $10^9$/l, (neutrophils 2.9 × $10^9$/l), platelets 331 × $10^9$/l
- ○ U&Es: $Na^+$ 179 mmol/l, $K^+$ 5.1 mmol/l, urea 45.8 mmol/l, creatinine 324 μmol/l
- ○ RBG: 73.1 mmol/l
- ○ LFTs: TBil 4.7mmol/l, ALT 21 iu/l, AST 13 iu/l, Alk Phos 161 iu/l, Alb 38 g/l
- ○ Clotting: INR 1.1; APTT 32 s
- ○ CRP 364 mg/l
- ○ ABGs on 2l/min: pH 7.22, $PaO_2$ 12.3 KPa, $PaCO_2$ 4.1 KPa, $HCO_3^-$ 16.0 mmol/l, BXS 4.9 mmol/l, lactate 6.9 mmol/l
- ○ Blood cultures sent.

    A   In this context the Hb and MCV are most likely explained by a megaloblastic anaemia.

    B   The haematocrit is in keeping with the underlying intravascular depletion.

    C   The Hb and MCV indicate a Coombs' test would be an appropriate second-line investigation.

    D   The white cell and differential are suggestive of an atypical pneumonia.

SCENARIO 11

E   The urea : creatinine ratio is consistent with obstructive nephropathy.

F   The calculated serum osmolality is 478.4 mOsmo/kg.

G   Given this patient's serum sodium, he should receive 3.0% saline solution.

H   Given the serum potassium, the patient should receive an additional 20 mmol/l potassium supplementation.

I   The random blood glucose is highly suggestive of a laboratory error.

J   The coagulation screen confirms the disseminated intravascular coagulopathy (DIC).

K   Given these results, this patient should be given VTE prophylaxis with low molecular weight heparin (LMWH) and TED stockings.

L   The ABGs suggest a severe mixed respiratory/metabolic acidosis.

M   The acidosis is exacerbated by the patient's oral hypoglycaemic agents.

N   This set of data is in keeping with diabetic keto-acidosis.

## Station 5

*Prescribing skills*                    *10-minute station*

Mr Bellows is admitted with a diagnosis of hyperosmolar, hyperglycaemic syndrome secondary to a severe community-acquired pneumonia. The on-call FY1 has written up Mr Bellows' drug chart.

■ Please check the charts below and answer the questions regarding the boarded medications, indicating whether they are TRUE (T) or FALSE (F).

1

A   The antibiotic regime chosen is appropriate for a severe community-acquired pneumonia.

B   Tazocin® is an appropriate drug for this particular patient.

C   In its present format the dose of Tazocin® can be given to the patient.

D   In view of the patient's AKI, the clarithromycin is written as a reduced dose.

E   Given the patient's previous medications and the degree of hyperglycaemia, it would have been appropriate to include a single, stat dose of a short-acting insulin.

| Allergies, sensitivities and adverse drug reactions | | | | Patient details/addressograph | |
|---|---|---|---|---|---|
| No known allergies ☐ | | Initials  AF | | NHS/ Hospital No:  609409 | |
| Not possible to ascertain ☐ | | Date | | | |
| Medicine/substance | Reaction & Severity | Initials & Date | Weight (kg)  81.5kg  Date | Surname:  BELLOWS | |
| PENICILLIN | SEVERE RASH | | Height  172cm | First name:  ADAM | |
| Alerts | | | Surface area (m²) | Date of birth:  13.09.58 | |

**IN-PATIENT MEDICATION PRESCRIPTION AND ADMINISTRATION RECORD**

PasTest HOSPITAL

| Consultant  GILL | Trainee Dr. Name and Bleep no.  DR SMITH 604 | Date of admission  27.02.12 | Date chart reboarded | Estimated date of discharge |
|---|---|---|---|---|
| This chart is no.  .............. of .......................... | Transcribing Check by Pharmacy  Sign .................. Date ............... | Ward  1. ........MAU............................  2. .......................... | | |

Supplementary Medication charts in use:  Other (please specify): 1 ...................................................  2 ..............................

| Epidural/PCA ☐ | Syringe driver ☐ | | TPN ☐ | Chemotherapy ☐ | Insulin sliding scale ☐ |
|---|---|---|---|---|---|

Once only medications – loading doses, pre-medication, PGDs  or surgical antibiotic propylaxis

| Date | Time to be given | Medicine (approved name) | Dose | Route | Signature and bleep no. | Pharmacy | Time given | Given by | Checked by |
|---|---|---|---|---|---|---|---|---|---|
| 27/02 | Stat | TAZOCIN | 4.5g | PO | MS 604 | | | | |
| 27/02 | Stat | CLARITHROMYCIN | 500mg | PO | MS 604 | | | | |
| | | | | | | | | | |
| | | | | | | | | | |

2

    A    If the patient has received the stat dose of Tazocin® with no ill effects, it would be appropriate to allow the patient to receive further doses of the drug.

    B    In view of the patient's AKI, this dose of Tazocin® is inappropriate.

    C    As charted, the clarithromycin regime is correct.

**Regular prescriptions continued**

Anti-infectives prescription   *prescribe long term prophylaxis and anti-tuberculosis medications in regular medications section*

| FOR 5 DAYS | Dose | | | Date | | | | | | | | | | | | |
|---|---|---|---|---|---|---|---|---|---|---|---|---|---|---|---|---|
| Date 27/02 | | | | Medication | | | Indication | | | Signature and bleep no. | | | Pharmacy | | | |
| Route | PO | | | TAZOCIN | | | C.A.P. | | | MS 604 | | | | | | |
| Signature | | | | | | | | | | | | | | | | |
| 06 | | | | | | | | | | | | | | | | |
| (09) | 4.5g | | | | | | | | | | | | | | | |
| (12) | 4.5g | | | | | | | | | | | | | | | |
| (18) | 4.5g | | | | | | | | | | | | | | | |
| (22) | 4.5g | | | | | | | | | | | | | | | |
| 24 | | | | | | | | | | | | | | | | |

**Regular prescriptions continued**

Anti-infectives prescription   *prescribe long term prophylaxis and anti-tuberculosis medications in regular medications section*

| FOR 5 DAYS | Dose | | | Date | | | | | | | | | | | | |
|---|---|---|---|---|---|---|---|---|---|---|---|---|---|---|---|---|
| Date 27/02 | | | | Medication | | | Indication | | | Signature and bleep no. | | | Pharmacy | | | |
| Route | PO | | | CLARITHROMYCIN | | | C.A.P. | | | MS 604 | | | | | | |
| Signature | | | | | | | | | | | | | | | | |
| 06 | | | | | | | | | | | | | | | | |
| (09) | 500mg | | | | | | | | | | | | | | | |
| (12) | 500mg | | | | | | | | | | | | | | | |
| 18 | | | | | | | | | | | | | | | | |
| (22) | 500mg | | | | | | | | | | | | | | | |
| 24 | | | | | | | | | | | | | | | | |

3

    A    The metformin should be given as charted.

    B    The sitagliptin should be given as charted.

    C    The ramipril should be given as charted.

    D    The simvastatin should be given as charted.

SCENARIO 11

SCENARIO 11

### Regular prescriptions continued

| | Dose | | | Date | 27 | 28 | 29 | 1 | 2 | 3 | 4 | 5 | | | | |
|---|---|---|---|---|---|---|---|---|---|---|---|---|---|---|---|---|
| Date 27/02 | | | | **Medication** | | | | **Indication** | | | | **Signature and bleep no.** | | | **Pharmacy** | |
| Route | PO | | | METFORMIN | | | | | | | | MS 604 | | | ☐ | |
| Signature | | | | | | | | | | | | | | | | |
| 06 | | | | | | | | | | | | | | | | |
| (09) | 500mg | | | | | | | | | | | | | | | |
| 12 | | | | | | | | | | | | | | | | |
| (18) | 500mg | | | | | | | | | | | | | | | |
| 22 | | | | | | | | | | | | | | | | |
| 24 | | | | | | | | | | | | | | | | |

### Regular prescriptions continued

**Anti-infectives prescription**   *prescribe long term prophylaxis and anti-tuberculosis medications in regular medications section*

| | Dose | | | Date | | | | | | | | | | | | |
|---|---|---|---|---|---|---|---|---|---|---|---|---|---|---|---|---|
| Date 27/02 | | | | **Medication** | | | | **Indication** | | | | **Signature and bleep no.** | | | **Pharmacy** | |
| Route | PO | | | SITAGLIPTIN | | | | | | | | MS 604 | | | ☐ | |
| Signature | | | | | | | | | | | | | | | | |
| 06 | | | | | | | | | | | | | | | | |
| (09) | 100mg | | | | | | | | | | | | | | | |
| 12 | | | | | | | | | | | | | | | | |
| (18) | 100mg | | | | | | | | | | | | | | | |
| 22 | | | | | | | | | | | | | | | | |
| 24 | | | | | | | | | | | | | | | | |

### Regular prescriptions continued

*Regular Medications*

| | Dose | | | Date | | | | | | | | | | | | |
|---|---|---|---|---|---|---|---|---|---|---|---|---|---|---|---|---|
| Date 27/02 | | | | **Medication** | | | | **Indication** | | | | **Signature and bleep no.** | | | **Pharmacy** | |
| Route | PO | | | RAMIPRIL | | | | | | | | MS 604 | | | ☐ | |
| Signature | | | | | | | | | | | | | | | | |
| 06 | | | | | | | | | | | | | | | | |
| (09) | 5mg | | | | | | | | | | | | | | | |
| 12 | | | | | | | | | | | | | | | | |
| 18 | | | | | | | | | | | | | | | | |
| 22 | | | | | | | | | | | | | | | | |
| 24 | | | | | | | | | | | | | | | | |

### Regular prescriptions continued

| | Dose | | | Date | | | | | | | | | | | | |
|---|---|---|---|---|---|---|---|---|---|---|---|---|---|---|---|---|
| Date 27/02 | | | | **Medication** | | | | **Indication** | | | | **Signature and bleep no.** | | | **Pharmacy** | |
| Route | PO | | | SIMVASTATIN | | | | | | | | MS 604 | | | ☐ | |
| Signature | | | | | | | | | | | | | | | | |
| 06 | | | | | | | | | | | | | | | | |
| (09) | 40mg | | | | | | | | | | | | | | | |
| 12 | | | | | | | | | | | | | | | | |
| 18 | | | | | | | | | | | | | | | | |
| 22 | | | | | | | | | | | | | | | | |
| 24 | | | | | | | | | | | | | | | | |

4
   A   The ibuprofen should be given as charted.
   B   The paracetamol should be given as charted.
   C   The metoclopramide is charted correctly.
   D   The Oramorph is charted correctly.

**As required medications**

| Medication IBRUPROFEN | | | | Date | | | | | | | | | | | | | | | | | | | | | | | |
|---|---|---|---|---|---|---|---|---|---|---|---|---|---|---|---|---|---|---|---|---|---|---|---|---|---|---|---|
| Indication PAIN | | | | Time | | | | | | | | | | | | | | | | | | | | | | | |

| Dose 600 mg | Route PO | Maximum frequency / dose 4 HOURLY | Start date 27/02 | Dose |
| Signature MS | | | Bleep no. 604 | Route |
| | | | | Given |

Additional instructions:         Pharmacy

**As required medications**

| Medication PARACETAMOL | Date |
| Indication PAIN | Time |
| Dose 1g | Route PO | Maximum frequency / dose 6 HOURLY | Start date 27/02 | Dose |
| Signature MS | | | Bleep no. 604 | Route |
| | | | | Given |

Additional instructions:         Pharmacy

**As required medications**

| Medication METOCLOPRAMIDE | Date |
| Indication VOMITING | Time |
| Dose 10 mg | Route PO | Maximum frequency / dose 8 HOURLY | Start date 27/02 | Dose |
| Signature MS | | | Bleep no. 604 | Route |
| | | | | Given |

Additional instructions:         Pharmacy

SCENARIO 11

### As required medications

| Medication ORO-MORPH | | | | Date | | | | | | | | | | | | | | | | | | | | |
|---|---|---|---|---|---|---|---|---|---|---|---|---|---|---|---|---|---|---|---|---|---|---|---|---|
| Indication PAIN | | | | Time | | | | | | | | | | | | | | | | | | | | |
| Dose 10g | Route IV | Maximum frequency / dose | Start date 27/02 | Dose | | | | | | | | | | | | | | | | | | | | |
| | | As Required | Stop date | Route | | | | | | | | | | | | | | | | | | | | |
| Signature MS | | | Bleep no. 604 | Given | | | | | | | | | | | | | | | | | | | | |
| Additional instructions: | | | | | | | | | | | | | | Pharmacy | | | | | | | | | | |

SCENARIO 11

5

    A    The volume of fluid is appropriate for this patient.
    B    The type of fluid is appropriate for this patient.
    C    The potassium supplementation is appropriate for this patient.
    D    If the patient weighs 81.5 kg, the FRIVII should be set at 0.82 ml/h.

### Infusion prescriptions continued

SC = subcutaneous  IVC = intravenous central  IVP = intravenous peripheral

| Date & time | Route | Infusion Fluid Name & strength | Volume | Medication Approved name with expiry / unit number | Dose | Duration | Rate | Prescriber's signature & bleep no. | Date given | Given by / Added by | Check by | Start time | Finish time | Pharmacy |
|---|---|---|---|---|---|---|---|---|---|---|---|---|---|---|
| 27/02 | | 0.45% Saline Exp: Batch/unit no: | 50ml | ACTRAPID INSULIN | 50 UNITS | | TO RUN IV AT 0.1 UNITS/kg/HOUR PATIENT'S WEIGHT = 81.5kg | MS 604 | | | | | | |
| 27/02 | | 5% Dextrose Exp: Batch/unit no: | 1l | + 20mmol KCL | | | 30 MINS | MS 604 | | | | | | |
| 27/02 | | 5% Dextrose Exp: Batch/unit no: | 1l | + 20mmol KCL | | | 1 HOUR | MS 604 | | | | | | |
| 27/02 | | 5% Dextrose Exp: Batch/unit no: | 1l | + 20mmol KCL | | | 2 HOURS | MS 604 | | | | | | |
| 27/02 | | 5% Dextrose Exp: Batch/unit no: | 1l | + 20mmol KCL | | | 4 HOURS | MS 604 | | | | | | |
| 27/02 | | 5% Dextrose Exp: Batch/unit no: | 1l | + 20mmol KCL | | | 6 HOURS | MS 604 | | | | | | |
| 27/02 | | 5% Dextrose Exp: Batch/unit no: | 1l | + 20mmol KCL | | | 8 HOURS | MS 604 | | | | | | |
| | | Exp: Batch/unit no: | | | | | | | | | | | | |
| | | Exp: Batch/unit no: | | | | | | | | | | | | |
| | | | | | | | | | | | | | | |

# Answers

## Station 1 – History

**Patient script**

You are Mr Adam Bellows (DOB 13 September 1958, 53 years old), who is attending the surgery this morning for your annual diabetes review. You are happy to talk to the 'young doctor' and are not in any rush, as you have taken a day of annual leave from work (you are a business manager in a large IT company).

You were diagnosed as being diabetic at 46 years old (7 years ago) 'just after my birthday – great birthday present!' It came as a bit of a shock as you'd always been healthy. Looking back now you hadn't been well for about 6 months. You had been feeling tired and listless and feeling generally 'quite awful'. 'I was so low I stopped playing golf' (which you normally do three times a week). Your weight had ballooned up over 18 months, ever since your mother became unwell. During that period you'd had lots of stress at work and your mother being ill meant you weren't looking after yourself, eating all the wrong foods and not doing any exercise.

Normally your weight is about 12 stone 7lb (80 kg) but during that period your weight was nearer 15 stone (95 kg). Your waist size went up to 38 inches (from 34 inches) and nothing seemed to fit or look good on you.

You came to see Dr Shah as you were feeling so bad. 'He was really shocked by my appearance' – 'told me how awful I looked – never one for beating around the bush. We occasionally play golf together but he hadn't seen me for about 6 months or so. He did a full physical on me and sent a whole lot of blood tests away. My blood pressure was high, my weight was huge and my blood sugar was well over 20. I was a mess.'

He sent you off to see a dietitian and to the local gym and signed you off work for a month while you got yourself back together again. Despite your weight coming down and feeling a lot better, you needed to go on several medications including metformin (now 500 mg twice a day), ramipril (5 mg once a day) and simvastatin 20 mg in the late evening. More recently he has added sitagliptin (100 mg once a day).

Since then you've felt 'better and better'; you've lost weight and stick to a far healthier lifestyle. You stopped smoking at diagnosis – 'best thing I ever did' – and now go swimming and dancing with your wife two to three times a week, as well as playing golf one to two times a week.

You see Dr Shah and his team at least twice a year and have so far not had any major problems. You monitor your own sugars once or twice a week by a fingerprick test, and the results usually show between 5 and 8 (very occasionally about 10 or 11). You take a keen interest in your blood results and the last yearly test (HbA1C) was 5.9%. The GP team check your urine and your eyes every visit and they have both been fine ('just a little wear and tear I believe').

As far as you know you've not suffered any major complications of the diabetes and have never been admitted to hospital with any serious illnesses or problems arising from your diabetes. If asked directly – no symptoms of macro, microvascular, neurological complications; good foot health – no trauma or ulcers. Now looking after yourself and feeling much better for it.

CV risk: ex-smoker – gave up at diagnosis, previously 20/day for 25 years, but occasional cigar at a golf club dinner; alcohol – one to two glasses of red wine with most evening meals, never during the day, occasional brandy or scotch at the golf club; cholesterol – now on simvastatin, last year your cholesterol was 5.1; blood pressure – previously 'very high' – now on ramipril usually between 120 and 130/70 or so; diet – stick to all the right foods again now – rarely stray!; weight this morning 78 kg, height 1.81 m, BMI 24; no other major illness – if asked no IHD, stroke or circulatory problems, but you're allergic to penicillin (rash).

Social history: married (wife a retired professional dancer); two children, both at university – daughter, Gemma, aged 22, studying Dance and Theatre at Middlesex; son, Richard, aged 19, studying Mechanical Engineering at Nottingham.

Diabetes complications: 'have really tried to look after myself once I was diagnosed'; eyes – last check, no problems, wear glasses for reading, watching TV and driving; hands and feet – no funny feelings (tingling or numbness), no ulcers; kidneys – last year was fine, nurse checked my water on arrival – 'all clear'; no symptoms of angina, heart failure, no stroke/TIA, no claudication; no admissions to hospital with any 'highs or lows', 'Dr Shah and the nurse look after my diabetes – don't see any hospital doctors'.

Ideas – Know I am much better since I was diagnosed and have been looking after myself.

Concerns – none really!

Expectations – 'I think you'll find I'm all in good working order doctor'.

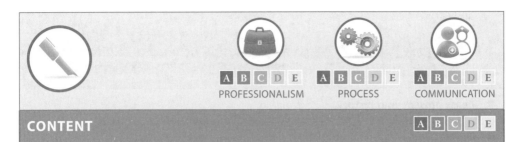

PROFESSIONALISM     PROCESS     COMMUNICATION

## CONTENT     A B C D E

### Identifies key information
- History of long-term condition: how, why and when was the condition diagnosed
- Progression since
- Normal control: self-monitoring; healthcare professionals involved – where; by whom, methods of monitoring; last review and outcome
- Best and worst health: acute deteriorations and exacerbations; admissions to hospital; serious complications.

### Includes important negatives, including systemic enquiry
- Specifically asks about diabetic complications
- Macrovascular: symptoms suggestive of angina, TIA or stroke, PVD
- Microvascular: visual and renal symptoms; symptoms of fluid overload (may also indicate CCF)
- Neurological: symptoms suggestive of peripheral sensory neuropathy; other problems – eg erectile dysfunction, dizziness and pre-syncope (autonomic)
- Feet and skin: ulcers; trauma and sores.

### Identifies key information from rest of history
- Cardiovascular risk
- Ex-smoker: gave up at diagnosis; previously 20/day for 25 years; but occasional cigar at a golf club dinner
- Alcohol: 1–2 glasses of red wine with most evening meals, never during the day; occasional brandy or scotch at the golf club
- Cholesterol: now on simvastatin; last cholesterol 5.1
- Blood pressure: previously 'very high'; now usually between 120 and 130/70 or so
- Diet: healthy now
- Weight this morning 78 kg, height 1.81 m, BMI 24
- No IHD, stroke or circulatory problems
- Relevant facts about employment, housing, social support, life stressors.

### Completing the patient history
- Drug and allergy history: ramipril 5 mg od, metformin 500 mg bd, simvastatin 20 mg od, sitagliptin 100 mg od; allergy to penicillin – severe rash
- Social and occupational history: as above.

### Summarises important areas of the history back to the patient

### Invites patient to ask questions and deals with them appropriately

### Establishes patient's ideas, concerns and expectations

SCENARIO 11

## CLINICAL DIAGNOSTIC REASONING

- **Please present your history**
  - Candidate offers a logical, well-structured account of the history.
- **How would you check his glycaemic control since he was last reviewed?**
  - HbA1C or similar (eg fructosamine).
- **What three essential bedside (clinical) investigations would you perform?**
  - Blood pressure: absolute, lying and standing
  - Ophthalmoscopy (pupils dilated with mydriatic eye drops)
  - Urinalysis
  - BMI: (height and weight). ± 5; ABPIs (if ulcers present or pulses were poorly palpable).

**Demonstrates safe, sensible and appropriate management plan**

**Demonstrates clear and logical diagnostic reasoning**

## GLOBAL HISTORY MARK

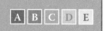

## Station 2 – Examination

**Patient script (see also page 385)**

You are a relatively fit and well 53-year-old man visiting the GP surgery today for your annual diabetes review; you are relaxed, chatty and are able to cooperate with the doctor in any way he/she wishes.

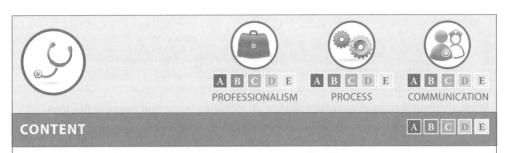

| A B C D E | A B C D E | A B C D E |
|---|---|---|
| PROFESSIONALISM | PROCESS | COMMUNICATION |

## CONTENT                                          A B C D E

**Exposes and positions patient correctly and maintains comfort**
- Patient's long-sleeved garments, trousers, shoes and socks to be removed.

**Comments on wellbeing of patient, ie well or unwell**

**'Feet to face'**
- Observes, and comments on patient and surroundings from foot of bed
- Evidence of obvious neurological deficit; mobility aids; stigmata of hyperlipidaemia, glycaemic control booklet
- Asks for height (1.81 m) and weight (81.5 kg ) – BMI 24.9 kg /m$^2$.

**Focussed examination**
- Cardiovascular system: tar staining, xanthelasma, HR, BP (lying and standing), palpates for all peripheral pulses, palpates AB and auscultates heart; assesses and comments on features of heart failure, bruits and aneurysms of central pulses (arteries), features of PVD
- Eyes: full assessment of eyes, including observation for gross abnormalities such as cranial nerve palsies, xanthelasma and corneal arcus, cataracts; visual acuity (both eyes) using Snellen chart
- If candidate attempts ophthalmoscopy – the examiner must stop him/her (see next station)
- Neurological system: assesses and comments on JPS, vibration, LT and pinprick sensation of upper and lower limbs – specifically examines for and excludes signs of peripheral sensory neuropathy
- Foot health: looks for and comments on any trauma, sores or ulcers of lower limbs and feet; specifically looks at webs between toe and comments on health of skin; palpates and notes presence of DP and PT pulses on both feet
- Urinalysis: should attempt to test urine (examiner to stop candidate).

**Thanks patient, offers assistance, maintains patient's dignity and privacy until they are dressed**

SCENARIO 11

## CLINICAL DIAGNOSTIC REASONING

**Correctly identifies the relevant physical signs, including important negative findings**

■ **Other than peripheral sensory neuropathy, can you tell me three neurological complications of diabetes?**

  • Autonomic neuropathy; impotence; diabetic amyotrophy; mononeuritis (multiplex); stroke.

■ **Given one of these complications is an autonomic neuropathy, how might you clinically assess for this?**

  • Pulse: resting tachycardia; but may have brady- or tachycardia and also arrhythmia
  • BP: lying/standing BP (postural hypotension)
  • Pupillary responses: may be sluggish (may also have Argyll–Robertson type pupils)
  • Palpable bladder; distended abdomen and abnormal bowel sounds
  • Excessive sweating.

**Demonstrates safe, sensible and appropriate management plan**

**Demonstrates clear and logical diagnostic reasoning**

## GLOBAL EXAMINATION MARK

## Station 3 – Procedural skills

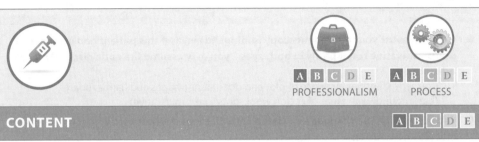

PROFESSIONALISM     PROCESS

### CONTENT

A B C D E

**Identifies and sets out equipment correctly; maintains aseptic technique throughout**
- Ophthalmoscope
- Pen torch
- Snellen chart
- Red pin.

**Correctly performs the procedure**

**Eye assessment**
- Observes the eyes: assesses and comments on any obvious cranial nerve lesions, symmetry of eyes and pupils; colour of sclera and cornea; peri-orbital lesions, eg xanthelasma
- Visual acuity: tests one eye at a time; if patient wears glasses, tests with (best) and without (worst) glasses; accurately records visual acuity for both eyes
- Visual fields: test all 4 x quadrants (nasal and temporal, upper and lower) for both eyes; tests for central scotoma using the red pin
- Extra-ocular muscles: tests CNS III, IV and VI for both eyes, using figure H procedure; comments on any diplopia or nystagmus
- Pupillary reflexes: comments on symmetry and size of pupils; using pen torch tests direct and consensual responses

**Ophthalmoscopy**
- Explains procedure and gains consent
- Correctly positions patient in chair or on edge of bed
- 'Fixes' patient's head with one hand, asking patient to fix stare into the distance
- Assesses and comments on red reflex in right/left eye
- Moves in towards patient (right/left eye) 'racking ophthalmoscope lens down' to focus in on retina
- Assesses and comments on: optic disc (colour and margin); macula; retinal vessels – integrity, pulsatility (veins) and tortuosity; retina – assesses for and comments on hard exudates, cotton wool spots, blot and dot haemorrhages, flame haemorrhages, new vessel formation, evidence of laser treatment.

**Does all in a fluent professional manner and uses appropriate techniques**

**Thanks patient, offers assistance, maintains patient's dignity and privacy throughout**

## CLINICAL DIAGNOSTIC REASONING

- **Please present your ophthalmoscopy findings to me, as if this patient had evidence of pre-proliferative retinopathy in both eyes – you may assume the optic disc and macula are normal**
  - Correctly identifies evidence of blot and dot haemorrhages and hard exudates (background) with areas of cotton wool spots (pre-proliferative).

- **Can you tell me the changes associated with diabetes mellitus that you might see at the macula and optic disc?**
  - Optic disc: optic atrophy (chronic change)
  - Macula: classically 'macula star' = hard exudates (maculopathy).

- **Can you tell me three reasons to refer a patient acutely to an ophthalmologist from the diabetic clinic?**
  - Apart from the obvious generic reasons (acute unilateral or bilateral blindness, acute red and /or painful eyes), the important reasons to refer a patient from diabetic clinic include: two or more line reduction (on the Snellen chart) in visual acuity between two reviews; evidence of pre- or proliferative retinopathy; maculopathy; cataracts.

**Demonstrates appropriate level of knowledge and skills**

**Demonstrates clear and logical diagnostic processes**

## GLOBAL PROCEDURE MARK

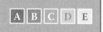

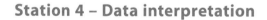

## Station 4 – Data interpretation

**A** **FALSE** – the data show Hb 8.3 g/dl, MCV 104 fl (ie a macrocytic anaemia). In the context of a previously fit and well, now acutely unwell, patient this is more likely to be due to a haemolytic anaemia, which may be associated with an atypical pneumonia. Megaloblastosis (the presence of large, immature red cells within the bone marrow) is a sign of erythrocyte DNA synthesis inhibition, principally caused by $B_{12}$ and folate deficiencies. Megaloblastic anaemia is also associated with hypersegmented neutrophils in the peripheral blood.

**B** **TRUE** – the normal haematocrit for men is approximately 0.45. In this patient's case it is elevated to a level of 0.56, consistent with gross intravascular depletion (ie dehydration).

**C** **TRUE** – in this case the macrocytosis is likely to be due to a Coombs' positive haemolytic anaemia, caused by an atypical pneumonia. Of this diverse group, haemolytic anaemia is most commonly associated with mycoplasma infection.

**D**      TRUE – the absolute white cell count is within normal limits but the differential shows a relative neutropenia (low neutrophil count); the rest of the count is unavailable. This relatively abnormal differential count is commonly seen with atypical pneumonias.

**E**      FALSE – urea 45.8 mmol/l, creatinine 324 $\mu$mol/l; the urea : creatinine ratio of this patient is approximately urea (11x normal) : creatinine (4x normal). Thus the urea has risen proportionally more than the creatinine, confirming pre-renal impairment, in keeping with gross dehydration.

**F**      FALSE – the calculated serum osmolality = 2(Na$^+$ + K$^+$)+ Urea + Glucose = 2(179 + 5.1) + 45.8 + 73.1 = 487.1 mOsmo/kg.

**G**      FALSE – there is gross hypernatraemia (Na$^+$ 179 mmol/l) present, and this needs careful and expert management. 'Normal' saline = 0.9% saline has a Na$^+$ of 150 mmol/l and is deemed isotonic with normal serum (although this is not really true, as the serum sodium should be between 135 and 145 mmol/l); 'half normal saline' = 0.45% saline is hypotonic and may be used (with caution) in patients with a very high serum sodium; 3.0%, 5.0%, 7.0% and 10% saline solutions are increasingly HYPERtonic to normal serum and are used in HYPOnatraemia. In both hyper- and hyponatraemia, large, and/or rapid changes in serum sodium need to be avoided at all cost, to avoid cerebral oedema and central pontine myelinolysis.

**H**      TRUE – (K$^+$ 5.1 mmol/l) – a normal adult requires approximately 40–60 mmol of potassium in 24 h. This patient has a potassium in the normal range and will require 20 mmol/l of K$^+$, given he/she will be on an intravenous insulin infusion.

**I**      FALSE – this patient has type 2 diabetes and will probably suffer hyperosmolar, hyperglycaemic syndrome (HHS) (previously known as hyperosmolar, non-ketotic (HoNK)) when acutely unwell. The principal metabolic derangements, ie hyperglycaemia and hypernatraemia, are often far more extreme than in the DKA, with glucose levels often climbing into ranges of 80–90 mmol/l c.f. DKA where they are around 50 mmol/l, and the serum sodium commonly climbing towards 200 mmol/l, c.f. DKA where it is commonly between 150 and 160 mmol/l.

**J**      FALSE – the patient's platelet count and clotting profile (INR and APTT) are within normal limits.

**K**      TRUE – all hospitalised patients should be treated with TED stockings and LMWH if there are no contraindications. Acute risk of bleeding and coagulopathy, eg DIC, will exclude the use of LMWH, but most patients should wear TED stockings. This patient has a very high risk of VTE disease because of his/her hyperosmolar state and, despite the haemolysis, LMWH should be given. In complex cases like this, one should seek the views of the haematologists before committing the patient to 24 h of anticoagulation with LMWH.

**L**      FALSE – this patient has a metabolic acidosis, as evidenced by the low bicarbonate, negative base excess and raised lactate. The PaCO$_2$ 4.1 KPa indicates some hyperventilation, either as a result of compensation, or more likely as a result of the underlying respiratory condition.

SCENARIO 11

**M**      TRUE – metformin should be stopped on admission in any diabetic patient with a significant metabolic acidosis. Metformin potentiates lactic acidosis, and this in turn is potentiated by failure to excrete metformin in severe AKI.

**N**      FALSE – this set of data is consistent with a patient suffering with hyperosmolar, hyperglycaemic syndrome (HHS). The patient is acidotic, but this is most likely as a result of the lactic acidodis present. Urinary or serum ketones need to be measured in all such cases, but they are rarely raised to sufficient levels to be considered DKA.

## GLOBAL DATA INTERPRETATION MARK

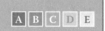

A B C D E

## Station 5 – Prescribing skills

**1**  **A**  False – community-acquired pneumonia (CAP) should be treated with an anti-streptococcal agent, eg amoxicillin or Augmentin, or levofloxacin, and an agent to cover haemophilus and atypicals, such as mycoplasma and chlamydia, eg a macrolide. Thus in the UK the first-line therapy should be amoxicillin and clarithromycin or levofloxacin and clarithromycin.

     **B**  False – Tazocin (piperacillin and tazobactam) is an anti-pseudomonal agent, reserved for serious Gram-negative, hospital-acquired infections. It should not be given to patients with penicillin allergy (as in this case), nor as a first-line agent in minor sepsis or in community-acquired respiratory infection.

     **C**  False – Tazocin is only manufactured as an intravenous preparation; this is written as an oral medication and therefore cannot be administered.

     **D**  False – clarithromycin is a macrolide that is normally given as a twice-daily preparation of 500 mg, either intravenously or as tablets. Only with an eGFR <30 ml/min the dose should be halved.

     **E**  False – giving a stat dose of long-acting insulin is recommended only for diabetic patients who are admitted with DKA or HHS already on a regular dose of long-acting insulin.

**2**  **A**  False – once a severe drug-associated allergy has been identified by a patient, relative or carer, then the drug should be stopped, even it has been given with no adverse effect.

     **B**  True – this prescription for Tazocin is wrong on several levels. The maximum dose is 4.5 g three times daily, reduced to 4.5 g twice daily in severe AKI (eGFR < 20 ml/min). The route of administration is also incorrect.

     **C**  False – clarithromycin is a twice-a-day medication (see above).

3  **A**  False – neither metformin nor sitagliptin should be given while the patient is on an intravenous insulin infusion. Both should be crossed through for the next 72 h, and 'not while on insulin infusion' written in the instruction box. Metformin should not be given with lactic acidosis and/or significant AKI.

    **B**  False – sitagliptin is written as a twice-a-day regime when it should be 100 mg once per day. It also should not be given with the insulin infusion.

    **C**  False – ramipril should be crossed through for 48–72 h until such time as the AKI has resolved. Hypotension is another contraindication common when patients are this unwell and dehydrated.

    **D**  False – statins should be given as an evening dose, not with breakfast. Theoretically, synthesis of cholesterol increases in the absence of dietary cholesterol, ie at night.

4  **A**  False – the prescriber has mistakenly written it up as 600 mg @ 4 hourly; the maximum dose is 600 mg @ 6 hourly, ie 2.4 g in 24 h.

    **B**  True – paracetamol may be given 0.5–1g @ 6 hourly, ie maximum of 4 g per 24 h.

    **C**  True – this is 'technically' true but should be regarded as nonsensical. The metoclopramide has been written as an oral preparation (used in unexplained nausea) but tablets will be redundant if the patient is actually vomiting. Anti-emetics should be written as subcutaneous, intravenous or intramuscular routes of administration.

    **D**  False – this is perhaps the most dangerous mistake on this chart. The prescriber has boarded Oramorph at 1000 times the normal dose. Opiates are commonly prescribed in milligrams; this prescription is for 10 g.

5  **A**  True – this patient is severely dehydrated and requires a minimum of 5–6 litres in the first 24 h. The rate may be increased or reduced depending on the patient's clinical response, as assessed by their blood pressure, heart rate and urine output.

    **B**  False – this is wrong on several levels:
      (a) Dextrose should be avoided in hyperglycaemic patients!
      (b) Dextrose contains NO sodium and so will precipitate a huge, rapid fall in serum sodium levels. This risks cerebral oedema and central pontine myelinolysis.

    **C**  True – hyperglycaemic patients receiving an intravenous insulin infusion require potassium supplementation of 20 mmol/l with each litre of fluid if their serum potassium is within normal limits. It may be necessary to give them 40 mmol/l if their potassium drops to sub-normal levels.

    **D**  False – the FRIVII is written to be set at 0.1 unit/kg/h. There are 50 units of actrapid insulin in 50 ml of 0.45% saline (this should be 0.9% saline), so there is 1 unit/ml. The patient weighs 81.5 kg, so the pump should be set at $81.5 \times 0.1 = 8.2$ ml/h.

**GLOBAL PRESCRIBING MARK**

# Scenario 11: Reflection and consolidation

## History

Mr Adam Bellows is a 53-year-old man who is attending the surgery this morning for his annual diabetes review.

He was originally diagnosed with type 2 diabetes mellitus 7 years ago (just after his 46th birthday) having been non-specifically unwell for several months. He describes feeling tired and listless and generally 'quite awful'. His weight had increased from his normal 12 and a half stone (80 kg) to about 15 stone (95 kg), and he was eating a very poor diet as he was having to visit his sick mother. He also admits to a lot of stress at work during this period. His GP diagnosed him as having hypertension and type 2 diabetes and he was placed on a weight reduction and exercise programme, and treated with several tablets including ramipril, simvastatin and metformin.

Since then he has felt 'better and better'; he has lost weight, stopped smoking and now goes swimming and dancing with his wife two to three times a week, as well as playing golf one to two times a week.

Mr Bellows sees the GP team at least twice a year and has so far not had any major problems. He monitors his own sugars once or twice a week by fingerprick testing, and the results usually show between 5 and 8 (very occasionally about 10 or 11). His last HbA1C was 5.9%. He has not suffered any major diabetic complications and has never been admitted to hospital with any serious illnesses or problems arising from his diabetes.

He apparently has no symptoms of macro- or microvascular, neurological complications; he has good foot health – no trauma or ulcers.

In his own words, 'he is now looking after himself and feeling much better for it'.

Of note is his CV risk:

- He is an ex-smoker, having given up at diagnosis; he previously smoked 20 cigarettes/day for 25 years; but still has the occasional cigar at a golf club dinner
- Alcohol – 1–2 glasses of red wine with most evening meals; never during the day; occasional brandy or scotch at the golf club
- Cholesterol – now on simvastatin; last check his cholesterol was 5.1.
- Blood pressure – previously 'very high' – now on ramipril usually between 120 and 130/70 or so
- Diet – has a healthy diet and has lost more than 10 kg in weight; today his weight was 78 kg and height 1.81 m (BMI 24 kg/m²)

Diabetes complications:

- Eyes – he wears glasses for reading, watching TV and driving but has had no new visual symptoms
- Hands and feet – no funny feelings (tingling or numbness); no ulcers
- Kidneys – last year was fine; urinalysis today – NAD
- Macrovascular disease – no symptoms of angina, heart failure, no stroke/TIA, no claudication
- Drug and allergy history – presently on ramipril 5 mg od, metformin 500 mg bd, simvastatin 20 mg od and sitagliptin 100 mg od; he is allergic to penicillin, which causes a severe rash
- Social history – he is a business manager in a large IT firm; he is married (his wife is a retired professional dancer) and has 2 children, both at university.

## Examination

Assessment of a patient with a long-term condition involves assessing the stability or progression of the condition, and assessing for long-term complications, associated disability and associated exacerbating factors.

For diabetic patients, this involves a sophisticated holistic assessment, including assessment of:

- Eyes – especially evidence of retinopathy and reduced visual acuity
- Cardiovascular disease – excluding evidence of cardiac dysfunction, central and peripheral vascular disease, hypertension and stigmata of hyperlipidaemia; cigarette smoking may be evidenced by tar staining of fingers
- Neurological complications – including peripheral sensory neuropathy
- Foot care (this is why it's essential to take off the patient's shoes and socks) – assessing for signs of PVD, trauma and neuropathy, and excluding ulcers.

At such reviews patients also require urinalysis to exclude microalbuminuria (a sign of microvascular disease) and weight/height (to assess for BMI).

## Data interpretation

In the latter part of this scenario Mr Bellows has been admitted to hospital with hyperglycaemic, hyperosmolar syndrome (HHS). His blood tests support a diagnosis of HHS secondary to an atypical pneumonia and AKI.

Other investigations that may prove to be useful in such cases include atypical antibody and antigen testing, blood and sputum cultures (although unlikely to culture 'atypical' microbes), ABG including lactate levels, CXR; and in middle-aged patients an ECG might be helpful (such severe stress may precipitate cardiac ischaemia and in less clear-cut cases may be the original clinical precipitant).

## Management

The initial management of such an acutely unwell patient will include:

- Nurse in high-dependency area
- Cardiac monitoring and regular observations
- Intravenous access and rapid rehydration with appropriate fluids (0.9% saline or Hartmann's solution), to include appropriate supplementation of potassium
- Fixed rate intravenous insulin infusion
- Intravenous antibiotics – levofloxacin and clarithromycin (can't have penicillin).

Once he is improving and eating and drinking again, Mr Bellows should be converted back to his regular oral hypoglycaemics. He should be reviewed by the diabetes nurse specialist to ensure compliance and full understanding of his condition.

**Further reading and web links**

http://www.nice.org.uk/nicemedia/live/11983/40803/40803.pdf

NICE guidelines on the management of type 2 diabetes

Vidyarthi M, Chowdhury TA. Diagnosis and early management of hyperglycaemic emergencies in the emergency department. QJM 2012; 105: 296-7.

http://emedicine.medscape.com/article/1914705-overview

# Scenario 12: 'All fall down'

## Station 1

*History*                                                  *10-minute station*

You are the FY1 on the Medical Admissions Unit (MAU). The next patient is Mrs Ravneeta Singh (DOB 27/01/31 – 81 years old) who has been brought into the Emergency Department having 'collapsed' this morning in the local supermarket.

■ Please take a focussed, diagnostic history with a view to presenting it to the MAU Consultant.

*You will be assessed on the following areas, as well as the content and diagnostic reasoning of your history – take them into account in your presentation.*

### Professionalism

- Professional appearance (NHS dress code) – including general appearance, hair and jewellery
- Maintains patient and personal safety
- Polite introduction; identifies patient or interviewee correctly; confirms patient's date of birth from name band or other source
- Obtains informal consent; maintains patient's privacy
- Displays empathetic and caring attitudes and behaviours throughout.

### Process

- Good organisation and structure; appropriate use of open and closed questions
- Appropriate fluency/rhythm/pace to the interview – this may change depending on environment and acute nature of the problem
- Appropriate time for the patient to respond/reply to questions
- Appropriate acknowledgement of difficult or emotional areas of the patient's history.

### Communication skills

- Demonstrates caring and sympathetic attitude
- Asks open questions
- Invites patient to ask questions and answers them appropriately
- Addresses patient's ideas, concerns and expectations.

## Station 2

*Examination*                    *10-minute station*

After presenting your history to the Consultant she asks you to perform a focussed, diagnostic assessment of Mrs Singh.

■ **Please make an appropriate clinical assessment of the patient with a view to confirming your diagnosis.**

**(If you do not have a model, please read and present the information given on page 386.)**

*You will be assessed on the following areas, as well as the content and skills of your examination – take them into account in your presentation.*

### Professionalism

- Professional appearance; maintains infection control standards, including hand cleaning and appropriate use of gloves and aprons
- Maintains patient and personal safety
- Polite introduction; identifies patient and confirms date of birth from name band or other source
- Obtains informal consent; maintains patient privacy and dignity
- Displays empathetic and caring attitudes and behaviours throughout.

### Process

- Appropriate fluency/rhythm/pace to the examination – this may change depending on environment and acute nature of the problem
- Organisation and structure of examination; sensitive and empathetic approach
- Uses appropriate clinical techniques throughout
- Maintains privacy and dignity throughout.

### Clinical communication

- Explains proposed examination/procedure: explains examination/procedure as it proceeds
- Offers information in a clear, structured and fluent manner, avoiding jargon
- Listens to patient and responds appropriately
- Demonstrates appropriate body language.

## Station 3

*Data interpretation*                    *10-minute station*

The MAU Consultant shows you Mrs Singh's ECG rhythm strip and the rhythm strips of several other recent admissions to the MAU.

- Please answer the questions below regarding each of the rhythm strips.

1       With regard to Mrs Singh's presentation:
  - A   What is the rhythm shown in this rhythm strip?
  - B   List three likely causes of this rhythm.
  - C   What is the definitive treatment for Mrs Singh?

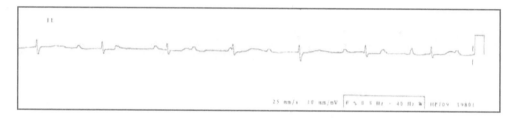

2   This is the rhythm strip of a 67-year-old man with known ischaemic heart disease (IHD) who was brought in by ambulance peri-arrest after collapsing at a friend's 65th birthday party.
  - A   What is the cardiac rhythm shown in this rhythm strip?
  - B   What is the likely cause of this rhythm?
  - C   What other exacerbating factors may be important in such cases?

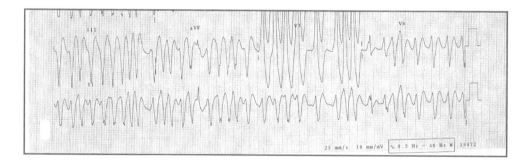

SCENARIO 12

3 This is the rhythm strip of a 78-year-old man with known IHD who was brought in by ambulance after falling off his grandson's skateboard, sustaining a suspected Colles' fracture to his right wrist.
   A What is the cardiac rhythm shown in this rhythm strip?
   B List the likely causes of this rhythm.
   C List three sinister symptoms that may convince you that this was not a 'simple accident'.

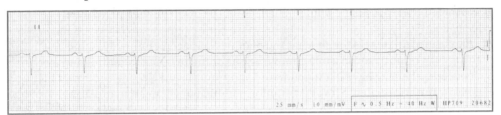

SCENARIO 12

4 This is the rhythm strip of a previously fit and well 73-year-old woman who was brought into hospital after being involved in a road traffic accident. She was a passenger in the front seat of a car hit side on by another car, after the other driver 'jumped the lights'.
   A What is the cardiac rhythm shown in this rhythm strip?
   B List three likely causes of this rhythm.
   C The patient is well after the accident, haemodynamically stable, and denies any associated cardiovascular or neurological symptoms. What would be your next management step?

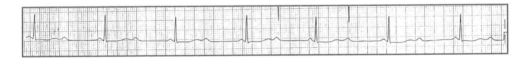

5 This is the rhythm strip of a 24-year-old woman who on examination appears to have clubbing of the fingernails, sweaty palms, palmar erythema, proximal limb weakness and a rash over both shins.
   A What is the cardiac rhythm shown in this rhythm strip?
   B What is the likely cause of this rhythm?
   C List three other possible causes of this rhythm.

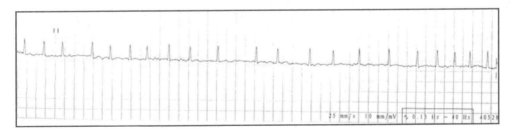

## Station 4

*Clinical communication skills*          *10-minute station*

You have an additional 5-minute preparation time to read the following information sheet and prepare your discussion.

It is decided that Mrs Singh would benefit from the insertion of a permanent pacemaker.

■ Please explain to Mrs Singh what the planned management involves, the alternatives, and any possible complications of the procedure, addressing any concerns she may have. First you have 5 minutes to read the patient leaflet below, which runs through the important information you will need to explain.

## Patient Information Regarding Permanent Pacemaker Insertion
## United Hospitals NHS Trust

### Normal electrical activity of the heart

The heart beat is normally maintained by an electrical circuit that runs from the smaller chambers (the atria) down through the larger chambers (ventricles). This electrical circuit starts at a special point at the top called the 'sino-atrial node' and runs down through a second special point called the atrio-ventricular node.

### Why you need a pacemaker

Unfortunately the electrical circuit in your heart has stopped working properly. This is causing your heart to beat too slowly, and this is most likely due to one of the special points (the nodes) not working properly.

### What is a pacemaker?

The pacemaker is a battery or generator connected to your heart by a series of small electrical cables (leads). This system bypasses your own electrical circuit and keeps the heart running smoothly and beating appropriately. The leads sense the heart beat and electrical activity and send electrical impulses to your heart. The battery is encased in a thin metal case and is the size of a book of matches, approximately 2.5 × 2.5cm and about 3–4 mm thick. The battery lasts for about 8–10 years before it needs changing.

### How is the procedure performed?

You will need to fast overnight (nothing to eat or drink from midnight before the procedure) and present yourself to the cardiology suite on the third floor of the Chest Centre, Frissley Park Road entrance (you may be brought here by ambulance if coming from one of the local hospitals or on pre-arranged transport).

You will be asked to put on a hospital gown, and a small needle (cannula) will be placed in the back of one of your hands. This is to allow us to give you medications if, and when, required. You will be told what time your procedure is and we will do our best to keep to this schedule; you will be told if anything delays your procedure (very rarely (less than 2% of procedures)) we may have to postpone your procedure until another day.

The procedure takes about 60–90 minutes; you will be taken down to the Cardiology Suite, where you will be met by your cardiologist (heart doctor) and the nursing team. They will give you an injection through the needle in your hand that will make you feel drowsy but will not put you to sleep. You will be placed on a special X-ray bed with a large camera above it, and a screen next to it; the top of your chest will be cleaned with a cold solution and then an area of about 2.5–5 cm will be injected with local anaesthetic (this is cold and initially stings a bit). The cardiologist will then identify an appropriate vein and will feed the leads of the pacemaker into your heart, guided by the camera. The leads are then connected to the battery casing and this is slotted under your skin, through the cut made in the top of your chest. The cardiologist will check the pacemaker is working correctly, and will then sew the battery in place. You will be left with a clean dressing over the site. You will be returned to the recovery area and allowed to go home or back to your original hospital normally within 6–8 hours.

### Common complications

You will experience mild to moderate pain at the site of the cut for the first few days after the procedure; you will be given painkillers to take during this period. The site is infiltrated with an antibiotic but simple infections (shown by the area becoming hot and red, excessive pain and/ or discharge) may occur – if this happens you will need to see your local doctor.

### Bleeding

There may be a small amount of bleeding associated with the pacemaker site; if you experience a large amount of bleeding or swelling below the skin, you should present yourself quickly to an emergency department, applying pressure with a towel or similar to the site.

### General advice

You should limit your use of the left arm for at least 4 weeks – no heavy lifting, pulling or pushing, and no activities such as swimming. Do not get the site wet for 7–10 days, and do not drive a motor vehicle until you have had your pacemaker checked and are given the OK by your doctor. Please ask if you have any other questions.

SCENARIO 12

## Station 5

*Prescribing skills*                    *10-minute station*

Mrs Singh is admitted to the day surgery unit at her local cardiac centre, where she has a pacemaker inserted under local anaesthetic. The procedure goes well and without complication, and it is decided that Mrs Singh should be discharged home to her family's care. You are the Cardiology FY1 and have been asked to write up the discharge summary (TTA) for Mrs Singh.

■ From the details you have gathered in the case so far, the details below and Mrs Singh's listed regular medications please write a TTA to the GP and referring consultant at the local general hospital.

### Details

- o Mrs Ravneeta Singh, DOB 27/01/1931, Hospital no. C2214533, Ward: CCU, Consultant: Dr Archibold
- o Admitted 23/03/2012, Discharge date: 30/03/2012
- o Medications:
- o Prednisolone 10 mg od for 5/7, reduce by 2 mg per day until back to normal dose over following 4 weeks
- o Thyroxine 125 μm od
- o AdcalD3 two tablets per day
- o Citalopram 20 mg od.

---

**Remember: DRUG DRs Don't Forget Signing Off** (page 396)

---

| GP<br>Name:<br>Address: | Date of Discharge<br>NHS No.<br>Hospital No.<br>DOB<br>Age (Years)<br>Gender | Patient Name<br><br>Address<br><br><br><br>Tel No: |
|---|---|---|
| Consultant at discharge: | | |
| Admission date: | Ward | |

| Acute Problem(s) | Chronic Problem(s) |
|---|---|
| | |

**Clinical presentation**

**Significant investigation / results**

**Clinical course**

**Drugs on Discharge**

| Medication | Dose | Frequecy | No. of days | To continue |
|---|---|---|---|---|
| | | | | |
| | | | | |
| | | | | |
| | | | | |
| | | | | |

Verified by pharmacist:   YES    NO

**Specific Follow up / Advice:**

Form completed by:

Date

Bleep No.

# Answers

## Station 1 – History

**Patient script**

You are Mrs Ravneeta Singh (DOB 27 January 1931 – 81 years old), a retired bank clerk who now lives with her oldest son and his family. Your husband of 63 years died last year and it has been a very traumatic and difficult year for you.

During this period of mourning you started to suffer 'funny turns' and episodes of collapse. Initially you thought it was due to the fact that you weren't eating very much, but they have persisted and even worsened despite your appetite and weight improving over the last few months.

The episodes started about 3 months ago. The first was in the garden of your son's house whilst you were hanging out the washing with your daughter-in-law. Without warning you suddenly felt very dizzy and came over 'all cold and sweaty' – you think you blacked out, because the next you thing remember is lying on the grass with your daughter-in-law trying to make sure you were OK. You do not remember any palpitations, chest pain or shortness of breath, and there were no pre-warning symptoms.

According to your daughter-in-law, the whole episode lasted about 5 minutes and you were conscious but 'groggy' for a few minutes after you fell to the floor. Once awake you could understand everything people were saying to you, and you were able to speak normally. There were no problems with your limbs (no weakness or pins and needles) and no features to suggest you had a seizure, although your daughter-in-law didn't specifically mention any shaking of your limbs. Your granddaughter brought you a glass of water and soon after you felt fine and was able to help with the preparation of the evening meal. Your family wanted to take you to hospital but you wouldn't hear of it.

The second episode (about 6 weeks later) was whilst getting ready for bed, and you hid this from your family as you didn't want to worry them. You were sitting on the side of the bath washing your face, when again, without warning, you suddenly felt very dizzy and 'sweaty' – 'like I was going to pass out'. Very similar to the previous episode – no specific cardiovascular or neurological symptoms, but you think you blacked out again, because you fell back into the bath, which fortunately was empty, and this cushioned your fall.

SCENARIO 12

You were woken by your grandson trying to use the bathroom but told him to wait a minute. You felt groggy and disorientated for a few more minutes but once this resolved you were able to get back to your bed without any help and immediately went to sleep. When you woke in the morning you were back to your normal self.

The episode today – you were out shopping with your granddaughter at the local supermarket. You were standing talking to her in the checkout queue, when the exact same thing happened. You had no warning but suddenly felt weak and unwell and according to your granddaughter and the checkout woman, you 'lost all your colour', 'became vacant and sweaty' and then collapsed to the floor. You were unconscious for a good few minutes and then slowly came around. There were no features of a seizure or any other neurological symptoms. You did not have any chest pains, palpitations or shortness of breath. Despite you feeling much better after about 10 minutes, the store manager had already called an ambulance and they insisted on bringing you here for a 'check-up'.

Otherwise you are very well, with no major health concerns at the present.

Cardiovascular risk – type 2 diabetes mellitus (T2DM) – dietary controlled; they check your sugars occasionally when you're at the GP surgery – 'usually 5–6'; no history of IHD, stroke or peripheral vascular disease (PVD), no high blood pressure; cholesterol – 'fine'; checked when I was diagnosed with diabetes; lifelong non-smoker, no alcohol.

Family history – father died in World War II; mother died in 'old age' (well over 90); two brothers (oldest died of bowel cancer aged 67 years old, younger still alive but has dementia).

Other medical problems – treated hypothyroidism (many years); polymyalgia rheumatica (PMR) (on steroids for 2 years); depression (after husband died).

Meds – citalopram 20 mg od, prednisolone 2 mg od, AdcalD3 2 tablets per day, thyroxine 125 µg od.

Allergies – nil known.

Social history – independent of activities of daily living (ADLs); occupation – retired bank clerk; 'won a scholarship to university in India but father wouldn't let me go'; married the next year. Came to UK in 1963, husband (local GP) got a job here. He retired in 1992. Three children – live with oldest son (lawyer) and his family; younger son lives in USA (NY state); daughter is married and lives nearby.

Ideas – 'I don't really know what are causing the funny turns but I'm worried they are serious.'

Concerns – 'Could be mini strokes or heart problems I suppose – I'm at that age aren't I?'

Expectations – 'I would hope you can give me something simple like aspirin to get rid of them.'

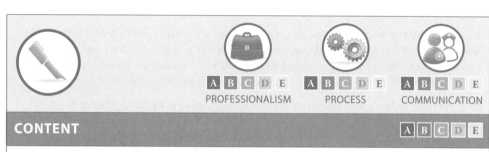

PROFESSIONALISM    PROCESS    COMMUNICATION

## CONTENT
A B C D E

**Identifies key information**
- Husband's death and prolonged period of mourning and depression
- History of presenting complaint
  - Onset; frequency of episodes
  - Characterises episodes – pre- (warning), intra- and post-collapse symptoms
  - Associated symptoms
  - Duration and time to complete resolution
  - Specifically asks about cardiac and neurological symptoms, including features of seizure.
- Cardiovascular risk including – IHD, stroke, PVD, DM, hypertension, smoking, alcohol, lipids
- Other exacerbating factors, eg medications – new or recent change in meds.

**Past medical history:** type 2 diabetes mellitus; hypoglycaemia; PMR; depression

**Completing the patient history**
- Drug and allergy history – prednisolone 2.5 mg od, adcal D3 two tablets per day, citalopram 20 mg od, thyroxine 125µg od; no known drug allergies
- Social and occupational history – ADLs, home; children, occupation.

**Summarises important areas of the history back to the patient**

**Invites patient to ask questions and deals with them appropriately**

**Establishes patient's ideas, concerns and expectations**

SCENARIO 12

## CLINICAL DIAGNOSTIC REASONING

- **Please present your history**
  - Candidate offers a logical, well-structured account of the history.

- **What is your diagnosis?**
  - This is a typical, relatively non-specific history of collapse in an older person. The most likely diagnosis from the history is probably cardiac arrhythmia (either tachy or brady arrhythmia, or indeed both (Tachy–brady syndrome)), but other possible causes should be considered, eg postural hypotension, with or without bradycardia
  - Neurological causes, eg transient ischaemic attacks or seizures are unlikely given the lack of supporting symptoms and the short recovery period but should be excluded by further investigation.

**Demonstrates safe, sensible and appropriate management plan**

**Demonstrates clear and logical diagnostic reasoning**

## GLOBAL HISTORY MARK

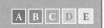

# Station 2 – Examination

**Patient script (see also page 386)**

You are a relatively fit and well 81-year-old woman who collapsed today in the supermarket. You are now feeling back to normal and are happy to cooperate with the young doctor's examination. You are slightly slow but able to do all the activities the doctor asks of you.

**SCENARIO 12**

A B **C** D E
PROFESSIONALISM

A B **C** D E
PROCESS

A B **C** D E
COMMUNICATION

## CONTENT

A B **C** D E

**Exposes and positions patient correctly and maintains comfort**

**Comments on wellbeing of patient, ie well or unwell**

**'Feet to face'**
- Observes and comments on patient and surroundings from foot of bed
- Evidence of obvious neurological deficit; mobility aids
- **A**VPU – Alert; AMTS = 10/10.

**Asks for appropriate/relevant clinical observations**
- HR 46 bpm, BP 122/73 mmHg, RR 14 bpm, $O_2$ sats 95% on air, temperature 36.4 °C, CBG 4.9 mmol/l

**General examination – including thyroid status**
- General examination – well, euthyroid; no signs of jaundice, anaemia, clubbing, cyanosis, oedema or lymphadenopathy

**Focussed examination**
- Pulse – rate and regularity; BP – lying/ sitting and standing (2 minutes)
- JVP and carotid pulse – including comment on character
- Auscultation
- Comments on signs of heart failure including chest crackles, pleural effusions and peripheral oedema
- Respiratory examination – specifically comments on chest crackles, pleural effusions
- Abdominal examination – assesses for organomegaly and masses but specifically comments on hepatomegaly and ascites (right heart failure)
- Neurological assessment – CNs I – XII (right and left); cerebellar assessment; PNS: upper and lower limbs – bulk/tone/power /coordination/reflexes/plantars; Romberg's test; gait.

**Thanks patient, offers assistance, maintains patient's dignity and privacy until they are dressed**

SCENARIO 12

## CLINICAL DIAGNOSTIC REASONING

A B C D E

**Correctly identifies the relevant physical signs, including important negative findings**

■ **Could you tell me five blood tests and five further investigations that you would organise for this patient, with a reason for each?**
  • Clinical tests – blood sugar, lying and standing blood pressure
  • Blood tests
    • FBC – Hb/MCV, anaemia/WCC and differential, lymphomas and leukaemias, incidental findings contributing to the collapses
    • U&Es – Na$^+$: (hyponatraemia, secondary to SSRI); K$^+$: hyper and hypo K$^+$ may promote arrhythmia; urea/creatinine: renal impairment may contribute to falls
    • RBG/HbA-1C – glycaemic control
    • Calcium and magnesium – hypocalcaemia and hypomagnesaemia promote prolonged QT syndrome
    • TFTs – known treated hypothyroidism (? over- or undertreated leading to arrhythmia)
  • Radiology
    • CXR – excludes underlying cardiac disease; incidental lesions, eg malignancy
    • CT head scan – excludes stroke disease
  • Cardiac investigation – 12-lead ECG; 24-hour tape; tilt table testing if others are unremarkable.

**Demonstrates safe, sensible and appropriate management plan**

**Demonstrates clear and logical diagnostic reasoning**

## GLOBAL EXAMINATION MARK

A B C D E

## Station 3 – Data interpretation

1

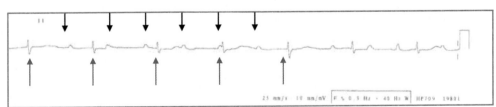

SCENARIO 12

A   The rhythm strip confirms that Mrs Singh has gone into third-degree or complete heart block. There is AV dissociation, as evidenced by the lack of association between the P waves (black arrows) and the QRS complexes (red arrows). There is a narrow escape rhythm, implying that the ventricular depolarisation originates from high in the bundle of His, leading to relatively normal depolarisation and ventricular contraction. Thus the patient is haemodynamically stable.

B   There are four generic causes of everything on the ECG – IHD, drugs, conduction system fibrosis and congenital heart disease. Given this patient's history, this may be due to conduction system disease, silent IHD or even congenital heart block, which may present in older asymptomatic patients, even in their very old age.

C   Given her presentation she requires a permanent pacemaker.

2

A   This is a broad complex tachycardia, most probably ventricular tachycardia (VT).

B   Given the patient's age (over 65), his history of IHD and his presentation, the most likely cause is IHD or possible conduction system disease following a myocardial infarction (MI).

C   Structural abnormalities of the heart (HOCM), drugs that prolong the QT interval (amiodarone, sotalol, haloperidol, venlafaxine and macrolide antibiotics) – digoxin is said to be able to cause all arrhythmia, especially in toxicity – and electrolyte disturbances (hypokalaemia, hypocalcaemia and hypomagnesaemia) may exacerbate or cause this and other tachyarrhythmia.

3

A   The rhythm strip shows sinus bradycardia (HR 55 bpm).

B   The patient has IHD so the probable cause is one of his medications, eg a beta blocker or calcium channel blocker, but this is excluded if he is not taking any rate-limiting medications.

C   Despite the relatively innocent presentation of this active older man, you need to exclude sinister causes of his fall. Sinister symptoms would include: pre-warning symptoms; chest pain; palpitations; loss of consciousness; feeling sweaty, clammy or nauseated; previous episodes of falls; or loss of consciousness.

SCENARIO 12

4

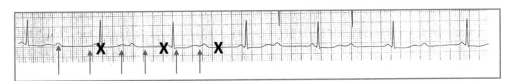

A   This is second-degree heart block with a 2 : 1 pattern. The strip shows P-QRS, P wave, no QRS, P-QRS, P wave no QRS (shown by the arrows and the crosses).

B   As with all arrhythmia, the causes include IHD (silent ischaemia may well be the cause in a trauma patient such as this), drugs, conduction system disease and congenital disease (unlikely in this case).

C   Second-degree heart block (both Mobitz type 1 and 2) can progress to third-degree heart block and haemodynamic collapse. Given the patient's trauma and the arrhythmia she should probably be admitted at least overnight and reviewed by a cardiologist. If her 12-lead ECG and tropinin are unremarkable after 24 hours and she remains haemodynamically stable she should be discharged with a 24 hour-tape and cardiology follow-up should be arranged.

5

A   The strip demonstrates fast atrial fibrillation, with a HR of 75 (slowest) – 200 (fastest) bpm.

B   This patient has several signs of thyrotoxicosis.

C   Cardiac causes – pericardial: pericarditis; myocardial: IHD and causes of cardiomyopathy; endocardial: mitral valve disease, conduction system disease. Extra-cardiac causes – pulmonary: pulmonary embolism, pneumonia, chronic obstructive pulmonary disease (cor pulmonale), severe sepsis or multi-organ failure.

**GLOBAL DATA INTERPRETATION MARK**

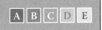

SCENARIO 12

## Station 4 – Clinical communication skills

**Patient script**

You are Mrs Ravneeta Singh, an 81-year-old Asian woman who was admitted last night after a collapse in a supermarket. You have met the junior doctor in the Emergency Department and are happy to talk to him or her.

What you've been told so far – 'I was told by the doctor last night that the electrics of my heart aren't working properly and may need a pacemaker'; 'To be honest I didn't really understand what she was talking about.'

Ideas – 'I know what a pacemaker is (my husband was a GP for 35 years) but I don't know much about how they work or how they are inserted into the heart.'

Concerns – 'I am worried that I won't be able to enjoy my grandchildren and lead a normal life if I have to rely on this pacemaker.'

Expectations – 'Not really sure what is happening or what will happen next but I really hope that this will stop these horrible funny turns.'

Questions you'd like to ask the doctor:

1 'Will this stop me helping my daughter-in-law around the house? – I don't want to be a burden to her.'

2 'It all sounds a bit of a fuss – aren't there any other alternatives, like medicines?'

3 'How long before it will need changing?'

SCENARIO 12

A B C D E
PROFESSIONALISM

A B C D E
PROCESS

## CONTENT

A B C D E

**Confirms reason for discussion**
- To talk to Mrs Singh about the investigation results, the need for a pacemaker and to answer any questions she may have.

**Establishes what patient wishes to know; gains agreement/informal consent to participate in the discussion**

**Investigates patient's present level of understanding of scenario**

**Summarises and confirms what has happened so far**

**Establishes patient's ideas, concerns and expectations**

**Explains the key, important information**
- The normal function of the conduction system of the heart
- The diagnosis – complete heart block: 'faulty electrics of the heart' causing the heart to beat too slowly
- Explains the management – insertion of a permanent pacemaker; explains no medication alternative
- Explains the procedure – avoids medical jargon, or explains appropriately when used
- Explains common complications – pain, infection and bleeding
- Gives general advice – activities to avoid, asks about driving, exercise, eg swimming.

**Invites patient to ask questions and is able to deal with them appropriately**

**Summarises important areas of the consultation back to the patient**

**Formally ends the consultation and ensures appropriate follow-up has been discussed**

SCENARIO 12

## GLOBAL COMMUNICATION MARK

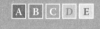
A B C D E

# Station 5 – Prescribing skills

**DISHARGE SUMMARY**      **PATIENT NAME:** Ravneeta Singh
THE CHEST CENTRE – HARLINGTON NHS TRUST
Discharge Information Summary

| GP | Date of Discharge: 30.03.12 | Patient Name |
|---|---|---|
| **Name:** Dr D.A. Gould | **NHS No:** 401-223-59223 | Ravneeta Singh |
| **Address:** The Surgery, | **Hospital No.** C2214533 | **Address** |
| 23, Bishop Avenue, | **DOB:** 27.01.31 | 6, The Drive, |
| Harlington, | **Age (Years):** 81 | Lower Harlington, |
| HE34-6LX | **Gender** FEMALE | HR21-9QT |
| | | **Tel No:**0612-344-8976 |

| Consultant at discharge: Dr Archibold | |
|---|---|

| Admission date: 23.03.12 | Ward: CCU | |
|---|---|---|

| Acute Problem(s) | Chronic Problem(s) |
|---|---|
| Collapse secondary to CHB – requiring insertion of PPM | Polymyalgia Rheumatica<br>Depression<br>Dietary controlled type 2 Diabetes<br>Treated hypothyroidism |

**Clinical presentation**

3-month history of episodes of collapse; First about 3-months ago whilst hanging out washing; second whilst sitting on edge of bath getting ready for bed. Third on day of admission – out shopping, standing at checkout – suddenly sweaty, unwell, 'lost all her colour', collapsed to the floor. Loss of consciousness for several minutes. Brought to emergency department where she was found to be in complete heart block (CHB)

**Significant investigation / results**

ECG on arrival – Complete heart block
Blood tests including FBC, U&Es, Glucose, Clotting, TFTs – all within normal limits
CXR – nil of note

**Clinical course**

On arrival HR 46bpm, BP 122/73 (lying = standing). ECG showed CHB
Admitted to CCU where she remained haemodynamically stable in CHB.
Transferred to Harlington Chest centre 30.03.12 for day care insertion of permanent pacemaker. (Discharge summary of procedure to be sent on)

SCENARIO 12

**Drugs on Discharge**

| Medication | Dose | Frequecy | No. of days | To con- tinue |
|---|---|---|---|---|
| Citalopram | 20mg | Once a day | 14 | YES |
| Thyroxine | 125mcg | Once a day | 14 | YES |
| Adcal D3 | T | Twice a day | 14 | YES |
| Prednisolone | 10mg | Once a day | 5 | YES |
| Prednisolone | 8mg - Reducing by 2mg per week until back to normal dose (2mg od) | Once a day | 7 | YES |
| **Verified by pharmacist:  YES   NO** | | | | |

**Specific Follow up / Advice:**
Dressing to be kept dry for 5 days
Sutures to be removed at day 5 by district nurses
Follow up: **Cardiology outpatient clinic – 28.05.12; Pacemaker check – BOOKED 28.05.12**

**Form completed by:** Dr Adam Feather                    **Bleep No.** 007
**Date** 30.03.12

**NOTE REGARDING TTA/TTOs**

The 'To Take Away' (TTA) or 'To Take Out' (TTO) is now a computer based form in most hospitals which makes them a lot easier to standardise and complete. They form an essential part of the FY1 / FY2's daily clerical duties but due to time pressures they are often sadly lost in the 'daily grind', especially when there are multiple TTAs to write.
They have several key roles including:
- Forms the essential communication between the hospital, the community teams, the patient and their carers.
- An essential record for future admitting teams to review – this is important in all patients but espe- cially those with long term conditions or recurrent admissions.
- Gives the doctor completing the TTA time to review the case and pull all the key diagnostic features together; this part of the TTA is often undervalued by junior doctors but is the way they start to develop their own methods of diagnostic reasoning.
- As well as diagnostic reasoning juniors also learn the art of therapeutics including monitoring, dos- ing, and review.
Like so much of the junior doctor's role this has major educational and training value and yet is poorly taught and poorly practised until graduation. We would recommend that you try to complete multiple TTAs during your clinical training. This helps the clinical team and gives you valuable insight into the skills and knowledge you will need as a FY1.

**GLOBAL PRESCRIBING MARK**

A B C D E

# Scenario 12: Reflection and consolidation

## History

Mrs Ravneeta Singh is a relatively fit and well 81-year-old woman who was brought to the Emergency Department today after collapsing whilst out shopping.

Of note she has had a very traumatic year. She lost her husband of 63 years, who died at the start of the year, and as a result became quite depressed, requiring treatment.

She now presents with a 3-month history of 3× episodes of collapse. All three episodes have been similar in duration and character. They come on suddenly with no pre-warning symptoms and have occurred at different times of the day and night.

The first was whilst she was hanging out some washing – there was a sudden onset of feeling dizzy and unwell. Mrs Singh collapsed to the floor and was groggy for a few minutes. The episode was witnessed by her daughter-in-law, who says she went pale and clammy and collapsed to the floor. She thought she remained conscious throughout and felt she was back to her normal self within 5 minutes or so. There were no features of a seizure, focal neurological deficit or cardiac symptoms.

The second episode (which she hid from her family) occurred about 6 weeks later. It was very similar but occurred as she was washing herself, sitting on the edge of the bath. She managed to get to her bed without her family noticing and was fine in the morning.

The third episode today occurred without warning whilst she was out with her granddaughter at the local supermarket. She became sweaty, pale and clammy and collapsed to the floor. The episode lasted about 5 minutes or so and she was 'fine' once she arrived here in the Emergency Department.

Mrs Singh has dietary-controlled T2DM but no other major risk for CV disease. She has long-standing treated hypothyroidism and PMR and has been on steroids for 2 years. She has been treated for depression for the last 6 months. Her regular medications are citalopram 20 mg od, prednisolone 2 mg o.d, AdcalD3 two tablets per day, thyroxine 125 µg od.

## Examination

On examination, Mrs Singh is a well, thin-looking elderly Asian woman. She was independently mobile and able to get on and off the bed unassisted. She was alert and had an AMTS = 10/10. Her observations on arrival were HR 46 bpm, BP 122/73 mmHg, $O_2$ sats 95% on air, RR 14 bpm, temperature 36.4 °C, CBG 4.9 mmol/l. The general examination was unremarkable, and of note she was clinically euthyroid. The CV examination showed her to be bradycardic with a HR of 44 bpm, which was regular and normal in character. She was haemodynamically stable with a BP 122/73 mmHg sitting and 125/80 mmHg standing (2 minutes). Auscultation was unremarkable, with no added sounds. There were no signs of heart failure. Respiratory and abdominal examinations were unremarkable, as was neurological assessment, with no focal neurological deficit detected.

## Investigations

The diagnosis in this case was made on the presenting ECG and rhythm strip. However, the history may be similarly non-specific and the examination unremarkable. Investigations should be initially directed to the two most likely causes: cardiac or neurological collapse. Such patients should have ECG (looking for structural abnormalities) and 24-hour tape (brady- and tachyarrhythmia), and if these are normal one should consider tilt table testing, looking for bradycardia and/or hypotension, and neurological, principally a CT head scan. Note: EEG is rarely if ever useful in such patients.

In this case iatrogenic causes may also be contributing. Thyroid replacement may be implicated, exacerbating bradycardia (under replacement) or tachycardia (over replacement), long-term steroids (collapse secondary to Addisonian symptoms), and antidepressants that cause dizziness and convulsions.

**Management**

This patient has an easily treatable cause of her collapse and should be 'cured' with insertion of a cardiac pacemaker. Another common presentation in this group of patients is 'tachy–brady' syndrome, in which patients suffer with episodes of severe bradycardia, leading to re-entry tachycardias, both causing episodes of collapse. Such patients require a 'belt and braces' approach with a pacemaker to stop the bradycardia and anti-arrhythmic (beta blocker or rate-limiting calcium channel blocker) to stop the tachyarrythmia. Patients who experience bradycardia and hypotension on tilt table testing may also derive great benefit from pacemaker insertion.

Patients with isolated hypotension or postural hypotension provide a far more difficult challenge. These patients require their anti-hypertensives removed (this may be difficult in patients with severe hypertension and associated postural symptoms), support stockings (often too difficult for them to put on without assistance), and in some cases a trial of fludrocortisone tablets. The major problem in elderly patients on fludrocortisone is fluid retention, secondary fluid overload and heart failure, and thus it should be used judiciously.

**Further reading and web links**

*NHS guide for patients regarding permanent pacemakers*:
www.nhs.uk/Conditions/PacemakerImplantation/Pages/howworkspage.aspx
*NICE guidelines for dual chamber pacemaker insertion*:
www.nice.org.uk/nicemedia/live/11552/33013/33013.pdf
*Excellent textbook for all budding geriatricians*:
Bracewell C, Gray R and Rai GS. (2010) *Essential Facts in Geriatric Medicine*, 2nd edition. Oxford: Radcliffe Publishing.

SCENARIO 12

# Scenario 13:
# 'Lose my breath'

## Station 1

*History*                                              *10-minute station*

You are a FY1 doctor in Respiratory Medicine. Mrs Gill has been referred to Outpatients with a 12-month history of increasing shortness of breath.

■ Please take a history from Mrs Gill and then present it to your Consultant together with your differential diagnosis.

*You will be assessed on the following areas, as well as the content and diagnostic reasoning of your history – take them into account in your presentation.*

### Professionalism

- Professional appearance (NHS dress code) – including general appearance, hair and jewellery
- Maintains patient and personal safety
- Polite introduction; identifies patient or interviewee correctly; confirms patient's date of birth from name band or other source
- Obtains informal consent; maintains patient's privacy
- Displays empathetic and caring attitudes and behaviours throughout.

### Process

- Good organisation and structure; appropriate use of open and closed questions
- Appropriate fluency/rhythm/pace to the interview – this may change depending on environment and acute nature of the problem
- Appropriate time for the patient to respond/reply to questions
- Appropriate acknowledgement of difficult or emotional areas of the patient's history.

### Communication skills

- Demonstrates caring and sympathetic attitude
- Asks open questions
- Invites patient to ask questions and answers them appropriately
- Addresses patient's ideas, concerns and expectations.

## Station 2

*Examination*                    *10-minute station*

After presenting your history, now complete a formal respiratory examination in front of your Consultant.

■ Please present your positive findings and differential diagnosis once you have completed your examination.

(If you do not have a model, please read and present the information given on page 386.)

*You will be assessed on the following areas, as well as the content and skills of your examination – take them into account in your presentation.*

### Professionalism

- Professional appearance; maintains infection control standards, including hand cleaning and appropriate use of gloves and aprons
- Maintains patient and personal safety
- Polite introduction; identifies patient and confirms date of birth from name band or other source
- Obtains informal consent; maintains patient privacy and dignity
- Displays empathetic and caring attitudes and behaviours throughout.

### Process

- Appropriate fluency/rhythm/pace to the examination – this may change depending on environment and acute nature of the problem
- Organisation and structure of examination; sensitive and empathetic approach
- Uses appropriate clinical techniques throughout
- Maintains privacy and dignity throughout.

### Clinical communication

- Explains proposed examination/procedure: explains examination/procedure as it proceeds
- Offers information in a clear, structured and fluent manner, avoiding jargon
- Listens to patient and responds appropriately
- Demonstrates appropriate body language.

SCENARIO 13

## Station 3

*Procedural skills*                                    *10-minute station*

You have been asked to perform an assessment of spirometry for Mrs Gill.

**Procedure**
- Please use the spirometer provided and demonstrate the correct technique.

**Equipment provided**
- Digital spirometer
- Disposable mouth pieces
- Antiseptic wipes.

## Station 4

*Data interpretation*                                  *10-minute station*

1. Below are the results of Mrs Gill's spirometry.
- Please describe the key abnormalities in these results.

|  | Actual | Predicted | % Predicted |
|---|---|---|---|
| FVC (L) | 1.32 | 4.1 | 32 |
| FEV1 (L) | 1.18 | 3.1 | 38 |
| FEV1/FVC (%) | 83 | 77 | |
| FRC | 1.73 | 3.80 | 45 |
| RV (L) | 1.12 | 2.59 | 43 |
| TLC (L) | 2.70 | 6.45 | 42 |
| RV/TLC (%) | 41 | 42 | |
| DLCO corr | 5.06 | 31.64 | 16 |

2. Mrs Gill has had a chest X-ray, which shows bilateral lower lobe interstitial shadowing, and so your Consultant has requested a high-resolution CT (HRCT) of her chest.

■ The images below are from other chest CTs. Please match the clinical scenarios to the CT images.

A

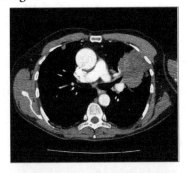

B

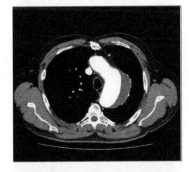

C

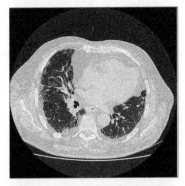

D

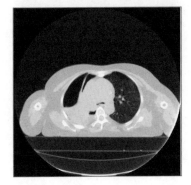

a. A 76-year-old man has presented with progressive shortness of breath and weight loss of 12 kg in 3 months.

b. A 28-year-old man presents with sudden-onset left-sided chest pain and shortness of breath.

c. A 42-year-old man presents with sever sepsis due to lower limb cellulitis and has developed progressive respiratory distress and hypoxia over the last 6 hours.

d. A 56-year-old man with a previous medical history of hypertension presents with sudden onset of tearing chest pain and collapse.

## Station 5

*Clinical communication skills*　　　　　*10-minute station*

Mrs Gill has returned for a follow-up appointment in the respiratory clinic. Your Consultant has made the diagnosis of idiopathic pulmonary fibrosis (IPF). As you have spent time with Mrs Gill, you have been asked to break this news to Mrs Gill under supervision.

■ Please explain the diagnosis and answer any questions Mrs Gill may have.

# Answers

## Station 1 – History

**Patient script**

You are Mrs Anne Gill (DOB 24 November 1952), a 59-year-old woman who has been referred to the chest clinic after presenting to your GP with increasing shortness of breath on exertion for the last 12 months. Prior to this you had been able to walk significant distance and enjoyed long walks in the Peak District most weekends with your husband.

You first noticed that you became short of breath on these walks. However, over the last 6 months you have been short of breath on climbing one flight of stairs or attempting to do the vacuuming. You feel lethargic and 'worn out.' You are not short of breath at rest. You have had no fever or sputum production. However, you have had a troublesome dry cough. You have had no haemoptysis or weight loss. You have not noticed any ankle swelling or difficulty lying flat. You have never smoked cigarettes.

You are a secondary school English teacher, and this is the only job you have ever had. You live with your husband. You have had a dog for the last 11 years but no other pets. You have no significant previous medical history, apart from a cholecystectomy after an episode of cholecystitis around 5 years ago. Specifically you have no symptoms of joint pains or colour changes in your hands, no dysphagia and no skin rashes.

You do not believe you have ever been exposed to asbestos and have never had any prescription drugs. You take cod liver oil, which you purchase over the counter, but no other medicines. You have no drug allergies.

A B C D E
PROFESSIONALISM

A B C D E
PROCESS

A B C D E
COMMUNICATION

## CONTENT

A B C D E

### Identifies key information
- Establishes duration of illness and insidious onset
- Establishes the presence of shortness of breath and decreased exercise tolerance
- Establishes the presence of non productive cough.

### Includes important negatives, including systemic enquiry
- Establishes the absence of wheeze, fever or sputum
- Establishes the absence of chest pain, haemoptysis or weight loss
- Establishes the absence of peripheral oedema or orthopnea.

### Identifies key information from rest of history
- Risk factors for respiratory disease
- Presence of pets and birds
- Exposure to asbestosis
  - Full and systematic review of systems to ascertain risk factors for interstitial lung disease
  - Symptoms of connective tissue disease including Raynaud's phenomenon and dysphagia
  - Exposure to chemotherapy
  - Occupational history.

### Completing the patient history
- Drug and allergy history: nil regular and no allergies
- Previous medical history: nil of note
- Social and occupational history: never smoked; secondary school teacher
- Family history: no relevant family history.

### Summarises important areas of the history back to the patient

### Invites patient to ask questions and deals with them appropriately

### Establishes patient's ideas, concerns and expectations

## CLINICAL DIAGNOSTIC REASONING

A B C D E

- **Please present your history**
  - Candidate offers a logical, well-structured account of the history.
- **What is your differential diagnosis at this point?**
  - A differential diagnosis of insidious onset breathlessness with no other respiratory symptoms includes: diffuse parencyhmal lung diseases such as idiopathic pulmonary fibrosis; diseases such as sarcoidosis or systemic sclerosis.

## GLOBAL HISTORY MARK

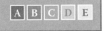

A B C D E

# Station 2 – Examination

**Patient script (see also page 386)**

You are not breathless at rest, but when taking a deep breath in you cannot expand your chest fully. You become breathless on minimal exertion.

A B C D E | A B C D E | A B C D E
PROFESSIONALISM | PROCESS | COMMUNICATION

## CONTENT

A B C D E

**Exposes and positions patient correctly and maintains comfort**

**Comments on wellbeing of patient, ie well or unwell**

**Asks for appropriate/relevant clinical observations**
- Observations: HR 60 bpm, BP 115/60 mmHg, RR 12 bpm, $O_2$ sats 94% on air, temperature 36.7 °C

SCENARIO 13

**General/systemic examination**

**Focussed examination**
- Inspection: assesses hands and nails for signs such as clubbing and palmar erythema; assesses neck for lymphadenopathy in all regions – supra-clavicular, cervical, sub-mental, pre- and post-auricular and occipital – right supra-clavicular lymph nodes; assesses trachea
- Palpation: assesses chest expansion anteriorly and posteriorly
- Percussion: in all zones, including apices; examines for any change in tactile vocal resonance
- Auscultation: auscultates in all areas; no breath sounds audible at right base.

**Completes examination by identifying relevant additional clinical signs**
- Listens to heart and assesses for apex beat and jugular venous pressure (JVP) – signs of pericardial tamponade/pericardial effusion
- Palpates for hepatosplenomegaly.

**Asks to examine for systemic lymphadenopathy**

**Thanks patient, offers assistance, maintains patient's dignity and privacy until they are dressed**

## CLINICAL DIAGNOSTIC REASONING

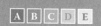

**Correctly identifies the relevant physical signs, including important negative findings**

- **What investigations you would like to request before the next outpatient appointment and why?**
  - Chest X-ray: looking for bilateral pulmonary infiltrates
  - Blood tests to include: FBC, for polycythemia as a result of hypoxia; inflammatory markers – C-reactive protein (CRP), erythrocyte sedimentation rate (ESR); test for connective tissue disorder – rheumatoid factor, ANA; arterial blood gas analysis
  - High-resolution chest CT, looking for pattern of pulmonary infiltrates
  - Spirometry – restrictive lung defect in interstitial lung disease.

## GLOBAL EXAMINATION MARK

## Station 3 – Procedural skills

**Procedure: Spirometry**

A B C D E
PROFESSIONALISM

A B C D E
PROCESS

### CONTENT

A B C D E

**Exposes and positions patient correctly and maintains comfort**
- Sitting up with feet uncrossed

**Identifies and sets out equipment correctly; maintains aseptic technique throughout**

**Explains the procedure to the patient**
- A test of how well the lungs function
- Patient will need to take deep breaths and blow out for as long as is able
- May make the patient feel dizzy.

**Correctly performs the procedure**
- Demonstrates the equipment to the patient
- Inputs patient's details onto spirometer
- Applies nose clips
- Instructs patient to take a deep breath and make a good seal around the mouthpiece
- Encourages patient to blow hard and for as long as they are able, using verbal prompts such as 'keep going, keep going'
- Checks results and repeats test three times to ensure three reproducible results.

**Obtains an acceptable/appropriate result**

**Ensures patient receives correct advice about what to do next and follow-up**

**Ensures nursing staff or other healthcare professionals receive correct information about the consequences/outcome of the procedure/task**

**Thanks patient, offers assistance, maintains patient's dignity and privacy until they are dressed**

### GLOBAL PROCEDURE MARK

A B C D E

SCENARIO 13

## Station 4 – Data interpretation

**1**

**Reduced FVC and reduced FEV1 with preserved FEV1/FVC, this is a restrictive lung pattern.**

**Reduced carbon monoxide diffusing capacity (DLCO), indicating that she has a reduced alveolar surface area for gas exchange, which suggests that the cause of her restrictive process lies within the lung parenchyma.**

**2**

|   |   |
|---|---|
| a | D |
| b | B |
| c | A |
| d | C |

**GLOBAL DATA INTERPRETATION MARK**

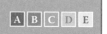

## Station 5 – Clinical communication skills

**Patient script**

You are a 59-year-old woman who is attending for follow-up after investigations for the shortness of breath you have been experiencing. You are attending alone as your husband is unwell and is at home.

You have been feeling just as short of breath since your last attendance and now it is becoming difficult for you to go to work. This is a major concern, as financially you cannot afford to give up work.

You are very worried that you have lung cancer, and when you hear that you do not have cancer you are very relieved. It takes significant time for you to take in the information regarding the diagnosis of IPF, and you are very concerned that incurable means there are no treatment options.

A B C D E  PROFESSIONALISM    A B C D E  PROCESS

## CONTENT  A B C D E

**Confirms reason for discussion**

**Establishes what patient wishes to know; gains agreement/informal consent to participate in the discussion**

**Investigates patient's present level of understanding of scenario**

**Summarises and confirms what has happened so far**

**Establishes patient's ideas, concerns and expectations**
- Establishes that patient is concerned that she believes that she has lung cancer.

**Explains the key important information**
- Gives warning that there is difficult information to be given
- Asks if any family members should be present
- Explains news in clear chunks of information, checking understanding throughout – explaining fibrosis, idiopathic and the treatment options to include trials of immunosuppression
- Explains that there is a range of outcomes and although it is not a curable disease some people live with the disease for many years
- Is empathetic and sensitive to patient throughout with good use of silence.

**Invites patient to ask questions and is able to deal with them appropriately**

**Summarises important areas of the consultation back to the patient**

**Formally ends the consultation and ensures appropriate follow-up has been discussed**
- Arranges further meeting with Consultant and meeting with the Respiratory Nurse Specialist.

SCENARIO 13

## GLOBAL COMMUNICATION MARK  A B C D E

## Scenario 13: Reflection and consolidation

### History

Mrs Gill is a 59-year-old woman who presents with a year-long history of increasing shortness of breath. This was insidious in its onset and progressed to the point where she is now breathless on minimal exertion. She also reports a dry cough but denies wheeze, sputum production, fever or haemoptysis. She has not lost weight. She denies chest pain, peripheral oedema and orthopnea. Her only medical history is a previous cholecystectomy.

She has only ever worked as a teacher and has never smoked. She denies exposure to asbestos. She has one pet, a dog. She takes no medication, has no allergies and has never had chemotherapy. She denies symptoms suggestive of connective tissue disease, including joint pain, dysphagia or Reynaud's phenomenon. The presentation of insidious onset of exertional shortness of breath without other respiratory symptoms raises the possibility of one of the diffuse parenchymal lung diseases (DPLD). The most likely is that of IPF.

### Examination

On examination of the respiratory system of Mrs Gill, she was comfortable at rest with no peripheral stigmata of respiratory disease. Her respiratory rate was 12 bpm and she had oxygen saturation of 94% on room air. On examination of her chest she had no scarring or asymmetry. She had bilaterally reduced chest expansion. Throughout the chest there was a normal percussion note. On auscultation there were fixed fine end inspiratory crackles at both bases.

There was no evidence of connective tissue disease such as sclerodactyly or arthritis. There was no evidence of lymphadenopathy.

The examination of a patient with suspected DPLD will reveal the fine crackles associated with the infiltrative process. However, the zones of the lungs can help to reveal the underlying cause of the fibrosis. The zones of the lungs affected by different fibrotic processes include: upper – ankylosing spondylitis, cancer, extrinsic allergic alveolitis, pneumoconiosis, old tuberculosis changes; middle – sarcoidosis; lower – IPF, asbestosis, connective tissue disease.

### Investigations

The chest X-ray in IPF typically shows diffuse interstitial shadowing, but this picture can be seen in a number of other diseases, including pneumonias, miliary tuberculosis, left ventricular failure or more rarely lymphangitis carcinomatosis or bronchoalveolar carcinoma.

The chest X-ray can also be near normal in IPF, so a low threshold for HRCT is required. The pattern of interstitial changes on HRCT may also give clues as the prognosis of patients with those who have a more diffuse ground glass opacification rather than honeycombing and traction bronchiectasis have a better response to treatment.

If the diagnosis of IPF cannot be made with a high degree of confidence, then a bronchoscopy and bronchoalveolar lavage may be required. Some patients may require a lung biopsy in order to confirm the diagnosis histologically. The histological appearance seen in IPF is described as usual interstitial pneumonia.

SCENARIO 13

## Management

The hypothesised pathological process behind IPF is that a repeated unknown stimulus provokes lung damage and subsequent abnormal healing and fibrosis. This may be related to the balance between the T1 and T2 helper T cells.

Treatments are aimed at modifying the inflammatory response; however, there is no treatment regime that has strong evidence of improving outcomes. Currently a treatment course with prednisolone, the immunosuppressant azathioprine and N-acetyl-cysteine have the best evidence.

The progression of this disease is relentless and without remission, with a mean prognosis of 2–4 years from diagnosis. Some patients can be considered for lung transplantation, but this is usually reserved for those under the age of 65 without significant co-morbidities. Therefore support with symptomatic relief with opiates and oxygen as well as community respiratory and palliative care support.

### Further reading and web links

*British Thoracic Society guide to diagnosis and treatment of IPF*:
www.brit-thoracic.org.uk/Portals/0/Guidelines/DPLDGuidelines/Thorax%20Sept%2008.pdf
*Patient.UK patient information site on IPF*:
www.patient.co.uk/health/Idiopathic-Pulmonary-Fibrosis.htm

# Scenario 14: 'Abdominal agony'

## Station 1

*History*        *10-minute station*

You are the FY1 doctor on call for the surgical take. A patient has been referred by a GP who was called to see a lady at home after she developed abdominal pain. The patient, Mrs Amanda Taylor, has arrived in the Emergency Department now and you have been called to assess her.

■ Please take a history, after which you will be asked to present to your Registrar.

*You will be assessed on the following areas, as well as the content and diagnostic reasoning of your history – take them into account in your presentation.*

### Professionalism

- Professional appearance (NHS dress code) – including general appearance, hair and jewellery
- Maintains patient and personal safety
- Polite introduction; identifies patient or interviewee correctly; confirms patient's date of birth from name band or other source
- Obtains informal consent; maintains patient's privacy
- Displays empathetic and caring attitudes and behaviours throughout.

### Process

- Good organisation and structure; appropriate use of open and closed questions
- Appropriate fluency/rhythm/pace to the interview – this may change depending on environment and acute nature of the problem
- Appropriate time for the patient to respond/reply to questions
- Appropriate acknowledgement of difficult or emotional areas of the patient's history.

### Communication skills

- Demonstrates caring and sympathetic attitude
- Asks open questions
- Invites patient to ask questions and answers them appropriately
- Addresses patient's ideas, concerns and expectations.

## Station 2

*Examination*                                    *10-minute station*

- Please perform a focussed abdominal examination, including assessment of specific signs related to acute hepatic/pancreatic/biliary pathology. A set of observations has been taken by the Emergency Department nurse, which you may ask for.
- (If you do not have a model, please read and present the information given on page 387.)

*You will be assessed on the following areas, as well as the content and skills of your examination – take them into account in your presentation.*

### Professionalism

- Professional appearance; maintains infection control standards, including hand cleaning and appropriate use of gloves and aprons
- Maintains patient and personal safety
- Polite introduction; identifies patient and confirms date of birth from name band or other source
- Obtains informal consent; maintains patient privacy and dignity
- Displays empathetic and caring attitudes and behaviours throughout.

### Process

- Appropriate fluency/rhythm/pace to the examination – this may change depending on environment and acute nature of the problem
- Organisation and structure of examination; sensitive and empathetic approach
- Uses appropriate clinical techniques throughout
- Maintains privacy and dignity throughout.

### Clinical communication

- Explains proposed examination/procedure: explains examination/procedure as it proceeds
- Offers information in a clear, structured and fluent manner, avoiding jargon
- Listens to patient and responds appropriately
- Demonstrates appropriate body language.

**SCENARIO 14**

## Station 3

*Data interpretation*                            *10-minute station*

The following day your Registrar has arranged some patient's blood test results for you to look at.

- Please answer the following questions.

A The patients below have all presented with weight loss. Please match the patient histories with the most appropriate investigation results and diagnosis.

| Patient history | Investigations | | Diagnosis |
|---|---|---|---|
| 1<br><br>A 67-year-old man with jaundice, pale stools and anorexia | A<br>Albumin<br>ALP<br>AST<br>Bili<br>Corr Ca$^{2+}$<br>Amylase | 23 g/l<br>232 iu/l<br>31 iu/l<br>13 mg/dl<br>1.80 mmol/l<br>23 units/l | a<br><br>Colonic carcinoma with multiple metastases |
| 2<br><br>A 52-year-old woman with palmar erythema, spider naevi and hepatosplenomegaly | B<br>Albumin<br>ALP<br>AST<br>Bili<br>Corr Ca$^{2+}$<br>Amylase | 24 g/l<br>454 iu/l<br>54 iu/l<br>32 mg/dl<br>2.42 mmol/l<br>43 units/l | b<br><br>Coeliac disease |
| 3<br><br>A 25-year-old woman with steatorrhoea and general malaise | C<br>Albumin<br>ALP<br>AST<br>Bili<br>Corr Ca$^{2+}$<br>Amylase | 35 g/l<br>321 iu/l<br>93 iu/l<br>124 mg/dl<br>1.92 mmol/l<br>1098 units/l | c<br><br>Carcinoma of the head of the pancreas |
| 4<br><br>A 59-year-old man with weight loss, constipation and rectal bleeding | D<br>Albumin<br>ALP<br>AST<br>Bili<br>Corr Ca$^{2+}$<br>Amylase | 26 g/l<br>607 iu/l<br>109 iu/l<br>45 mg/dl<br>3.05 mmol/l<br>32 units/l | d<br><br>Acute pancreatitis |
| 5<br><br>A 43-year-old obese woman with generalised abdominal pain and fever | E<br>Albumin<br>ALP<br>AST<br>Bili<br>Corr Ca$^{2+}$<br>Amylase | 21 g/l<br>644 iu/l<br>245 iu/l<br>308 mg/dl<br>2.56 mmol/l<br>204 units/l | e<br><br>Primary biliary cirrhosis |

SCENARIO 14

B  The following patients have presented to the hepatology clinic with deranged liver function tests (LFTs). Please match the patient histories with the most appropriate diagnosis and disease marker.

| Patient history | Diagnosis | Marker |
|---|---|---|
| 1<br><br>A 47-year-old man who has known chronic hepatitis B disease now presenting with hepatomegaly and weight loss | A<br><br>Wilson's disease | a<br><br>Raised serum ferritin |
| 2<br><br>A 58-year-old woman with recent weight loss and constipation | B<br><br>Primary biliary cirrhosis | b<br><br>Anti-smooth muscle antibody |
| 3<br><br>A 34-year-old man with diabetes, a 'suntan' and jaundice | C<br><br>Colonic carcinoma with metastases | c<br><br>Antimitochondrial antibody |
| 4<br><br>A 56-year-old woman with signs of chronic liver disease and periorbital xanthelasma | D<br><br>Hepatoma | d<br><br>Low serum copper and caeruloplasmin |
| 5<br><br>A 33-year-old woman with signs of chronic liver disease, jaundice and a cushingoid appearance | E<br><br>Haemochromatosis | e<br><br>Alpha fetoprotein |
| 6<br><br>A 39-year-old man with tremor, gait problems and Kyser-Fleischer rings | F<br><br>Autoimmune hepatitis | f<br><br>Markedly raised carcinoembryonic antigen |

## Station 4

*Clinical communication skills*          *10-minute station*

Mrs Taylor is admitted to the Surgical High-dependency Unit (HDU). Over the course of the next few hours she develops a fever and becomes more pyrexial, tachycardic and hypotensive in spite of fluid resuscitation and treatment with antibiotics. She has an ultrasound scan, which demonstrates features of cholangitis and confirms the diagnosis of gallstone pancreatitis. A decision is made to take her for urgent endoscopic retrograde cholangiopancreatography (ERCP) with stone extraction and sphincterotomy.

■ Your Registrar goes to the Endoscopy Unit to book the case and asks you to explain to Mrs Taylor about the ERCP procedure, why it is necessary, and what will be involved. She may have several questions to ask as well. He will come to take consent from her and answer any further questions that she may have once he returns from the Endoscopy Unit.

# Answers

## Station 1 – History

**Patient script**

You are Amanda Taylor, DOB 14 April 1961. You developed severe abdominal pain about 6 hours ago. The pain started during the night, waking you up, and you were unable to sleep again as the pain continued to get worse. You took both paracetamol and ibuprofen at home, but had no relief from the pain. Since getting up this morning you have been sick four or five times. The pain is sharp and severe (9/10). It seems to be in the centre of your abdomen, and feels like it bores through to your back. You can't get comfortable, but found that lying in bed seemed to make it worse, and so you have been sitting up as this seems slightly more tolerable.

You have not had any diarrhoea or constipation lately, and opened your bowels normally yesterday. You didn't feel unwell at all yesterday, and had spent the day with your family, shopping and going to the cinema in the evening. You have not noticed any fever. You have not had any urinary symptoms at all.

You have never had any pain as severe as this, and have never had any similar episodes. You did see your GP after a few episodes of milder right-sided abdominal pain about 6 months ago. You only noticed these pains a couple of times, and they went away on their own. Your GP told you that it could have been indigestion, or possibly 'biliary colic', and arranged for you to have some sort of a scan. However, you had been on holiday when the appointment was sent for, and had cancelled it as the pains had settled.

You are otherwise healthy, and have never had any medical or surgical problems other than an appendicectomy when you were in your twenties. You take no regular medications, and do not have any allergies.

You work as a court clerk, and are married with two teenage children. You drink alcohol occasionally, usually a glass or two of wine but rarely more. You have never smoked. You feel you probably aren't as fit as you should be, as you do not regularly exercise, and you would like to lose a few pounds of weight that you have put on in the past few years since going through the menopause.

There is no family history of any medical problems that you are aware of.

SCENARIO 14

# 'ABDOMINAL AGONY'

PROFESSIONALISM — A B C D E

PROCESS — A B C D E

COMMUNICATION — A B C D E

## CONTENT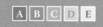

A B C D E

### Identifies key information
- Severe, sudden onset, sharp abdominal pain
- Radiates to back
- Eased by sitting position
- Vomited 4–5 times

### Includes important negatives, including systemic enquiry
- No diarrhoea or constipation
- No urinary symptoms
- Denies a fever
- Well until onset of pain.

### Identifies key information from rest of history
- Few episodes of undiagnosed pain several months ago – possibly biliary colic/dyspepsia.

### Completing the patient history
- Drug and allergy history: took paracetamol and ibuprofen at home; no allergies
- Previous medical history: previous biliary colic/dyspepsia – diagnosis not made; cancelled ultrasound scan; post-menopausal
- Social and occupational history: occasional alcohol; non-smoker; feels slightly overweight; works as court clerk; married with children
- Family history: nil reported.

### Summarises important areas of the history back to the patient

### Invites patient to ask questions and deals with them appropriately

### Establishes patient's ideas, concerns and expectations

SCENARIO 14

## CLINICAL DIAGNOSTIC REASONING

- ■ **Please present your history**
  - • Candidate offers a logical, well-structured account of the history.

- ■ **What is the likely cause of this patient's symptoms?**
  - • Candidate offers the correct diagnosis and appropriate differentials
  - • Acute severe central abdominal pain, radiating to back and eased by sitting – this is classical of acute pancreatitis
  - • Differential diagnoses: acute cholecystitis; perforated peptic/duodenal ulcer; severe gastritis; high intestinal obstruction; ruptured abdominal aortic aneurysm; acute myocardial infarction.

- ■ **This lady presented to her GP with episodes of right-sided abdominal pains about 6 months ago. What is likely to have been the cause of those episodes, and what would have been revealed on her ultrasound scan?**
  - • These episodes are consistent with bouts of biliary colic; gallstones represent the most common cause of acute pancreatitis in the UK (about 50% of all cases); ultrasound would presumably have demonstrated evidence of gallstones (or sludge in the gallbladder) without features of cholecystitis (ie gallbladder thickening, pericholecystic fluid, gallbladder distension, common bile duct distension).

## GLOBAL HISTORY MARK

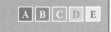

## Station 2 – Examination

---

**Patient script (see also page 387)**

You should appear in severe pain, especially when lying flat. You have a generally tender abdomen, but exquisite tenderness when examined in the epigastric region, where you also have muscle rigidity and rebound tenderness.

SCENARIO 14

PROFESSIONALISM A B **C** D E

PROCESS A B **C** D E

COMMUNICATION A B **C** D E

## CONTENT
A B **C** D E

**Exposes and positions patient correctly and maintains comfort**
- Supine position.

**Comments on wellbeing of patient, ie well or unwell**
- In moderate/severe pain.

**'Feet to face'**
- Observes and comments on patient and surroundings from foot of bed
- Sweaty and ill-looking.

**Asks for appropriate/relevant clinical observations**
- Observations: HR 108 bpm, BP 89/48 mmHg, RR 22 bpm, $O_2$ sats 96% on air, temperature 37.9 °C, CBG 11.1 mol/l, height 1.62 m, weight 81 kg, BMI 30.9.

**General/systemic examination**
- Hands, face and neck: cool hands, clammy skin, dry mucous membranes; inspects for jaundice.

**Focussed abdominal examination**
- Inspection:
    - Appendicectomy scar noted
    - Observes for masses, assymetry, pulsations.
    - Observes for ecchymosis at: flank (Grey-Turner's sign); peri-umbilical region (Cullen's sign); inguinal ligament (Fox's sign); these can all occur in retroperitoneal haemorrhage, as may be seen in haemorrhagic pancreatitis.
- Palpation:
    - Systematic palpation beginning at site remote from area of pain
    - Light followed by deep palpation
    - Palpates liver edge, moving fingers towards costal margin with patient's inspiration – attempting to elicit Murphy's sign as seen in acute cholecystitis
    - Attempts to palpate gall-bladder
    - Identifies area of maximal tenderness at epigastric region
    - Examines for features of localised or generalised peritonitis: rebound tenderness and guarding
    - Palpates spleen and ballots kidneys.
- Percussion: systematic percussion, including percussion for upper border of liver
- Auscultation: auscultates for bowel sounds – not heard.

**Completes examination by asking to perform digital rectal examination**

**Thanks patient, offers assistance, maintains patient's dignity and privacy until they are dressed**

SCENARIO 14

## CLINICAL DIAGNOSTIC REASONING

**Correctly identifies the relevant physical signs, including important negative findings**

- ■ **What are the causes of pancreatitis?**
  - • **G**   Gallstones
  - • **E**   Ethanol
  - • **T**   Trauma
  - • **S**   Steroids
  - • **M**   Mumps (also Coxsackie virus)
  - • **A**   Autoimmune
  - • **S**   Scorpion bites
  - • **H**   Hypercalcaemia; hypothermia; hyperlipidaemia
  - • **E**   ERCP; emboli
  - • **D**   Drugs.

- ■ **What criteria can be used to predict severity in acute pancreatitis, and what blood tests are required to be measured?**
  - • Glasgow criteria or Ranson's criteria
  - • Glasgow: 3 or more factors within 48 hours = severe pancreatitis
  - • **P** – $PaO_2$ <8k Pa
  - • **A** – Age >55 years
  - • **N** – Neutrophils: WBC >15 × $10^9$/l
  - • **C** – Calcium <2 mmol/l
  - • **R** – Renal function: urea > 16 mmol/l
  - • **E** – Enzymes: LDH > 600 iu/l; AST >200 iu/l
  - • **A** – Albumin <32g/l
  - • **S** – Sugar: blood glucose >10 mmol/l
  - • Or
  - • Ranson's criteria: 3 or more within 48 hours – severe pancreatitis
  - • At presentation:
  - • **G** – Glucose >10 mmol/l
  - • **A** – Age >55 years (or >70 if gallstones)
  - • **L** – LDH >350 iu/l
  - • **A** – AST >250 iu/l
  - • **W** – WBC >16 × $10^9$/l
  - • At 48 hours:
  - • **C** – Calcium <2.0 mmol/l
  - • **O** – Oxygen ($PaO_2$) <8 kPa
  - • **U** – Urea increase >10 mmol/l in spite of IV fluids
  - • **C** – Concealed (sequestered) fluid estimated >6l
  - • **H** – Haematocrit increase > 10%.

- ■ **What other blood tests would you want to perform?**
  - • FBC; U&E; LFT; amylase; CRP; bone profile; blood sugar; ABG; group and save (if haemorrhage suspected); lipid profile (to rule out hyperlipidaemia as a cause).

**Demonstrates safe, sensible and appropriate management plan**

**Demonstrates clear and logical diagnostic reasoning**

SCENARIO 14

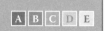

**GLOBAL EXAMINATION MARK**

A B C D E

## Station 3 – Data interpretation

**A**

**1     E     c**

Carcinoma of the head of pancreas causes an obstructive jaundice, the patient often presenting 'severely' jaundiced both clinically and biochemically.

**2     B     e**

Primary biliary cirrhosis is an autoimmune disorder of the liver, which principally affects middle-aged women. It is suggested that there is a cross-antigen reaction in childhood between *E. coli* and hepatocytes. Patients present with signs of chronic liver disease and may have a hepatic jaundice.

**3     A     b**

Coeliac disease is also an autoimmune disease of the small bowel. It may present at any age but principally affects young female adults. It rarely causes derangement of the liver function tests but causes general malabsorption leading to folate deficiency, hypocalcaemia, hypomagnesaemia and hypoalbuminaemia.

**4     D     a**

Colonic carcinoma commonly metastases to the liver and the skeleton. There is derangement of the liver function tests with a raised alkaline phosphatase. This may indicate both liver and bony metastases as it is produced in both tissues, but the raised calcium infers bony metastases as well.

**5     C     d**

Gallstones within the lower common bile duct may produce an obstructive jaundice with an acute pancreatitis. An amylase over 1000 may be caused by an acute pancreatitis, a perforated viscus or a leaking abdominal aortic aneurysm. The low calcium is indicative of acute pancreatitis.

**B**

**1     D     e**

Chronic viral hepatitis is the principal risk factor for developing a hepatoma. All patients with decompensating chronic disease should be screened for a hepatoma using the marker alpha fetoprotein and ultrasound scan. Hepatoma may be amenable to surgical resection or radiological embolisation.

**2    C    f**

This patient has developed liver metastases from a primary colonic carcinoma. Although carcinoembryonic antigen (CEA) is requested in many hospitals as a screening tool for colonic carcinoma, the pick-up rate has been disappointingly low. It should be mainly used after surgical resection as a marker of secondary disease, so that aggressive therapy may be instituted.

**3    E    a**

This patient has developed primary haemachromatosis, an autosomal recessive disorder of iron metabolism. Excess iron is laid down in the liver leading to cirrhosis and its secondary sequelae. The suntanned appearance is due to melanin excess in the skin and not iron. Treatment is by regular venesection, some patients also requiring the chelating agent desferrioxamine. All first degree relatives should undergo screening.

**4    B    c**

The patient has primary biliary cirrhosis, an autoimmune disorder of the liver that principally affects middle-aged women. It is thought to be a cross-antigen reaction between *E. coli* and hepatocytes, as these patients have been shown to be susceptible to *E. coli* urinary tract infections in childhood. Immune markers of the disease include antimitochondrial antibodies and, less commonly, anti-smooth muscle and anti-nuclear antibodies.

**5    F    b**

Autoimmune hepatitis (previously termed autoimmune or lupoid chronic active hepatitis) has now been divided into two separate disorders by the different autoantibodies present.

Type 1 is characterised by non-organ-specific autoantibodies and liver-specific autoantibodies. Non-organ-specific autoantibodies are a heterogeneous group, the most common being the dsDNA antibodies. The principal of these antismooth muscle antibodies with anti-actin specificity. The most specific of the liver antibodies is anti-ASGP-R (asiaglycoprotein receptor).

Type 2 is characterised by the presence of circulating anti-liver/kidney microsomal antibodies (anti-LKM), which have been subdivided into three distinct antibodies, anti LKM 1, 2 and 3.

**6    A    d**

Wilson's disease is a rare autosomal recessive disorder that leads to an inability to metabolise copper normally. The copper is deposited in various sites, the liver (leading to cirrhosis), the brain (particularly the basal ganglia), and the cornea (leading to the pathognomic Kayser-Fleischer ring). The disorder leads to a dyskinetic syndrome or bradykinetic/rigidity syndrome (Parkinsonism). There is an associated progressive cognitive impairment. The progression of the disease may be 'retarded' by the use of oral penicillamine. All relatives should have genetic counselling and screening.

SCENARIO 14

## GLOBAL DATA INTERPRETATION MARK

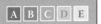

## Station 4 – Clinical communication skills

**Patient script**

You are feeling very unwell, and don't feel any better since being admitted to the ward and being given all of these 'drips', although the pain is slightly better than it was owing to all the morphine that you have been given. You have been told that you had pancreatitis, but are now confused because the ultrasound scan that you have just had showed gallstones, and you are not sure which (or both) is causing all the symptoms.

You are concerned about having any procedure done but understand that it may be necessary.

Question: 'Will I be asleep for the procedure? Will I have a general anaesthetic?'

Question: 'If the stone is extracted does this mean that I won't need any further surgery?'

Question: 'Will I feel better straight afterwards?'

SCENARIO 14

## CONTENT

A B C D E

**Confirms reason for discussion**

**Establishes what patient wishes to know; gains agreement/informal consent to participate in the discussion**

**Investigates patient's present level of understanding of scenario**

**Summarises and confirms what has happened so far**
- Cause of abdominal pain is inflammation of the pancreas – pancreatitis
- The pancreatitis has been caused by gallstones, and the ultrasound scan has confirmed this, and shown that there is a stone causing obstruction of the biliary system
- Antibiotics, intravenous fluids and painkillers have been given so far, but will not treat the underlying problem.

**Establishes patient's ideas, concerns and expectations**

**Explains the key, important information**
- Obstruction from the stone means that the problem is not likely to get better on its own
- ERCP is advised to remove the stone and to relieve the obstruction, helping to clear the infection
- Performed under sedation but not a general anaesthetic
- May have a sore throat afterwards
- Informs that she is unlikely to feel markedly different immediately after the procedure has been performed; however, because the obstruction will hopefully be relieved, the pancreas will begin to recover and the inflammation will begin to settle
- She will need to remain in hospital for a while and will continue to need treatments, including intravenous fluids, antibiotics and painkillers until she is well enough
- Removal of the gallbladder (laparoscopic cholecystectomy) will be advised once she has recovered – this is necessary to prevent further problems related to the gallstones from occurring again in the future
- Informs patient that registrar will come to explain the procedure further and take consent.

**Invites patient to ask questions and is able to deal with them appropriately**

**Summarises important areas of the consultation back to the patient**

**Formally ends the consultation and ensures appropriate follow-up has been discussed**

## GLOBAL COMMUNICATION MARK

A B C D E

SCENARIO 14

# Scenario 14: Reflection and consolidation

### History

Mrs Amanda Taylor, a 51 year old court clerk presents with a six hour history of severe central abdominal pain. She was awoken when the pain started during the night. The pain is 9/10 severity, central, and radiates through to the back. She feels restless and has found that lying still makes the pain seem worse, and that sitting up makes the pain better. The pain has not been alleviated by paracetemol and ibuprofen. She has also vomited approximately five times. She has not reported any fever, urinary or lower gastrointestinal symptoms, having opened her bowels yesterday. She has never had any episodes of similar pains in the past. However, she has seen her GP approximately six months ago after several episodes of mild right-sided abdominal pain. She was diagnosed with biliary colic, and a scan was arranged, which she cancelled as the pains had settled.

She is generally healthy, her only medical history being an appendicectomy in her twenties. She does not take regular medications, nor have any allergies. She is married, does not smoke or drink heavily, but feels that she is slightly overweight. She does not report any family history.

### Examination

This lady is overweight with a BMI of 30.9. She is in moderate pain and appears unwell, and she is tachycardic at 108 bpm, hypotensive at 89/48 mmHg, tachypnoeic at 22/min, with a mild pyrexia at 37.9°. She has cool peripheries, clammy skin and dry mucous membranes. There is no sign of jaundice.

Inspection of the abdomen reveals an appendicectomy scar. There is no asymmetry, no pulsations or visible masses, and no evidence of flank, periumbilical or inguinal ecchymosis. She has severe tenderness with localised peritonism at the epigastric region, characterised by rebound tenderness and guarding, including percussion tenderness. Her abdomen is otherwise generally tender, but soft and without features of generalised peritonitis. She does not display any organomegaly; Murphy's sign is negative. On auscultation, bowel sounds are of normal pitch and frequency.

### Investigations

A full set of bloods should be sent if pancreatitis is suspected. A markedly raised amylase will clinch the diagnosis, but a normal amylase does not rule it out, and lipase is increasingly used as a more sensitive and specific serum marker. Amylase does not correlate to disease severity, and other parameters should be measured according to the Glasgow or Ranson's criteria:

**Glasgow: 3 or more factors within 48hrs = severe pancreatitis**

**P** – $PaO_2 < 8$ kPa

**A** – Age > 55 yrs

**N** – Neutrophils: WBC > 15 x $10^9$/L

**C** – Calcium <2 mmol/L

**R** – Renal function: Urea > 16 mmol/L

**E** – Enzymes: LDH > 600iu/L; AST > 200 iu/L

**A** – Albumin < 32 g/L

**S** – Sugar: blood glucose > 10 mmol/L

Or

**Ranson's Criteria: 3 or more within 48 hours = severe pancreatitis**

**At presentation:**

**G** – Glucose > 10 mmol/L

**A** – Age > 55 yrs (or >70 if gallstones)

**L** – LDH >350 iu/L

**A** – AST - >250 iu/L

**W** – WBC > 16 x $10^9$/L

**At 48 hours:**

**C** – Calcium < 2.0 mmol/L

**O** – Oxygen (PaO$_2$) < 8 kPa

**U** – Urea increase > 10 mmol/L in spite of IV fluids

**C** – Concealed (sequestered) fluid estimated >6 L

**H** – Haematocrit increase > 10%

Imaging investigations in pancreatitis include erect chest x-ray – to rule out perforated viscus and identify pleural effusions; abdominal x-ray – sentinel loop, gallstones, or calcification may be seen in chronic pancreatitis; USS – gallstones, pseudocyst, abscess or necrosis; CT – pseudocyst, abscess or necrosis possible; ERCP – in gallstone pancreatitis.

## Management

Pancreatitis is a serious disease with significant total mortality. Severe disease with features of multi-organ failure lasting more than 48 hours is associated with over 50% mortality. Early complications include shock, multi-organ failure (including respiratory (ARDS), renal), disseminated intravascular coagulopathy, hypocalcaemia, hyperglycaemia.

Late complications include pancreatic necrosis and pseudocyst formation. Psuedocysts are encapsulated collections of necrotic material and pancreatic fluid that usually collect in the lesser sac (between posterior wall of stomach and pancreas). Depending on the size of collection, pseudocysts may need to be drained, either percutaneously or laparoscopically. Other late complications include abscess formation, gastrointestinal or vascular injury due to elastase erosion, and thrombosis leading to bowel necrosis.

Management of pancreatitis is aimed at halting the progression of the disease and preventing failure of remote organs. Patients require very close monitoring, and a low threshold for suspecting complications and deterioration. HDU/intensive therapy unit (ITU) care is often necessary, with central venous catheter, urinary catheter and arterial lines often needed to enable close monitoring of fluid input/output and intravascular volume. Patients require supplementary oxygen and aggressive fluid resuscitation, and regular blood tests to monitor for disease progression.

**Further reading and web links**

*British Society of Gastroenterology: UK Working Party on Acute Pancreatitis, 2005 Guidelines*:
www.bsg.org.uk/clinical-guidelines/pancreatic/index.html
*Several excellent resources including: Acute pancreatitis; Chronic pancreatitis; ERCP*:
www.patient.co.uk

SCENARIO 14

# Scenario 15:
## 'Weaker and weaker'

## Station 1

*History*                                                    *10-minute station*

You are the FY1 working on the acute Medical Admissions Unit (MAU). A GP has been on a home visit and referred the following patient, Mr Gerald Paterson, to your Registrar. The patient has now arrived on the ward.

■ Please take a history from the patient and present it as if presenting on the mid-take or post-take ward round.

*You will be assessed on the following areas, as well as the content and diagnostic reasoning of your history – take them into account in your presentation.*

### Professionalism

- Professional appearance (NHS dress code) – including general appearance, hair and jewellery
- Maintains patient and personal safety
- Polite introduction; identifies patient or interviewee correctly; confirms patient's date of birth from name band or other source
- Obtains informal consent; maintains patient's privacy
- Displays empathetic and caring attitudes and behaviours throughout.

### Process

- Good organisation and structure; appropriate use of open and closed questions
- Appropriate fluency/rhythm/pace to the interview – this may change depending on environment and acute nature of the problem
- Appropriate time for the patient to respond/reply to questions
- Appropriate acknowledgement of difficult or emotional areas of the patient's history.

### Communication skills

- Demonstrates caring and sympathetic attitude
- Asks open questions
- Invites patient to ask questions and answers them appropriately
- Addresses patient's ideas, concerns and expectations.

## Station 2

*Examination*                    *10-minute station*

■ Please perform a general systematic examination of the patient. You should particularly consider the context of this gentleman's presentation – 'advanced prostate cancer' – and assess for features of disease progression. You will then be asked to present your findings as if presenting on the mid-take or post-take ward round.

(If you do not have a model, please read and present the information given on page 387.)

*You will be assessed on the following areas, as well as the content and skills of your examination – take them into account in your presentation.*

### Professionalism

- Professional appearance; maintains infection control standards, including hand cleaning and appropriate use of gloves and aprons
- Maintains patient and personal safety
- Polite introduction; identifies patient and confirms date of birth from name band or other source
- Obtains informal consent; maintains patient privacy and dignity
- Displays empathetic and caring attitudes and behaviours throughout.

### Process

- Appropriate fluency/rhythm/pace to the examination – this may change depending on environment and acute nature of the problem
- Organisation and structure of examination; sensitive and empathetic approach
- Uses appropriate clinical techniques throughout
- Maintains privacy and dignity throughout.

### Communication skills

- Explains proposed examination/procedure: explains examination/procedure as it proceeds
- Offers information in a clear, structured and fluent manner, avoiding jargon
- Listens to patient and responds appropriately
- Demonstrates appropriate body language.

SCENARIO 15

## Station 3

*Prescribing skills*                    *10-minute station*

- Blood results show that Mr Paterson is hypercalcaemic, and the Medical Registrar asks you to demonstrate how you would prescribe a pamidronate infusion. A BNF is provided.

> **Remember: DRUG DR**s **D**on't **F**orget **S**igning **O**ff (page 396)

## Station 4

*Data interpretation*                    *10-minute station*

The patients listed below have abnormal bone and/or calcium metabolism.

- Please rearrange the table to match the histories with the correct data set and diagnoses.

| | Patient history | Corrected calcium (Ca²⁺) | Phosphate (PO₄) | Alkaline phosphatase (ALP) | Diagnosis |
|---|---|---|---|---|---|
| | Normal range: | (2.20–2.60 mmol/l) | (0.70–1.40 mmol/l) | (30–130 iu/l) | |
| 1 | 29-year-old Asian woman with proximal limb weakness | A 2.32 | 1.02 | 3033 | a Osteoporosis |
| 2 | 31-year-old Black woman from Missouri, with lupus pernio | B 1.82 | 1.30 | 107 | b Multiple myeloma |
| 3 | 73-year-old woman with premature menopause, now presenting with back pain | C 3.45 | 1.02 | 421 | c Paget's disease of the bone |
| 4 | 71-year-old man with an enlarged skull, deafness and hip and back pain | D 2.25 | 0.76 | 135 | d Pseudohypo-parathyroidism |
| 5 | 81-year-old man with multiple lytic lesions of the skull and bone pain | E 1.65 | 0.57 | 678 | e Sarcoidosis |
| 6 | 16-year-old woman with low IQ, short stature and short 4th and 5th metacarpals | F 2.98 | 0.92 | 104 | f Osteomalacia |

SCENARIO 15

## Station 5

*Clinical communication skills*          *10-minute station*

■ After 24 hours, a bone scan is arranged. The scan shows several areas of high uptake of radioisotope at the spine, pelvis, ribs, and both femora. Your registrar has suggested that he observes you explaining to Mr Paterson what the scan shows and answer any questions he may have. He has told nurses on the ward that he 'fears the worst'.

# Answers

## Station 1 – History

**Patient script**

Your name is Gerald Paterson (DOB 15 March 1932). You have been visited by your GP at home this afternoon, as your daughter called the surgery after she came to visit you and found you still in bed.

You have prostate cancer, which was diagnosed about 3 years ago, and were offered an operation at the time but decided that you would prefer not to have any surgery. You declined chemotherapy as well, as you were worried about taking such strong medicines.

You have been feeling increasingly tired and weak over the past few weeks. You have not been eating very much at all and have had barely any appetite. You try to keep drinking juice and tea.

You found it difficult to get up out of bed for the past few days because of terrible pain in your back. You have not injured yourself but find the pain is very severe, sharp and in the middle of the lower back, and worse when you try and move. You cannot get comfortable. You have not noticed any weakness or numbness in your legs.

You are also very uncomfortable with constipation, having struggled to open your bowels properly for a few days (last bowel movement 3 days ago), partly because of the back pain, and partly because you have struggled with constipation for at least 6 months. The laxatives that you occasionally take don't really seem to help very much.

You have occasional abdominal pains, which come and go. You also feel quite nauseous and 'gassy' and are drinking milk to try and take away the acid feeling in your throat. You think it is probably due to not eating well.

You have not had any particular worsening in terms of being able to pass urine, and have not been up in the night to pass urine more than before. You have not been aware of any change in the urinary stream, which was already poor, or dribbling.

Apart from the prostate cancer you don't have any other medical problems except for an irregular heart beat.

You take atenolol (40 mg od), tramadol (50–100 mg qds prn), paracetamol (1 g qds prn) and lansoprazole (30 mg od) as a regular prescription. You have no allergies.

You live on your own in a ground floor flat. Your daughter lives nearby and visits most days. She helps with shopping and cleaning, and you prepare simple meals that she buys for you. You used to work as a civil servant. You smoked 20/day for about 50 years but stopped about 10 years ago when your wife died. You don't drink alcohol.

You are not aware of any family history.

A B C D E   A B C D E   A B C D E
PROFESSIONALISM   PROCESS   COMMUNICATION

## CONTENT

A B C D E

### Identifies key information
- Increasingly tired and weak for several weeks
- Poor appetite – reduced oral intake
- Severe back pain for last few days – middle lower back, sharp and worse on movement
- Not opened bowels for several days – and has been chronically constipated in the past.

### Includes important negatives, including systemic enquiry
- No history of injury
- No weakness or numbness to lower limbs
- No progressive symptoms of prostatism (difficulty passing urine, nocturia, terminal dribbling, frequency).

### Identifies key information from rest of history
- Occasional abdominal pains, acidic in nature, and associated with nausea; eased by drinking milk
- Lives alone in ground-floor flat – widower
- Support from daughter – assistance with shopping, cleaning.

### Completing the patient history
- Drug and allergy history: atenolol, tramadol, lansoprazole, paracetamol; no allergies
- Previous medical history: prostate cancer, diagnosed 3 years ago; declined surgery and chemotherapy; atrial fibrillation
- Social and occupational history: smoked 20/day for 50 years, stopped 10 years ago (50 pack years); no alcohol.

### Summarises important areas of the history back to the patient

### Invites patient to ask questions and deals with them appropriately

### Establishes patient's ideas, concerns and expectations

SCENARIO 15

## CLINICAL DIAGNOSTIC REASONING

- **Please present your history**
  - Candidate offers a logical, well-structured account of the history.

- **What is your diagnosis?**
  - Candidate offers the correct diagnosis and appropriate differentials.

- **What do you suspect is the cause of this patient's symptoms?**
  - Symptoms of progressive cancer, with high suspicion of bony metastasis to lumbar spine and associated hypercalcaemia.

- **What is likely to be the cause of this patient's complaint of abdominal pains with acidic discomfort in his throat?**
  - Hypercalcaemia predisposes patients to formation of peptic ulcers as a result of elevated production of gastrin.

## GLOBAL HISTORY MARK

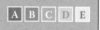

## Station 2 – Examination

**Patient script (see also page 387)**

You are an 80 year-old gentleman who is weak, tired and remarkably thin. You are generally uncomfortable, but have no specific tenderness when examined except for at your lower back.

SCENARIO 15

A B C D E PROFESSIONALISM A B C D E PROCESS A B C D E COMMUNICATION

## CONTENT
A B C D E

**Exposes and positions patient correctly and maintains comfort**
- Supine position.

**Comments on wellbeing of patient, ie well or unwell**
- Thin and cachectic gentleman, appears pale and weak.

**'Feet to face'**
- Observes and comments on patient and surroundings from foot of bed.

**Asks for appropriate/relevant clinical observations**
- Observations: HR 58 bpm irregularly irregular, BP 95/48 mmHg, RR 20 bpm, $O_2$ sats 97% on air, temperature 35.9 °C, CBG 7.9 mmol/l, height 1.78 m, weight 59 kg, BMI 18.6.

**General/systemic examination**
- Hands, face and neck: reduced skin turgor, dry, coated tongue and dry mucous membranes; jugular venous pressure not seen
- Cardiovascular examination: pulses – irregularly irregular; heart sounds normal
- Respiratory examination: normal vesicular breath sounds; percussion tenderness to lateral chest wall bilaterally
- Abdominal examination: irregular, enlarged liver edge
- Musculoskeletal examination: examines for tenderness at long bones (humeri and femurs); inspects spine for swellings, deformities, pressure sores; elicits tenderness by palpating length of spine and identifies region of tenderness at lumbar region; grossly assesses motor and sensory function of lower limbs.

**Completes examination by identifying relevant additional clinical signs**
- Request to perform digital rectal examination
- Performs full neurological examination.

**Thanks patient, offers assistance, maintains patient's dignity and privacy until they are dressed**

SCENARIO 15

## CLINICAL DIAGNOSTIC REASONING

**Correctly identifies the relevant physical signs, including important negative findings**

- **Mr Paterson has several features consistent with advanced metastatic prostate cancer. Justifying your answers from your assessment so far, what blood tests would you like to arrange?**
  - Blood tests: FBC: anaemia, infection
  - U&E: features of dehydration and renal impairment (raised urea and creatinine)
  - Bone profile: hypercalcaemia
  - LFTs: irregular liver edge raises suspicion of liver metastasis.

- **An ECG is also performed – what ECG changes may you expect to find in hypercalcaemia?**
  - Most commonly – shortened QT interval
  - J waves (Osborn wave) may also be seen – also seen in hypothermia.

- **What radiological investigation would help to assess the extent of bony metastatic spread?**
  - Nuclear scintigraphy (also known more commonly as a bone scan).

## GLOBAL EXAMINATION MARK

SCENARIO 15

## Station 3 – Prescribing skills

| Infusion prescriptions continued | | | | | | | | | SC = subcutaneous | | IVC = intravenous central IVP = intravenous peripheral | | |
|---|---|---|---|---|---|---|---|---|---|---|---|---|---|
| Date & time | Route | Infusion Fluid | | Medication | | Duration | Rate | Prescriber's signature & bleep no. | Date given | Given by / Added by | Check by | Start time | Finish time | Pharmacy |
| | | Name & strength | Volume | Approved name with expiry / unit number | Dose | | | | | | | | | |
| 7/05 | IV | 0.9% Saline Exp: Batch/unit no: | 250ml | PAMIDRONATE | 60mg | TO RUN OVER 1XHOUR ≡ 60 MINS | | AF 201 | | | | | | |
| | | Exp: Batch/unit no: | | | | | | | | | | | | |
| 7/05 | IV | 0.9% Saline Exp: Batch/unit no: | 1l | | | | 6⁰ | AF 201 | | | | | | |
| 7/05 | IV | 0.9% Saline Exp: Batch/unit no: | 1l | + 20mmol KCL | | | 6⁰ | AF 201 | | | | | | |
| 7/05 | IV | 0.9% Saline Exp: Batch/unit no: | 1l | | | | 6⁰ | AF 201 | | | | | | |
| 7/05 | IV | 0.9% Saline Exp: Batch/unit no: | 1l | + 20mmol KCL | | | 6⁰ | AF 201 | | | | | | |
| | | Exp: Batch/unit no: | | | | | | | | | | | | |
| | | Exp: Batch/unit no: | | | | | | | | | | | | |
| | | Exp: Batch/unit no: | | | | | | | | | | | | |
| | | | | | | | | | | | | | | |
| | | | | | | | | | | | | | | |

**GLOBAL PRESCRIBING MARK**   A B C D E

SCENARIO 15

273

## Station 4 – Data interpretation

**1      E      f**

This woman has symptoms consistent with osteomalacia, ie proximal muscle weakness and pain. In childhood the lack of vitamin D and its metabolites lead to bone deformity, particularly of the lower limb bones, leading to the classical appearance of rickets. The bone abnormality arises as a result of ineffective osteoid mineralization.

**2      F      e**

This is a classic history of sarcoidosis. Black American women, particularly in the southern states of the USA, have a very high incidence of the disorder. Sarcoid causes hypercalcaemia and hypercalciuria, leading to renal tract calcification and stones.

**3      D      a**

The premature menopause suggests long-term oestrogen deficiency, a primary risk factor for the development of osteoporosis. The disorder per se does not affect calcium levels, and a raised calcium should make the physician think of associated malignancy, particularly myeloma, which may present in a similar fashion.

**4      A      c**

This is a classic history of Paget's disease of the bone. The calcium and phosphate are unchanged by the disorder but the alkaline phosphatase is often greatly raised. This reflects the excessive bone turnover and increased osteoclastic activity. Complications of the disease include: bone pain, pathological fractures, the classic anterior bowing of the tibia, cranial nerve compression, high-output cardiac failure and, rarely, osteosarcoma formation.

**5      C      b**

Multiple myeloma is one of the most common causes of hypercalcaemia in the elderly. Clinically it presents with bone pain. As well as hypercalcaemia, the patient has a raised erythrocyte sedimentation rate (ESR), often over 100, and a normochromic, normocytic anaemia. Other markers include the presence of a paraprotein in the serum, shown by plasma electrophoresis, and Bence-Jones proteins in the urine. Lytic lesions are present radiologically.

**6      B      d**

Pseudohypoparathyroidism is a rare disorder that occurs as a result of end-organ resistance to the effects of parathyroid hormone. The patients are dysmorphic, with a low IQ, and have shortened 4th and 5th metacarpals. Biochemically the patient appears to have hypoparathyroism, but the parathyroid hormone levels are normal. Pseudo-pseudohypoparathyroidism is the disorder of abnormal phenotype with normal calcium metabolism.

**GLOBAL DATA INTERPRETATION MARK**

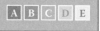

SCENARIO 15

## Station 5 – Clinical communication skills

**Patient script**

You have been feeling very unwell over the past few weeks and are grateful to your daughter for calling the doctor today – to be honest you had been afraid to call the doctor yourself because you have been scared that all this is because the cancer has progressed. You don't, however, understand why the pain in the back has now started and become so severe.

You would like to receive any treatments that will help you feel better, and reduce the pain. You don't expect that very much can be done to help as you knew that things were likely to get worse when the cancer was originally diagnosed 3 years ago, at which time you didn't feel surgery or chemotherapy would have been right. You do not regret that.

You are unsure what will happen now. You are worried because you would like to go home rather than spend a long time in hospital but are worried that you may not be able to cope even though your daughter is very supportive. You are not aware of the Palliative Care team and are grateful when told about the services that may be available, including hospice care if needed in due course.

Your main concern is that you do not become a burden for your daughter and you do not want her to suffer as you become more unwell. You think she will find it very difficult.

Question: 'Is there any treatment to help with pain in the back where the metastases seem to be?'

Question: 'What can I expect now? How long do you think I may have left?'

Question: 'Will support be available for my daughter as well, especially after I die?'

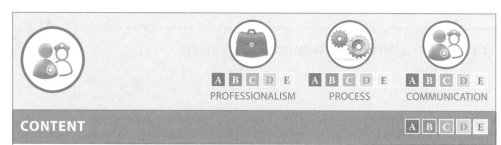

PROFESSIONALISM     PROCESS     COMMUNICATION

## CONTENT

A B C D E

**Confirms reason for discussion**

**Establishes what patient wishes to know; gains agreement/informal consent to participate in the discussion**

**Investigates patient's present level of understanding of clinical scenario**
- Patient understands that he has prostate cancer and he suspects that the reason that he has become more unwell over the past few weeks is because the cancer has progressed.

**Summarises and confirms what has happened so far**

**Establishes patient's ideas, concerns and expectations**
- Patient would like to be offered treatments that will help improve the pain
- Patient understands that deterioration is likely
- Patient is concerned about not being able to cope when he goes home
- Patient is concerned about his daughter, and how she will find it difficult, both looking after him and after he dies.

**Explains the key, important information**
- Explains that the cancer is advanced, and establishes understanding that he will not get better from this
- Explains that various medicines and other treatments are available to help with the symptoms that he is getting
- Treatments include radiotherapy for the pain in his spine; strong painkillers including morphine; anti-sickness medications; medications to help reduce his calcium levels; laxatives, and many others.
- Discusses palliative care and what it means
- Discusses the Palliative Care team, including specialist doctors, nurses, physiotherapists, and full range of hospital and community-based services
- Discusses hospice as a possibility if he is unable to manage at home in spite of community palliative services
- Explains that it is difficult to anticipate how long he is likely to live
- Explains that plenty of support will be available for his daughter, both now and after he dies.

**Invites patient to ask questions and is able to deal with them appropriately**

**Summarises important areas of the consultation back to the patient**

**Formally ends the consultation and ensures appropriate follow-up has been discussed**
- Advises that he talk things through openly with his daughter and offers to help explain the situation to her as well.

## GLOBAL COMMUNICATION MARK

# Scenario 15: Reflection and consolidation

### History

Mr Paterson is an 80-year-old retired civil servant who was diagnosed with prostate cancer 3 years ago, at which he point he declined surgical or medical intervention.

He attends via his GP today having been increasingly weak and tired over the past few weeks. He has had a very poor appetite and reduced oral intake. He has also developed severe, sharp, non-radiating lower back pains over the past few days, although he has not had any history of trauma.

He has also not been able to open his bowels for the past 3 days, and has been suffering from constipation for about 6 months. He also reports occasional abdominal discomfort and acid reflux, which is relieved by drinking milk.

Mr Paterson has not developed any further symptoms of prostatism.

He has been previously fit and well other than atrial fibrillation. His regular medications are atenolol, tramadol, paracetamol and lansoprazole. He has no allergies.

He is an ex-smoker of 50 pack years, but does not drink alcohol.

His wife died 10 years ago and he now lives alone in a ground-floor flat but is well supported by his daughter, who lives locally and who helps him with shopping and cleaning.

### Examination

When faced with a clinical situation such as this one, in which a patient clearly has significant illness but whose symptoms are diverse and affect several systems of the body, a full and thorough examination is important. However, the time constraints of an OSCE exam do not afford ample opportunity to perform a full, detailed physical examination, and so intention to examine further should be demonstrated, eg reporting that a full neurological examination would be indicated given the high clinical suspicion of lumbar spine pathology (metastasis) and further possibility of cerebral metastasis.

In this OSCE station, the history highlights several concerning symptoms that could either indicate potential metastatic spread or be caused by hypercalcaemia: back pain and rib pain (bony metastasis), constipation, acid reflux, lethargy. Physical assessment should help to establish the degree of progression of his cancer, and help to delineate the symptoms from their likely cause.

### Management

A variety of different treatments are used to manage the wide variety of symptoms encountered in end-of-life care:

Pain: the analgesic ladder:

1 – Non-opioid, eg aspirin, paracetamol, nonsteroidal anti-inflammatrory drug (NSAID)

2 – Weak opioid, eg codeine, dihydrocodeine

3 – Strong opioid, eg morphine, diamorphine, fentanyl.

Radiotherapy has an important role in easing bone pain, and can also be used to reduce other symptoms such as haemoptysis, dyspnoea and cough.

Nausea: eg cyclizine, metoclopramide, ondansetron, haloperidol

Constipation: eg co-danthrusate, bisacodyl, enemas (eg arachis oil), lactulose

Coated tongue: eg hydrogen peroxide 6%, pineapple chunks (release proteolytic enzymes)

Mass effect (eg superior vena cava obstruction): steroids eg dexamethasone (also may stimulate appetite)

Bronchial secretions: eg hyoscine hydrobromide, glycopyrrolate, atropine.

### Further reading and web links

*Guideline: Control of pain in adults with cancer.*

www.sign.ac.uk/guidelines/fulltext/106/index.html

www.macmillan.org.uk

www.palliativecareguidelines.scot.nhs.uk/

**SCENARIO 15**

# Scenario 16:
# 'The pit of despair'

## Station 1

*History*                                                    *10-minute station*

You are the FY1 on call with the Acute Medical Team. The next patient is Mr James Tan (DOB 07/04/1968 – 44 years old) who has been brought to the Emergency Department by ambulance with increasing confusion, drowsiness and a chest infection. The Medical ST6 has asked you to get a corroborative history from Mr Tan's wife, Jenni, whilst she reviews Mr Tan in the resus room.

■ Please take a full history of this patient's condition with a view to presenting it to the ST6.

*You will be assessed on the following areas, as well as the content and diagnostic reasoning of your history – take them into account in your presentation.*

### Professionalism

- Professional appearance (NHS dress code) – including general appearance, hair and jewellery
- Maintains patient and personal safety
- Polite introduction; identifies patient or interviewee correctly; confirms patient's date of birth from name band or other source
- Obtains informal consent; maintains patient's privacy
- Displays empathetic and caring attitudes and behaviours throughout.

### Process

- Good organisation and structure; appropriate use of open and closed questions
- Appropriate fluency/rhythm/pace to the interview – this may change depending on environment and acute nature of the problem
- Appropriate time for the patient to respond/reply to questions
- Appropriate acknowledgement of difficult or emotional areas of the patient's history.

### Communication skills

- Demonstrates caring and sympathetic attitude
- Asks open questions
- Invites patient to ask questions and answers them appropriately
- Addresses patient's ideas, concerns and expectations.

## Station 2

*Examination*                                    *10-minute station*

On hearing your presentation of the history, Dr Rook, the ST6, agrees that this patient may be presenting in Addisonian crisis secondary to a chest infection. However, she is also concerned that Mr Tan may be poorly adherent with his hormone replacement therapy. According to his GP prescription he should be on hydrocortisone 10 mg, 5 mg, 5 mg, thyroxine 125 μg od, monthly testosterone injections and amlodipine 10 mg od.

■ Please perform a diagnostic assessment of Mr Tan, focussing on an assessment:
   1. Of his wellbeing
   2. For signs of under/over-replacement of his hormone therapy
   3. Of his respiratory system.

You do not need to examine any other systems, as Mr Tan has already been assessed by Dr Rook.

(If you do not have a model, please read and present the information given on page 388.)

*You will be assessed on the following areas, as well as the content and skills of your examination – take them into account in your presentation.*

---

### Professionalism

- Professional appearance; maintains infection control standards, including hand cleaning and appropriate use of gloves and aprons
- Maintains patient and personal safety
- Polite introduction; identifies patient and confirms date of birth from name band or other source
- Obtains informal consent; maintains patient privacy and dignity
- Displays empathetic and caring attitudes and behaviours throughout.

---

### Process

- Appropriate fluency/rhythm/pace to the examination – this may change depending on environment and acute nature of the problem
- Organisation and structure of examination; sensitive and empathetic approach
- Uses appropriate clinical techniques throughout
- Maintains privacy and dignity throughout.

---

### Clinical communication

- Explains proposed examination/procedure: explains examination/procedure as it proceeds
- Offers information in a clear, structured and fluent manner, avoiding jargon
- Listens to patient and responds appropriately
- Demonstrates appropriate body language.

SCENARIO 16

## Station 3

*Procedural skills*                    *10-minute station*

Given how acutely unwell Mr Tan appears to be, the Senior Nursing Sister in the Emergency Department asks you to show her how you would set up and monitor an acutely ill patient.

### Procedure

- Using the equipment provided please set up the monitoring of the patient as if you were the only person present and obtain and record a complete set of observations on the chart provided.
- Now please telephone the Senior Nursing Sister and relay Mr Tan's observations (provided in the station below) as if handing over the patient to a colleague.

### Equipment provided

- A volunteer to perform the observations on
- Cardiac monitoring with ECG
- Oxygen sats probe
- Aural thermometer
- Capillary blood glucose kit
- Urinalysis kit
- Dynamap blood pressure cuff
- Observation charts.

### PATIENT DETAILS

- Mr James Tan, DOB 07/04/1968, Hospital no. 6619432
- Hospital: Redfern Hospital NHS Trust, Ward: Emergency Department, Consultant: Dr Ghafor

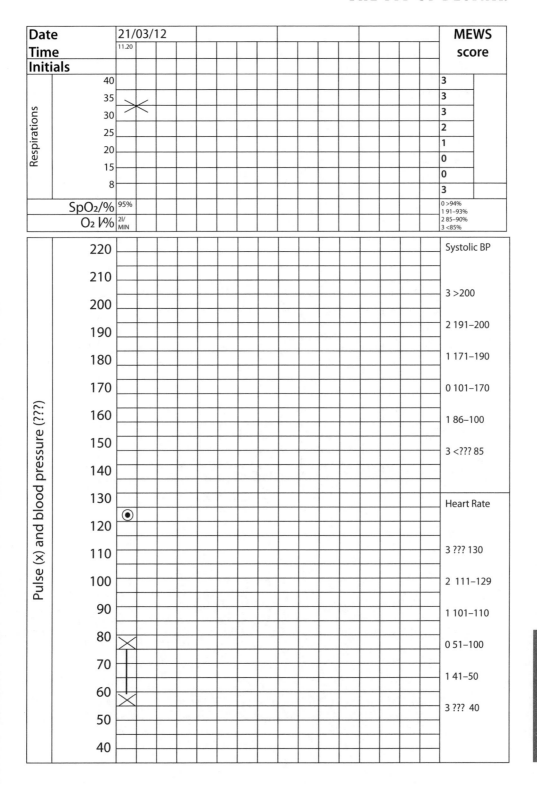

| Date | 21/03/12 | | | | | | | | | | | MEWS |
|---|---|---|---|---|---|---|---|---|---|---|---|---|
| Time | 11.20 | | | | | | | | | | | score |
| Initials | | | | | | | | | | | | |

Respirations

| | | | | | | | | | | | | MEWS score |
|---|---|---|---|---|---|---|---|---|---|---|---|---|
| 40 | | | | | | | | | | | | 3 |
| 35 | ✗ | | | | | | | | | | | 3 |
| 30 | | | | | | | | | | | | 3 |
| 25 | | | | | | | | | | | | 2 |
| 20 | | | | | | | | | | | | 1 |
| 15 | | | | | | | | | | | | 0 |
| | | | | | | | | | | | | 0 |
| 8 | | | | | | | | | | | | 3 |

| SpO₂/% | 95% | | | | | | | | | | | 0 >94% / 1 91–93% / 2 85–90% / 3 <85% |
| O₂ l/% | 2l/MIN | | | | | | | | | | | |

Pulse (x) and blood pressure (???)

Systolic BP
- 3 >200
- 2 191–200
- 1 171–190
- 0 101–170
- 1 86–100
- 3 <??? 85

Heart Rate
- 3 ??? 130
- 2 111–129
- 1 101–110
- 0 51–100
- 1 41–50
- 3 ??? 40

SCENARIO 16

281

| | | | | | | | | | | | | | | | | | | | | | |
|---|---|---|---|---|---|---|---|---|---|---|---|---|---|---|---|---|---|---|---|---|---|
| **Neurological** | Alert | | | | | | | | | | | | | | | | | | 0 | |
| | Voice | ⊗ | | | | | | | | | | | | | | | | | 1 | |
| | Confused | | | | | | | | | | | | | | | | | | 2 | |
| | Pain | | | | | | | | | | | | | | | | | | 3 | |
| | Unresponsive | | | | | | | | | | | | | | | | | | 3 | |
| | Eye | | | | | | | | | | | | | | | | | | | |
| | Voice | | | | | | | | | | | | | | | | | | | |
| | Motor | | | | | | | | | | | | | | | | | | | |
| | Total | | | | | | | | | | | | | | | | | | | |
| | Pupils L | | | | | | | | | | | | | | | | | | | |
| | Pupils R | | | | | | | | | | | | | | | | | | | |
| **Temperature** | 39.5 | | | | | | | | | | | | | | | | | | 3 | |
| | 39.0 | ⊗ | | | | | | | | | | | | | | | | | 3 | |
| | 38.5 | | | | | | | | | | | | | | | | | | 1 | |
| | 38.0 | | | | | | | | | | | | | | | | | | 1 | |
| | 37.5 | | | | | | | | | | | | | | | | | | 0 | |
| | 37.0 | | | | | | | | | | | | | | | | | | 0 | |
| | 36.5 | | | | | | | | | | | | | | | | | | 0 | |
| | 36.0 | | | | | | | | | | | | | | | | | | 0 | |
| | 35.5 | | | | | | | | | | | | | | | | | | 2 | |
| | 35.0 | | | | | | | | | | | | | | | | | | 2 | |
| | 35.0 | | | | | | | | | | | | | | | | | | 3 | |

| | | | | | | | | | | | | | | | | | | | |
|---|---|---|---|---|---|---|---|---|---|---|---|---|---|---|---|---|---|---|---|
| **MEWS** | Respirations | | | | | | | | | | | | | | | | | Urine Output | |
| | SpO₂ | | | | | | | | | | | | | | | | | (ml/hr) | |
| | BP | | | | | | | | | | | | | | | | | | |
| | Heart Rate | | | | | | | | | | | | | | | | | **0** 31–199 | |
| | Neurological | | | | | | | | | | | | | | | | | **3** ??? 200 | |
| | Temperature | | | | | | | | | | | | | | | | | **3** ??? 30 | |
| | Urine Output | 3ml | | | | | | | | | | | | | | | | | |
| | Total | | | | | | | | | | | | | | | | | | |
| **Team called** | | | | | | | | | | | | | | | | | | | |

O – Outreach Support Team   M – Medical Team   P – Patient Team   C – Cardiac Arrest Team

## Station 4

*Data interpretation*                                    *10-minute station*

1. Shown below is a gadolinium-enhanced MRI scan of the pituitary fossa.
■ Please label the structures on the scan labelled A–H.

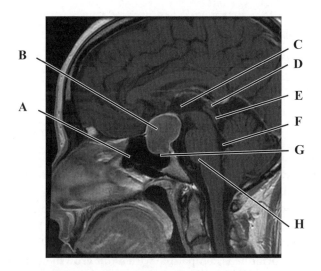

2. The ST5 in Endocrinology comes to see Mr Tan on the ward you work on. Whilst reviewing his old notes she comes across a previous set of dynamic pituitary testing results that Mr Tan had whilst under the care of Professor Watkins at St Hilda's Teaching Hospital in 2003.
■ Please look at the data and answer the questions overleaf, indicating whether they are TRUE (T) or FALSE (F).

Details
- o Mr James Tan, DOB 07/04/1968, Hospital no. 213433
- o Department of Endocrinology – St Hilda's University Hospital NHS Trust
  Consultant: Professor J Watkins
- o Date: 12/03/2003
- o Protocol: insulin tolerance test (ITT)
- o Patient fasted from midnight – YES / NO
- o Patient arrived at 0832 h
- o Test started at 0845 h
- o Aim: blood glucose must be below 2.2 mmol/l for test to be considered valid
- o Blood samples taken at 0, 15, 30, 60, 90 and 120 minutes after administration of 0.1 u/kg actrapid insulin
- o Patient's weight – 76.9 kg
- o Dose of actrapid given = 7.7 units

SCENARIO 16

|  | Normal values | Baseline |
|---|---|---|
| Glucose | 3.5–5.5 mmol/l | 4.9 |
| Cortisol (0900 h) | 140–500 nmol/l | 125 |
| ACTH | 4.4–20 pmol/l | <1.5 |
| IGF-1 | 114–492 ng/ml | 58.3 |
| fT4 | 11–22 pmol/l | 14.7 |
| TSH | 0.17–3.2 mu/l | 0.59 |

| As per protocol 0.1 units/kg Actrapid given | Baseline cortisol nmol/l | Minimum blood glucose (mmol/l) | Peak cortisol Nmol/l | Peak growth hormone (mU/l) |
|---|---|---|---|---|
| Levels | 125 | 1.2 | 189 | 5.7 |
| Diagnostic of deficiency |  |  | <500 | <9.0 |

A This was a suboptimal ITT test.

B The baseline thyroid function indicates sufficient thyroxine replacement.

C The baseline cortisol and ACTH indicate cortisol deficiency.

D Normal growth hormone secretion is under hypothalamic control by GnRH.

E IGF-1 is secreted from the anterior pituitary in parallel with growth hormone.

F The peak cortisol demonstrates hypopituitary–adrenal insufficiency.

G The peak growth hormone is compatible with adult growth hormone deficiency.

H Adults with growth hormone deficiency require treatment with growth hormone replacement.

I Hydrocortisone replacement should be given as equal, divided doses through the day, eg breakfast 10 mg, afternoon 10 mg, evening 10 mg.

J Given these results, this patient should be given a medi-alert bracelet to wear at all times.

## Station 5

*Prescribing skills*                    *10-minute station*

You are the FY1 looking after Mr Tan and have been asked by one of the third-year medical students to review the practice chart she has written out for Mr Tan. She admits that 'she wasn't very familiar with many of the medications she was asked to prescribe', and 'this was the first time she had used this 'new' drug chart'.

■ Please check the charts for errors, listing any you may find and rewrite the charts correctly.

### Details

- o Mr James Tan, DOB 07/04/1968, Hospital no. 6619432
- o Consultant: Dr Ghafor, FY1: Dr Burt 068
- o Height 1.65 m, weight approx 80 kg
- o Allergies: penicillin – 'all over body swelling'
- o Most recent U&Es: Na$^+$ 126 mmol/l, K$^+$ 3.3 mmol/l, urea 23.6 mmol/l, creatinine 131 µmol/l

---

**Remember: DRUG DRs Don't Forget Signing Off (page 396)**

---

| Allergies, sensitivities and adverse drug reactions | | | | Patient details/addressograph | |
|---|---|---|---|---|---|
| No known allergies ✓ | | Initials AF | Gender (M)/ F | NHS/ Hospital No: 6619432 | |
| Not possible to ascertain ☐ | | Date 7/05 | Weight (kg) | Date | |
| Medicine/substance | Reaction & Severity | Initials & Date | 80kg | | Surname: TAN |
| | | | Height | | First name: JEREMY |
| | | | 165 | | |
| Alerts | | | Surface area (m²) | | Date of birth: 07.04.58 |
| | | | | | |

| IN-PATIENT MEDICATION PRESCRIPTION AND ADMINISTRATION RECORD | | | | PasTest HOSPITAL | |
|---|---|---|---|---|---|
| Consultant | Trainee Dr. Name and Bleep no. | Date of admission | Date chart reboarded | Estimated date of discharge | |
| GHAFOR | DR BURT 068 | 21.03.12 | | | |
| This chart is no. | Transcribing Check by Pharmacy | Ward | | | |
| .........1........ of .........1......... | Sign ............. Date ............ | 1. .................................................. | | 2. ................................... | |

## Thromboprophylaxis please prescribe treatment regimens in the regular medications section

| Choice of mechanical prophylaxis and leg(s) to be applied to | | | | | | Enter Time | Enter details below | | | | | | | | | | |
|---|---|---|---|---|---|---|---|---|---|---|---|---|---|---|---|---|---|
| Graduated elastic compression stockings | Intermittent pneumatic compression device (IPC) | | Leg | | | | | | | | | | | | | | |
| | | | Left | Right | Both | | | | | | | | | | | | |
| ☐ Start Date: 21/3 | End Date: | ☐ | Signature and Bleep No. | ☐ | ☐ | ☐ | | | | | | | | | | | | |
| ☐ Start Date: | End Date: | ☐ | Signature and Bleep No. BB | ☐ | ☐ | ☐ | | | | | | | | | | | | |

| Medication | | Dose | | Dose Change | Enter Time | Enter details below | | | | | | | | | | | |
|---|---|---|---|---|---|---|---|---|---|---|---|---|---|---|---|---|---|
| ENOXAPARIN | | 40mg | | | | | | | | | | | | | | | |
| Please ensure you have completed the VTE risk assessment form | Date | 21/3 | | | | | | | | | | | | | | | |
| | Route | SC | | | | | | | | | | | | | | | |
| | Signature | BB | | | Instructions | | | | | | | | Pharmacy | | | | ☐ |
| | Bleep no. | 068 | | | | | | | | | | | | | | | |

## Regular prescriptions continued

### Regular Medications

| | Dose | | | Date | | | | | | | | | | | | |
|---|---|---|---|---|---|---|---|---|---|---|---|---|---|---|---|---|
| | | | | | 21 | 22 | 23 | 24 | | | | | | | | |
| Date | 21/3 | | | Medication | | | Instructions | | | Signature and bleep no. | | | Pharmacy | | | |
| Route | IV | | | HYDROCORTISONE | | | | | | BB 068 | | | ☐ | | | |
| Signature | BB | | | | | | | | | | | | | | | |
| 06 | | | | | | | | | | | | | | | | |
| (09) | 10mg | | | | | | | | | | | | | | | |
| (12) | 5mg | | | | | | | | | | | | | | | |
| (18) | 5mg | | | | | | | | | | | | | | | |
| 22 | | | | | | | | | | | | | | | | |
| 24 | | | | | | | | | | | | | | | | |

## Regular prescriptions continued

| | Dose | | | Date | | | | | | | | | | | | |
|---|---|---|---|---|---|---|---|---|---|---|---|---|---|---|---|---|
| | | | | | | | | | | | | | | | | |
| Date | 21/3 | | | Medication | | | Instructions | | | Signature and bleep no. | | | Pharmacy | | | |
| Route | PO | | | THYROXINE | | | | | | BB 068 | | | ☐ | | | |
| Signature | BB | | | | | | | | | | | | | | | |
| 06 | | | | | | | | | | | | | | | | |
| (09) | 125mg | | | | | | | | | | | | | | | |
| 12 | | | | | | | | | | | | | | | | |
| 18 | | | | | | | | | | | | | | | | |
| 22 | | | | | | | | | | | | | | | | |
| 24 | | | | | | | | | | | | | | | | |

**Regular prescriptions continued**

Anti-infectives prescription  *prescribe long term prophylaxis and anti-tuberculosis medications in regular medications section*

| | Dose | | | Date | | | | | | | | | | | | | |
|---|---|---|---|---|---|---|---|---|---|---|---|---|---|---|---|---|---|
| Date | 21/3 | | | Medication | | | | Indication | | | | Signature and bleep no. | | | | Pharmacy | |
| Route | LM | | | TESTOSTERONE | | | | | | | | BB 068 | | | | ☐ | |
| Signature | BB | | | | | | | | | | | | | | | | |
| 06 | | | | | | | | | | | | | | | | | |
| (09) | 1g | | | | | | | | | | | | | | | | |
| 12 | | | | | | | | | | | | | | | | | |
| 18 | | | | | | | | | | | | | | | | | |
| 22 | | | | | | | | | | | | | | | | | |
| 24 | | | | | | | | | | | | | | | | | |

**Regular prescriptions continued**

Anti-infectives prescription  *prescribe long term prophylaxis and anti-tuberculosis medications in regular medications section*

| | Dose | | | Date | | | | | | | | | | | | | |
|---|---|---|---|---|---|---|---|---|---|---|---|---|---|---|---|---|---|
| Date | 21/3 | | | Medication | | | | Indication | | | | Signature and bleep no. | | | | Pharmacy | |
| Route | PO | | | AMANTADINE | | | | | | | | BB 068 | | | | ☐ | |
| Signature | BB | | | | | | | | | | | | | | | | |
| 06 | | | | | | | | | | | | | | | | | |
| (09) | 10mg | | | | | | | | | | | | | | | | |
| 12 | | | | | | | | | | | | | | | | | |
| 18 | | | | | | | | | | | | | | | | | |
| 22 | | | | | | | | | | | | | | | | | |
| 24 | | | | | | | | | | | | | | | | | |

**Regular prescriptions continued**

Anti-infectives prescription  *prescribe long term prophylaxis and anti-tuberculosis medications in regular medications section*

| FOR 10 DAYS | Dose | | | Date | | | | | | | | | | | | | |
|---|---|---|---|---|---|---|---|---|---|---|---|---|---|---|---|---|---|
| Date 21/3 | | | | Medication | | | | Indication | | | | Signature and bleep no. | | | | Pharmacy | |
| Route IV | | | | AUGMENTIN | | | | | | | | BB 068 | | | | ☐ | |
| Signature | | | | | | | | | | | | | | | | | |
| (06) | 1.2g | | | | | | | | | | | | | | | | |
| 09 | | | | | | | | | | | | | | | | | |
| 12 | | | | | | | | | | | | | | | | | |
| (18) | 1.2g | | | | | | | | | | | | | | | | |
| 22 | | | | | | | | | | | | | | | | | |
| 24 | | | | | | | | | | | | | | | | | |

**Regular prescriptions continued**

Anti-infectives prescription  *prescribe long term prophylaxis and anti-tuberculosis medications in regular medications section*

| FOR 10 DAYS | Dose | | | Date | | | | | | | | | | | | | |
|---|---|---|---|---|---|---|---|---|---|---|---|---|---|---|---|---|---|
| Date 21/3 | | | | Medication | | | | Indication | | | | Signature and bleep no. | | | | Pharmacy | |
| Route IV | | | | CLARITHROMYCIN | | | | | | | | BB 068 | | | | ☐ | |
| Signature | | | | | | | | | | | | | | | | | |
| (06) | 500mg | | | | | | | | | | | | | | | | |
| 09 | | | | | | | | | | | | | | | | | |
| 12 | | | | | | | | | | | | | | | | | |
| (18) | 500mg | | | | | | | | | | | | | | | | |
| 22 | | | | | | | | | | | | | | | | | |
| 24 | | | | | | | | | | | | | | | | | |

SCENARIO 16

287

## Infusion prescriptions continued

| | | | | | | | | SC = subcutaneous | | IVC = intravenous central | | |
| | | | | | | | | | | IVP = intravenous peripheral | | |

| Date & time | Route | Infusion Fluid | | Medication | | Duration | Rate | Prescriber's signature & bleep no. | Date given | Given by / Added by | Check by | Start time | Finish time | Pharmacy |
|---|---|---|---|---|---|---|---|---|---|---|---|---|---|---|
| | | Name & strength | Volume | Approved name with expiry / unit number | Dose | | | | | | | | | |
| 21/3 | IV | 5% Dextrose Exp: Batch/unit no: | 1L | | | | 6° | BB 068 | | | | | | |
| 21/3 | IV | 5% Dextrose Exp: Batch/unit no: | 1L | | | | 6° | BB 068 | | | | | | |
| 21/3 | IV | 5% Dextrose Exp: Batch/unit no: | 1L | | | | 6° | BB 068 | | | | | | |
| 21/3 | IV | 5% Dextrose Exp: Batch/unit no: | 1L | | | | 6° | BB 068 | | | | | | |
| | | Exp: Batch/unit no: | | | | | | | | | | | | |
| | | Exp: Batch/unit no: | | | | | | | | | | | | |
| | | Exp: Batch/unit no: | | | | | | | | | | | | |
| | | Exp: Batch/unit no: | | | | | | | | | | | | |
| | | Exp: Batch/unit no: | | | | | | | | | | | | |

## As required medications

| Medication PARACETAMOL | | | | Date | | | | | | | | | | | | | | | |
|---|---|---|---|---|---|---|---|---|---|---|---|---|---|---|---|---|---|---|---|
| Indication | | | | Time | | | | | | | | | | | | | | | |
| Dose 0.5 - 1mg | Route PO | Maximum frequency / dose QDS | Start date 21/3 | Dose | | | | | | | | | | | | | | | |
| | | | Stop date | Route | | | | | | | | | | | | | | | |
| Signature BB 068 | | | | | | | | | | | | | | | | | | | |
| | | | Bleep no. | Given | | | | | | | | | | | | | | | |
| Additional instructions: | | | | | | | | | | | | Pharmacy | | | | | | | |

## As required medications

| Medication TEMAZEPAM | | | | Date | | | | | | | | | | | | | | | |
|---|---|---|---|---|---|---|---|---|---|---|---|---|---|---|---|---|---|---|---|
| Indication | | | | Time | | | | | | | | | | | | | | | |
| Dose 10 mg | Route PO | Maximum frequency / dose QDS | Start date 21/3 | Dose | | | | | | | | | | | | | | | |
| | | | Stop date | Route | | | | | | | | | | | | | | | |
| Signature BB 068 | | | | | | | | | | | | | | | | | | | |
| | | | Bleep no. | Given | | | | | | | | | | | | | | | |
| Additional instructions: | | | | | | | | | | | | Pharmacy | | | | | | | |

SCENARIO 16

288

| As required medications | | | | | | | | | | | | | | | | | | | | | | | | | | |
|---|---|---|---|---|---|---|---|---|---|---|---|---|---|---|---|---|---|---|---|---|---|---|---|---|---|---|
| **Medication** METOCLOPRAMIDE | | | **Date** | | | | | | | | | | | | | | | | | | | | | | | |
| **Indication** | | | **Time** | | | | | | | | | | | | | | | | | | | | | | | |
| **Dose** 50 mg | **Route** IV/ IM | **Maximum frequency / dose** QDS | **Start date** 21/3 | **Dose** | | | | | | | | | | | | | | | | | | | | | | |
| | | | **Stop date** | **Route** | | | | | | | | | | | | | | | | | | | | | | |
| **Signature** BB 068 | | | **Bleep no.** | **Given** | | | | | | | | | | | | | | | | | | | | | | |
| **Additional instructions:** | | | | | | | | | | | | **Pharmacy** | | | | | | | | | | | | | | |

| As required medications | | | | | | | | | | | | | | | | | | | | | | | | | | |
|---|---|---|---|---|---|---|---|---|---|---|---|---|---|---|---|---|---|---|---|---|---|---|---|---|---|---|
| **Medication** CYCLIZINE | | | **Date** | | | | | | | | | | | | | | | | | | | | | | | |
| **Indication** | | | **Time** | | | | | | | | | | | | | | | | | | | | | | | |
| **Dose** 50 mg | **Route** IV/ IM | **Maximum frequency / dose** QDS | **Start date** 21/3 | **Dose** | | | | | | | | | | | | | | | | | | | | | | |
| | | | **Stop date** | **Route** | | | | | | | | | | | | | | | | | | | | | | |
| **Signature** BB 068 | | | **Bleep no.** | **Given** | | | | | | | | | | | | | | | | | | | | | | |
| **Additional instructions:** | | | | | | | | | | | | **Pharmacy** | | | | | | | | | | | | | | |

## Station 6

*Clinical communication skills*          *10-minute station*

Mr Tan has made a speedy recovery, and the Consultant has asked you to accompany him to see Mr Tan to explain his future management and the importance of his medications. He decides that this would be an excellent opportunity to observe your counselling skills and asks you to lead the session.

■ Please:
    1    Investigate how much Mr Tan understands about his condition
    2    Explain his medications and their importance
    3    Address any concerns Mr Tan may have.

**SCENARIO 16**

# Answers

## Station 1 – History

**Patient script**

You are Mrs Jenni Tan, the wife of Mr James Tan. He was recently brought into the Emergency Department by ambulance after becoming increasingly unwell over the last 48 hours.

Mr Tan is 44 years old and is originally from Hong Kong. He and his family came to the UK in 1991 during the hand back of Hong Kong to China. You have been married for 15 years this spring and you live with your three children in a flat above your local newsagent business.

'It's very important that you know that James had 'brain surgery' in his late teens for a large tumour. It wasn't exactly in the brain but a little structure below the brain. They operated by going up through his nose and he ended up with no hormones. Surgery was performed in Hong Kong, when he was about 18 years old (you don't know any more). (If the student mentions 'pituitary gland', you may confirm 'yes – I'm pretty sure that's it'.)

You know that your husband was under the care of Professor Watkins at St Hilda's Hospital in Birmingham (that's where his family emigrated to) as you've seen letters from the Professor, but when you got married, you decided to move here to Norwich (to be near your family) and James didn't see anyone except his GP after that. You're not really sure why.

He has to take special tablets and injections all the time to remain well, although you're pretty sure he often misses doses. He hasn't managed to take any of his regular medications for at least 4 days or so.

Previous medical history: he has high blood pressure but no other serious illness; he has had one previous admission to hospital, about 10 years or so ago: 'He got in a muddle with his tablets but that was years ago and he's been really well since then.'

If the candidate asks about 'Addisonian crisis' – you don't know what this is; you've never heard James mention it.

You have brought the GP repeat prescription, which shows
  • Hydrocortisone 10 mg (am), 5 mg (afternoon), 5 mg (evening)
  • Thyroxine 125 μg od
  • Nebido® IM 1 g once every 10 weeks
  • Amlodipine 10 mg od

If asked, your husband is allergic to penicillin – 'his whole body swells up'.

If asked about medi-alert bracelet, 'Oh yes he used to wear it when we first met but I haven't seen him wear it for years.' You have never seen a blue steroid card.

Your husband has now been unwell for about 2 weeks. It started as a head cold and then went to his chest. He has been increasingly confused over the last 3 or 4 days and over yesterday became increasingly drowsy and sleepy. This morning he was really unwell, and that's when you called the GP, who told you to call an ambulance.

Over the last 3–4 days he has had a really 'nasty cough' with thick green sputum. You haven't noticed any blood in the sputum. He has been wheezy and short of breath and has had high fevers with sweats day and night (he's soaked the bed sheets on several occasions).

He lives with you and your three children in a three-bedroom flat above the newsagent shop. You have three sons, aged 13, 11 and 7 – all doing well at school.

Your husband is a non-smoker (lifelong); he drinks occasional whisky and beer – rarely if ever more than one or two per week. He is a keen badminton player – plays for a club in town. 'He was a national standard player at school.'

He works 'too hard' in the newsagents (up at 0530 h every morning – 7 days a week) but is very generous and generally a very happy man.

Ideas – 'I know James is seriously ill. He looked terrible this morning and was so confused... I just hope you can get him better quickly.'

Concerns – 'I'm always reminding him to take his medications. Is it anything to do with that?'

Expectations – 'I'm hoping now he's in the hospital you will get him better. He is going to be alright isn't he?'

| A | B | C | D | E | | A | B | C | D | E | | A | B | C | D | E |
PROFESSIONALISM     PROCESS     COMMUNICATION

## CONTENT      | A | B | C | D | E |

**Identifies key information**

- History of pituitary disease
  - Identifies pituitary tumour in the past – timing of operation (where and when); details of endocrine follow-up
  - Hormone replacement regime (see below); adherence
  - Previous complications and admissions to hospital; asks specifically about Addisonian crisis – offers explanation when wife says she doesn't understand the term
  - Asks about medi-alert bracelet/blue steroid card.
- Present illness
  - Duration and progression
  - Respiratory symptoms – cough, sputum, haemoptysis, shortness of breath, wheeze, orthopnoea
  - Systemic symptoms – fevers and sweats, confusion, drowsiness
  - Notes patient hasn't taken his medications for at least 4 days.

**Completing the patient history**

- Drug and allergy history: hydrocortisone 10 mg, 5 mg, 5 mg; thyroxine 125 mg, Nebido® (testosterone) IM 1 g every 10 weeks, amlodipine 10 mg od; allergic to penicillin – 'body swells up'
- Previous medical history: hypertension; nil else of note
- Social and occupational history: married with three children (sons aged 13, 11 and 7 years); owns a newsagents – works very hard; non smoker; occasional beer and whisky; keen badminton player.

**Summarises important areas of the history back to the patient's wife**

**Invites patient's wife to ask questions and deals with them appropriately**

**Establishes patient's wife's ideas, concerns and expectations**

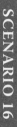
SCENARIO 16

## CLINICAL DIAGNOSTIC REASONING

A B C D E

- **Please present your history**
  - Candidate offers a logical, well-structured account of the history.

- **What is your diagnosis?**
  - Chest infection leading to secondary Addisonian crisis.

- **Could you tell me two clinical (bedside tests) you would wish to perform on this patient to confirm that the patient may have developed an Addisonian crisis?**
  - Blood pressure – absolute, lying and standing
  - Capillary blood glucose – hypoglycaemia.

**Demonstrates safe, sensible and appropriate management plan**

**Demonstrates clear and logical diagnostic reasoning**

## GLOBAL HISTORY MARK

A B C D E

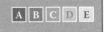

# Station 2 – Examination

**Patient script (see also page 388)**

You are a confused and unwell middle-aged man; you are not able to cooperate easily with the doctor's examination but should not be aggressive or obstructive as they try to assess you.

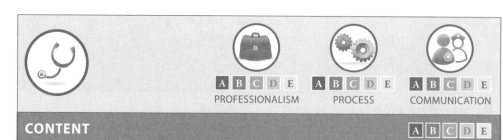

PROFESSIONALISM   PROCESS   COMMUNICATION

## CONTENT

**Exposes and positions patient correctly and maintains comfort**

**Comments on wellbeing of patient, ie well or unwell**

**'Feet to face'**
- Observes and comments on patient and surroundings from foot of bed
- Not overtly panhypopituitary; no obvious hormone excess or deficiency.

**Asks for appropriate/relevant clinical observations**
- Observations: HR 119 bpm, BP 87/56 mmHg (lying), 68/44 mmHg (sitting) RR 26 bpm, $O_2$ sats 95% on 2 l/min, temperature 39.6 °C, CBG 2.4 mmol/l (treated in the ambulance)
- Peripheries – cold and shut down.

**General/systemic examination**
- GCS or AVPU – responding to voice.

**Hormone replacement assessment**
- Not overtly panhypopituitary; no obvious hormone excess or deficiency
- Normal facies – hair: normal; skin: no hyper- or hypopigmentation
- Thyroid status – no features of thyrotoxicosis or hypothyroidism
- Steroid status – no overt features of Addison's or Cushing's BUT has features of Addisonian crisis, including hypotension and postural drop, and hypoglycaemia
- Testosterone– normal distribution of adult male hair: evidence of a few days' facial growth; penis and testes normal.

**Focussed examination of respiratory system**
- Assesses all elements of the respiratory system (anterior and posterior; one side vs the other; appropriate technique)
- Trachea – expansion; percussion; TVF/VF; auscultation.

**Thanks patient, offers assistance, maintains patient's dignity and privacy until they are dressed**

SCENARIO 16

## CLINICAL DIAGNOSTIC REASONING

A B C D E

**Correctly identifies the relevant physical signs, including important negative findings**

- **What are the features that confirm Mr Tan is suffering with an Addisonian crisis?**
  - Hypotension with postural drop
  - Initial hypoglycaemia.

- **Given these findings, can you tell me five essential therapeutic interventions for this patient?**
  - Hypoglycaemia – glucagon and dextrose infusion
  - Hypotension – intravenous fluids (possible colloid and then crystalloid infusion)
  - Suspected Addisonian crisis – intravenous hydrocortisone
  - Severe chest infection – intravenous antibiotics (must avoid penicillin, eg levofloxacin and clarithromycin)
  - High temperature – remove excess clothing and blankets; antipyretics – paracetamol and fanning
  - Oxygen via nasal prongs or mask – oxygen sats being maintained at 95% on 2 l/min.

**Demonstrates safe, sensible and appropriate management plan**

**Demonstrates clear and logical diagnostic reasoning**

## GLOBAL EXAMINATION MARK

A B C D E

## Station 3 – Procedural skills

**Procedure**

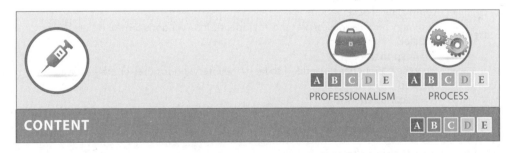

A B C D E
PROFESSIONALISM

A B C D E
PROCESS

### CONTENT

A B C D E

### Identifies and sets out equipment correctly
- Cardiac monitoring
- Sats probe
- Dynamap blood pressure cuff
- Urinalysis
- Capillary blood glucose monitoring kit
- Aural thermometer.

### Correctly performs the elements of the observations
- Cardiac monitoring - places leads on correctly: red = right arm ; yellow = left arm; black or green = left leg (abdomen or lower chest)
- Obtains and records valid cardiac trace and HR reading
- Oxygen saturation – places oxygen probe correctly on finger or thumb and obtains and records valid pulse oximetry reading
- Temperature – uses the aural thermometer appropriately and obtains and records valid aural temperature
- Blood pressure – uses the dynamap blood pressure cuff and obtains and records a valid blood pressure reading
- Capillary blood glucose (CBG) (if volunteer allows) – uses blood monitoring kit and correctly obtains and records CBG
- Urinalysis (using tap water or similar) – demonstrates how to perform and record urinalysis.

### Thanks patient, offers assistance, maintains patient's dignity and privacy until they are dressed

### Correctly relays observations to a colleague
- Correctly identifies the abnormalities of Mr Tan's observations and calculates his MEWS score = 15–16, ie VERY HIGH
- Uses SBARR or similar methodical presentation to handover the patient:
  - **S = Situation**
  - Identifies – who they are, where they and the patient are, and the patient's details; why they are calling and their major concerns
  - **B= Background**
  - Explains – patient's reason for admission, significant previous medical history and presents clinical status, including latest blood or other investigation results
  - **A = Assessment/Action**
  - Latest clinical observations
  - Summary and diagnoses; presents therapeutic interventions they or others have initiated
  - **R = Response**
  - How the patient has responded so far to the interventions they or others have commenced
  - **R = Recommendations**
  - Explains what they need and when – is specific in terms of expectations of the other person, including a time frame.

### Agrees on plan; thanks colleague

### Records conversation accurately in notes

| PATIENT NAME: | HOSPITAL NUMBER: |
|---|---|
| WARD | DOB |
| CONSULTANT | |

Handover of Patient to Sister (Name)          TIME

Used SBARR handover

Agreed plan:

Sister (Name) will ensure patient is nursed in HDU / ITU environment; I will notify ITU registrar of patient's present status and ask for review

Patient to continue on 30 minute observations

Patient presently on 2 hourly litre of saline; urine output to be monitored

Handover to night registrar via handover meeting at 10pm – for regular review over next 24 hours

I will discuss with wife present serious clinical condition of Mr Tan – Registrar (Dr Hook) to confirm CPR status.

Sister (name) will ensure handover to nursing staff and will not allow transfer of Mr Tan from resus unless all parties agree on destination and ongoing care.

Name - PRINTED

Signature

Bleep number

| DATE: | SIGNATURE | BLEEP NUMBER |
|---|---|---|

**GLOBAL PROCEDURE MARK**

A B C D E

SCENARIO 16

## Station 4 – Data interpretation

**1.**

A       Spenoidal air sinus

B       Large pituitary tumour, with suprasellar extensions

C       Third ventricle

D       Pineal body

E       Tectum of midbrain

F       Fourth ventricle

G       Distorted pituitary fossa

H       Pons

**2.**

A       False – the blood glucose dropped to 1.9 mmol/l, below the 2.2 mmol/l required for a valid hypoglycaemic stress response. Patients are often given oral dextrose after the test or may require intravenous dextrose if they suffer severe or prolonged hypoglycaemia. In addition, patients with a poor cortisol response are often given hydrocortisone at the end of the test.

B       False – the patient has a normal thyroid-stimulating hormone (TSH) and free T4 (fT4), indicating adequate thyroxine replacement.

C       True – the baseline cortisol and adrenocorticotrophic hormone (ACTH) are very low and indicate the patient to be cortisol-deficient.

D       False – normal growth hormone secretion is under hypothalamic control by growth-hormone-releasing hormone (GHRH). Gonadotrophin-releasing hormone (GnRH) controls the release of FSH and LH.

E       False – insulin-like growth factor 1 (IGF-1) is mainly secreted from the liver under the stimulant control of GH secretion from the pituitary.

F       True – the peak cortisol is very low, and well below the 500 nmol threshold required to diagnose hypopituitary–adrenal insufficiency.

G       True – the peak growth hormone (5.7 mU/l) is compatible with adult growth hormone deficiency, diagnosed at a peak <9 mU/L.

H       False – by the NICE guidelines for replacement of GH in adults (over 25 years old) patients must:
- (a) Have demonstrable GH levels below 9 mU/l on the ITT
- (b) Undergo a questionnaire ('Quality of life assessment of growth hormone deficiency in adults') and score at least 11
- (c) Already be on hormone replacement therapy of other hormones if suffering from hypopituitarism, before they are eligible for GH treatment.

**I**      False – physiological cortisol secretion normally peaks in the early morning and is lower at night. In view of this most patients were previously prescribed a twice daily regime of 20 mg (morning) and 10 mg (evening). However, more recently an additional dose in the afternoon has proven to be more effective; thus most patients receive a triple dose regime of 10 mg (morning), 5 mg (lunchtime), 5 mg (evening). Some patients require an afternoon dose of 10 mg, making their regime 10 mg, 10 mg, 5 mg.

**J**      True – all patients taking regular steroids, especially for hypopituitarism should wear a medi-alert bracelet and carry a blue steroid card.

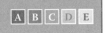

**GLOBAL DATA INTERPRETATION MARK**     A B C D E

## Station 5 – Prescribing skills

NOTE: Whilst many of these prescribing errors seem far-fetched, we speak from bitter experience when we say that they are all too common in the workplace. When you are tired, in a rush, trying to multitask, or being distracted, small but often important errors creep in to your work. These charts demonstrate some common prescribing errors – don't be the one who makes them!

Wrong patient details – common mistake when filling in multiple charts or when one is distracted or tired.

Omission of important information – drug allergies and oxygen treatment – these may be fatal.

Writing drugs without taking into account acute kidney injury (AKI) or other potential hazards – THINK: Do any of these drug doses need to be modified for this patient? This may also include drug interactions.

Writing inappropriate antibiotics –make sure you know what drugs are contained in trade preparations; if you are the prescriber it's your duty to look up uncommon or unknown drug preparations in the BNF or on the web. There are no excuses for writing contraindicated drugs on the chart!

Writing sub-optimal doses and incorrect frequency of a drug, eg hydrocortisone; this patient is in Addisonian crisis and writing up their normal dose of steroids will be ineffectual and life-threatening in this case. Remember: 'If in doubt give them the 'roids' (The Fatman in *The House of God* by Samuel Shem, 1978).

Writing incorrect or illegible doses/units (thyroxine) – this can be fatal.

Testosterone is given once every 10 weeks – such medications rarely have a place in the acute management of a sick patient.

SCENARIO 16

Writing the wrong drug (amantadine rather than amlodipine) is a common error by novice prescribers who are tired, multitasking or distracted. The amlodipine should not be given if the patient is hypotensive. **TREAT THE PATIENT IN FRONT OF YOU.**

It is common practice amongst FY doctors to have a menu of commonly prescribed 'as required/prn' drugs that they write for each patient. Whilst this works for many patients, it can be a recipe for disaster – **BE A THINKING CLINICIAN.**

Prescribing fluids is as much an art as a science and demands lots of practice. Until such time think about the following factors – how much (VOLUME), which type (VARIETY), over how long (RATE) and supplements (ADDITIONS).

**Fluids should be tailored to the patient's fluid balance, BP, HR and blood biochemistry.**

| Allergies, sensitivities and adverse drug reactions | | | | | | Patient details/addressograph | |
|---|---|---|---|---|---|---|---|
| No known allergies ✓ | | Initials BB | | Gender ⓜ/ F | | NHS/ Hospital No: 6619432 | |
| Not possible to ascertain ☐ | | Date 7/05 | | Weight (kg) | Date | | |
| Medicine/substance | Reaction & Severity | Initials & Date | | 80kg | | Surname: TAN | |
| | | | | Height | | First name: JEREMY | |
| | | | | 165 | | | |
| Alerts | | | | Surface area (m²) | | Date of birth: 07.04.58 | |

no reaction stated,
leading to prescription/
possible administration
of augmentin

wrong name

wrong DOB

| IN-PATIENT MEDICATION PRESCRIPTION AND ADMINISTRATION RECORD | | | | PasTest HOSPITAL | |
|---|---|---|---|---|---|
| Consultant | Trainee Dr. Name and Bleep no. | Date of admission | Date chart reboarded | | Estimated date of discharge |
| GHAFOR | DR BURT 068 | 21.03.12 | | | |
| This chart is no. | Transcribing Check by Pharmacy | Ward | | | |
| ........1........ of ........1........ | Sign ............... Date ............ | 1. .................................................. | | 2. .................................. | |

**Thromboprophylaxis please prescribe treatment regimens in the regular medications section**

| Choice of mechanical prophylaxis and leg(s) to be applied to | | | | | | Enter Time | Enter details below | | | | | | | | | | | |
|---|---|---|---|---|---|---|---|---|---|---|---|---|---|---|---|---|---|---|
| Graduated elastic compression stockings | Intermittent pneumatic compression device (IPC) | | Leg | | | | | | | | | | | | | | | |
| | | | Left | Right | Both | | | | | | | | | | | | | |
| ☐ Start Date: 21/3 | End Date: | ☐ Signature and Bleep No. | ☐ | ☐ | ☐ | | | | | | | | | | | | | |
| ☐ Start Date: | End Date: | ☐ Signature and Bleep No. BB | ☐ | ☐ | ☐ | | | | | | | | | | | | | |

| Medication | Dose | | Dose Change | Enter Time | Enter details below | | | | | | | | | | |
|---|---|---|---|---|---|---|---|---|---|---|---|---|---|---|---|
| ENOXAPARIN | 40mg | | | | | | | | | | | | | | |
| Please ensure you have completed the VTE risk assessment form | Date | 21/3 | | | | | | | | | | | | | |
| | Route | SC | | | | | | | | | | | | | |
| | Signature | BB | | Instructions | | | | | | | Pharmacy | | | ☐ | |
| | Bleep no. | 068 | | | | | | | | | | | | | |

dose doesn't take
into account renal
impairment

**Regular prescriptions continued**

*Regular Medications*

| | Dose | | | Date | 21 | 22 | 23 | 24 | | | | | | | | | | |
|---|---|---|---|---|---|---|---|---|---|---|---|---|---|---|---|---|---|---|
| Date | 21/3 | | | Medication | | | | Instructions | | | | | Signature and bleep no. | | | Pharmacy | | |
| Route | IV | | | HYDROCORTISONE | | | | | | | | | BB 068 | | | ☐ | | |
| Signature | BB | | | | | | | | | | | | | | | | | |
| 06 | | | | | | | | | | | | | | | | | | |
| 09 | 10mg | | | | | | | | | | | | | | | | | |
| 12 | 5mg | | | | | | | | | | | | | | | | | |
| 18 | 5mg | | | | | | | | | | | | | | | | | |
| 22 | | | | | | | | | | | | | | | | | | |
| 24 | | | | | | | | | | | | | | | | | | |

written as 10 mg, 5 mg,
5 mg – IV BUT in
Addisonian crisis

**Regular prescriptions continued**

| Date | Dose | | | Date | | | | | | | | | | | |
|------|------|--|--|------|--|--|--|--|--|--|--|--|--|--|--|
| Date 21/3 | | | | Medication THYROXINE | | Instructions | | Signature and bleep no. BB 068 | | Pharmacy | | | | | |
| Route PO | | | | | | | | | | | | | | | |
| Signature BB | | | | | | | | | | | | | | | |
| 06 | | | | | | | | | | | | | | | |
| (09) | 125mg | | | | | | | | | | | | | | |
| 12 | | | | | | | | | | | | | | | |
| 18 | | | | | | | | | | | | | | | |
| 22 | | | | | | | | | | | | | | | |
| 24 | | | | | | | | | | | | | | | |

unclear as to mcg or mg

**Regular prescriptions continued**

Anti-infectives prescription *prescribe long term prophylaxis and anti-tuberculosis medications in regular medications section*

| Date | Dose | | | Date | | | | | | | | | | | |
|------|------|--|--|------|--|--|--|--|--|--|--|--|--|--|--|
| Date 21/3 | | | | Medication TESTOSTERONE | | Indication | | Signature and bleep no. BB 068 | | Pharmacy | | | | | |
| Route LM | | | | | | | | | | | | | | | |
| Signature BB | | | | | | | | | | | | | | | |
| 06 | | | | | | | | | | | | | | | |
| (09) | 1g | | | | | | | | | | | | | | |
| 12 | | | | | | | | | | | | | | | |
| 18 | | | | | | | | | | | | | | | |
| 22 | | | | | | | | | | | | | | | |
| 24 | | | | | | | | | | | | | | | |

written as IM injection daily – should be testosterone 1 g IM once/10 weeks

**Regular prescriptions continued**

Anti-infectives prescription *prescribe long term prophylaxis and anti-tuberculosis medications in regular medications section*

| Date | Dose | | | Date | | | | | | | | | | | |
|------|------|--|--|------|--|--|--|--|--|--|--|--|--|--|--|
| Date 21/3 | | | | Medication AMANTADINE | | Indication | | Signature and bleep no. BB 068 | | Pharmacy | | | | | |
| Route PO | | | | | | | | | | | | | | | |
| Signature BB | | | | | | | | | | | | | | | |
| 06 | | | | | | | | | | | | | | | |
| (09) | 10mg | | | | | | | | | | | | | | |
| 12 | | | | | | | | | | | | | | | |
| 18 | | | | | | | | | | | | | | | |
| 22 | | | | | | | | | | | | | | | |
| 24 | | | | | | | | | | | | | | | |

should be crossed off as patient hypotensive

SCENARIO 16

302

**Regular prescriptions continued**

**Anti-infectives prescription**   *prescribe long term prophylaxis and anti-tuberculosis medications in regular medications section*

| FOR 10 DAYS | Dose | | | Date | | | | | | | | | | | | | | |
|---|---|---|---|---|---|---|---|---|---|---|---|---|---|---|---|---|---|---|
| Date 21/3 | | | | Medication AUGMENTIN | | | | | Indication | | | | | Signature and bleep no. BB 068 | | | Pharmacy ☐ | |
| Route IV | | | | | | | | | | | | | | | | | | |
| Signature | BB | | | | | | | | | | | | | | | | | |
| (06) | 1.2g | | | | | | | | | | | | | | | | | |
| 09 | | | | | | | | | | | | | | | | | | |
| 12 | | | | | | | | | | | | | | | | | | |
| (18) | 1.2g | | | | | | | | | | | | | | | | | |
| 22 | | | | | | | | | | | | | | | | | | |
| 24 | | | | | | | | | | | | | | | | | | |

**allergic to penicillin – potentially fatal
especially when patient is Addisonian
and unable to mount stress response**

**Regular prescriptions continued**

**Anti-infectives prescription**   *prescribe long term prophylaxis and anti-tuberculosis medications in regular medications section*

| FOR 10 DAYS | Dose | | | Date | | | | | | | | | | | | | | |
|---|---|---|---|---|---|---|---|---|---|---|---|---|---|---|---|---|---|---|
| Date 21/3 | | | | Medication CLARITHROMYCIN | | | | | Indication | | | | | Signature and bleep no. BB 068 | | | Pharmacy ☐ | |
| Route IV | | | | | | | | | | | | | | | | | | |
| Signature | BB | | | | | | | | | | | | | | | | | |
| (06) | 500mg | | | | | | | | | | | | | | | | | |
| 09 | | | | | | | | | | | | | | | | | | |
| 12 | | | | | | | | | | | | | | | | | | |
| (18) | 500mg | | | | | | | | | | | | | | | | | |
| 22 | | | | | | | | | | | | | | | | | | |
| 24 | | | | | | | | | | | | | | | | | | |

**Oxygen – none written up**

| Infusion prescriptions continued | | | | | | | | | | | | SC = subcutaneous | | IVC = intravenous central IVP = intravenous peripheral | |
|---|---|---|---|---|---|---|---|---|---|---|---|---|---|---|---|
| Date & time | Route | Infusion Fluid | | Medication | | Duration | Rate | Prescriber's signature & bleep no. | Date given | Given by / Added by | Check by | Start time | Finish time | Pharmacy | |
| | | Name & strength | Volume | Approved name with expiry / unit number | Dose | | | | | | | | | | |
| 21/3 | IV | 5% Dextrose Exp: Batch/unit no: | 1l | | | | 6⁰ | | | | | | | | |
| 21/3 | IV | 5% Dextrose Exp: Batch/unit no: | 1l | | | | 6⁰ | | | | | | | | |
| 21/3 | IV | 5% Dextrose Exp: Batch/unit no: | 1l | | | | 6⁰ | | | | | | | | |
| 21/3 | IV | 5% Dextrose Exp: Batch/unit no: | 1l | | | | 6⁰ | | | | | | | | |
| | | Exp: Batch/unit no: | | | | | | | | | | | | | |
| | | Exp: Batch/unit no: | | | | | | | | | | | | | |
| | | Exp: Batch/unit no: | | | | | | | | | | | | | |
| | | Exp: Batch/unit no: | | | | | | | | | | | | | |
| | | Exp: Batch/unit no: | | | | | | | | | | | | | |
| | | | | | | | | | | | | | | | |
| | | | | | | | | | | | | | | | |

no signature

| As required medications | | | | | | | | | | | | | | | | | | | | | | | |
|---|---|---|---|---|---|---|---|---|---|---|---|---|---|---|---|---|---|---|---|---|---|---|---|
| Medication PARACETAMOL | | | | Date | | | | | | | | | | | | | | | | | | | |
| Indication | | | | Time | | | | | | | | | | | | | | | | | | | |
| Dose 0.5 – 1mg | Route PO | Maximum frequency / dose QDS | Start date 21/3 | Dose | | | | | | | | | | | | | | | | | | | |
| Signature BB 068 | | | Stop date | Route | | | | | | | | | | | | | | | | | | | |
| | | | Bleep no. | Given | | | | | | | | | | | | | | | | | | | |
| Additional instructions: | | | | | | | | | | | | | | | Pharmacy | | | | | | | | |

wrong units

| As required medications | | | | | | | | | | | | | | | | | | | | | | | | |
|---|---|---|---|---|---|---|---|---|---|---|---|---|---|---|---|---|---|---|---|---|---|---|---|---|
| **Medication** TEMAZEPAM | | | **Date** | | | | | | | | | | | | | | | | | | | | | |
| **Indication** | | | **Time** | | | | | | | | | | | | | | | | | | | | | |
| **Dose** 10 mg | **Route** PO | **Maximum frequency / dose** QDS | **Start date** 21/3 | **Dose** | | | | | | | | | | | | | | | | | | | | |
| | | | **Stop date** | **Route** | | | | | | | | | | | | | | | | | | | | |
| **Signature** BB 068 | | | **Bleep no.** | **Given** | | | | | | | | | | | | | | | | | | | | |
| **Additional instructions:** | | | | | | | | | | | | | | | | | **Pharmacy** | | | | | | | |

wrong frequency and dangerous drug to
be writing up in confused/drowsy patient

| As required medications | | | | | | | | | | | | | | | | | | | | | | | | |
|---|---|---|---|---|---|---|---|---|---|---|---|---|---|---|---|---|---|---|---|---|---|---|---|---|
| **Medication** METOCLOPRAMIDE | | | **Date** | | | | | | | | | | | | | | | | | | | | | |
| **Indication** | | | **Time** | | | | | | | | | | | | | | | | | | | | | |
| **Dose** 50 mg | **Route** IV/ IM | **Maximum frequency / dose** QDS | **Start date** 21/3 | **Dose** | | | | | | | | | | | | | | | | | | | | |
| | | | **Stop date** | **Route** | | | | | | | | | | | | | | | | | | | | |
| **Signature** BB 068 | | | **Bleep no.** | **Given** | | | | | | | | | | | | | | | | | | | | |
| **Additional instructions:** | | | | | | | | | | | | | | | | | **Pharmacy** | | | | | | | |

wrong dose and frequency

| As required medications | | | | | | | | | | | | | | | | | | | | | | | | |
|---|---|---|---|---|---|---|---|---|---|---|---|---|---|---|---|---|---|---|---|---|---|---|---|---|
| **Medication** CYCLIZINE | | | **Date** | | | | | | | | | | | | | | | | | | | | | |
| **Indication** | | | **Time** | | | | | | | | | | | | | | | | | | | | | |
| **Dose** 50 mg | **Route** IV/ IM | **Maximum frequency / dose** QDS | **Start date** 21/3 | **Dose** | | | | | | | | | | | | | | | | | | | | |
| | | | **Stop date** | **Route** | | | | | | | | | | | | | | | | | | | | |
| **Signature** BB 068 | | | **Bleep no.** | **Given** | | | | | | | | | | | | | | | | | | | | |
| **Additional instructions:** | | | | | | | | | | | | | | | | | **Pharmacy** | | | | | | | |

wrong frequency

**GLOBAL PRESCRIBING MARK**

 A B C D E

**SCENARIO 16**

305

## Station 6 – Clinical communication skills

### Patient script

You are Mr James Tan (DOB 07/04/1968 – aged 44 years old). You don't remember the young doctor as you were too unwell on admission but are pleased to make his/her acquaintance. You are happy to talk to the doctor about your condition and the treatment.

**What you've been told** – your wife has told you that you were very unwell on admission and that this was due to a serious chest infection.

**Ideas** - you don't think it was anything to do with your underlying condition or your poor adherence to your medications. You are really looking forward to going home and are slightly irritated with the doctor for implying it was a problem with your medications that may have caused you to get so unwell.

**Concerns** – you are concerned that the doctor is blaming you for getting unwell and that really it's the doctor's fault for not being able to explain things properly.

**Expectations** – you are going to carry on as you did before as you've 'been 'totally well' without too much help for over 10 years'.

**In the past** – you have been very well since your operation and have had only one admission to hospital due to 'a mix up with your drugs'. 'It was the GP's fault as he didn't prescribe the right things for me and that made me ill.' You remember when you had your operation in Hong Kong and after when you were looked after at St Hilda's that several people sat you down and explained the importance of your medicines. 'I've never really been bothered to find out very much as they seem to keep me well.'

**If asked** – you admit that you often miss doses of the tablets and occasionally your injections (of testosterone) as 'it never really seems to affect me one way or another whether I take them or not'. ' I work very hard and as long as I have enough energy to work and play badminton I'm happy.'

You haven't been to see a hospital doctor in over 10 years since you moved here from Birmingham. Professor Watkins did explain that it would be important to see a new doctor to look after you but you see the GP regularly and she never seems to think it's an issue.

You are happy to listen to the doctor about the medications but should not be inquisitive or particularly interested in their explanation. You should agree to follow the doctor's advice, including agreeing to come to follow-up under Dr Mills, the Endocrinologist.

However, if the doctor is judgemental, unsupportive, or explains things poorly then you should not co-operate and ask to speak to a more senior doctor who may be able to 'do a better job'.

| A | B | C | D | E |   | A | B | C | D | E |   | A | B | C | D | E |
PROFESSIONALISM      PROCESS      COMMUNICATION

## CONTENT

| A | B | C | D | E |

**Confirms reason for discussion**
- To talk to the patient about his diagnosis, the medications he is taking, and the follow-up process once he leaves hospital.

**Establishes what patient wishes to know; gains agreement/informal consent to participate in the discussion**

**Investigates patient's present level of understanding of scenario**
- What he's been told by other healthcare professionals in the past and on this admission.

**Summarises and confirms what has happened so far**

**Establishes patient's ideas, concerns and expectations**

**Explains the key, important information**
- The diagnosis of hypopituitarism (in an appropriate/empathetic manner)
- Normal physiology of the pituitary gland and the hormones
- Explains what has happened as a result of James' surgery, ie now hypopituitary
- Explains hormone replacement therapy
- Hydrocortisone/steroids – essential for normal function of the major systems within the body and particularly in stress-related situations; normally produced by the adrenal glands next to the kidneys
- Thyroxine – normally produced by the thyroid gland and essential for normal functioning of many important systems within the body
- Testosterone – normally produced by the adrenal glands and the testicles and essential for sexual development and maintaining 'men as men': hair, testicle and penis development and function
- Explains why it's essential to take medications on a regular rather than ad hoc basis – danger of Addisonian crisis (as occurred on this admission); poor control of testosterone and thyroid levels may damage bones and other structures in the body; should wear medi-alert bracelet and carry blue steroid card.

**Invites patient to ask questions and is able to deal with them appropriately**

**Summarises important areas of the consultation back to the patient**

**Formally ends the consultation and ensures appropriate follow-up has been discussed**

## GLOBAL COMMUNICATION MARK

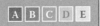
| A | B | C | D | E |

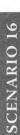
SCENARIO 16

## Scenario 16: Reflection and consolidation

| History |
| --- |

This is a complex case and one that may require you to do some preparatory reading in textbooks and old case notes (if available) prior to seeing the patient. If old notes are available it is very useful to summarise the patient's medical history and record the results of any previous complex investigations such as dynamic pituitary testing and previous MRI scans.

According to the patient's wife, Mr Tan is a 44-year-old Hong Kong Chinese man who has lived in the UK since 1991. He had a transphenoidal excision of a pituitary tumour removed in Hong Kong aged 18 years old, leaving him panhypopituitary. After he and his family immigrated to the UK he lived in Birmingham, where he was cared for by Professor Watkins at St Hilda's Hospital. After getting married he and his wife moved to Norwich to be near her family, and unfortunately it appears he was lost to hospital follow-up but is still seeing his local GP.

Of note he has had one previous hospital admission due to some confusion with his medications, but his wife was unclear as to whether this was associated with an Addisonian crisis.

Previous medical history – Mr Tan has high blood pressure but no other serious illness of note.

His wife provided us with a GP repeat prescription which shows: hydrocortisone 10 mg (am), 5 mg (afternoon), 5 mg (evening), thyroxine 125 μg od, Nebido® IM 1 g once every 10 weeks, amlodipine 10 mg od. According to his wife, Mr Tan misses doses of his tablets from time to time but on the whole is pretty adherent with his medications. He is allergic to penicillin, which leads to 'total body swelling'. He does not wear his medi-alert bracelet or carry his blue steroid card.

Mr Tan has now been unwell for about 2 weeks. It started as a head cold and then went to his chest. Over the last 3–4 days he has had a cough with thick green sputum. There has been no haemoptysis. He has also been wheezy and short of breath and has had high fevers with sweats day and night, soaking the bed sheets on several occasions.

During this acute period he has been increasingly confused and during the last 24 hours increasingly drowsy and sleepy. His wife became concerned about him this morning and called the GP, who told her to call an ambulance.

Mr Tan lives with his wife and three sons in a three-bedroom flat above their newsagent shop. He is a lifelong non-smoker and drinks occasional whisky and beer – rarely if ever more than one or two per week. He is a keen badminton player.

Mrs Tan is very concerned that her husband is very ill and that this may be due to him forgetting his tablets from time to time.

## Examination

On examination of this middle-aged man with known treated hypopituitarism, he is acutely unwell. He was confused and drowsy but easily rousable. His observations on arrival showed HR 119 bpm, BP 87/56 mmHg (lying); 68/44 mmHg (sitting to 90 degrees); temperature 39.6 °C, $O_2$ sats 95% on 2 l/min, RR 26 bpm, CBG 2.4 mmol/l (treated in the ambulance) and his peripheries were poorly perfused.

On assessment of his endocrine status he was not overtly panhypopituitary and there were no signs of obvious hormone excess or deficiency.

On examination of his chest there were signs consistent with a left lower lobe pneumonia, including dullness to percussion and coarse crackles at the left base.

In summary, this is a middle-aged Chinese man with known treated hypopituitarism who now presents with features of Addisonian crisis secondary to a severe left lower lobe pneumonia.

Being asked to examine such a patient can be daunting and slightly bemusing to the novice clinician. If one thinks about the history and 'worst case scenario' one should be thinking about:

- Addisonian crisis – this is true for any patient on long-term steroid therapy, but especially the acutely ill patient who is on steroid replacement therapy
- Significant sepsis – given the history this patient sounds to have a serious community-acquired pneumonia; in certain areas of the country this history may be suggestive of tuberculosis
- Hormone status – given the patient's 'poor' adherence to his medications and lack of specialist follow-up one needs to assess the patient for signs of hormone excess or deficiency; this is a sophisticated part of the assessment and one could forgive the junior clinician for not thinking about this part of the assessment in such a seriously ill man.

Regardless of his underlying condition, Mr Tan, like all acutely unwell patients, requires a comprehensive assessment, including cardiovascular, respiratory, abdominal and neurological examination. It is important that you don't lose sight of the overarching themes and get bogged down in the complexity of his underlying condition.

## Investigations

In the acute setting this man would require a comprehensive set of blood tests, including full blood count (signs of sepsis), urea and electrolytes (significant hyponatraemia would be consistent with his Addisonian presentation), random blood glucose (to demonstrate hypoglycaemia), C-reactive protein (would be de rigueur in most hospitals but really not very useful here), blood cultures and arterial blood gases (given his relative hypoxia). He should also have a chest X-ray and electrocardiogram (given his tachycardia).

Baseline and dynamic pituitary testing would be indicated once he has recovered from his acute illness. These would be best performed in an endocrine day unit several weeks after discharge.

## Management

This patient personifies the old adage of 'if they are sick – give them the 'roids'. Any patient on long-term steroid therapy who presents acutely unwell should receive an intravenous dose of steroids (hydrocortisone 100–200 mg) immediately. This should be repeated every 6 hours until such time as their steroid status can be properly assessed.

In this case the patient should receive:

- Intravenous hydrocortisone
- Intravenous fluids – he should have 2 to 3 litres of 0.9% saline or Hartmann's solution over 1–2 hours, with a further 3–4 litres, titrated against his BP, HR and urine output
- Intravenous antibiotics – because he is allergic to penicillin, he should receive levofloxacin and clarithromycin (but this may vary in different regions, and one should always treat according to local antibiotic policy)
- Anti-pyretics – paracetamol and cooling by fan, removing any excess clothing
- Oxygen via a mask or nasal cannulae.

His amlodipine should be stopped until such time as his BP recovers.

SCENARIO 16

**Further reading and web links**

*Simple but useful overview of hypopituitarism*:
www.ncbi.nlm.nih.gov/pubmedhealth/PMH0001383/
*Comprehensive guide to diagnosis and treatment of hypopituitarism*:
http://emedicine.medscape.com/article/122287-overview
*NICE guidelines on GH replacement in adults*:
www.nice.org.uk/nicemedia/live/11504/32665/32665.pdf
*Nicely set out guide to the patient with hypopituitarism*:
www.endobible.com/condition/hypopituitarism/
*The House of God* by Samuel Shem, 1978, ISBN 0-440-13368-8.

# Scenario 17: 'A little rash'

## Station 1

*History*                                    *10-minute station*

You are the FY1 on the Medical Admissions Unit (MAU). You've been asked by the Consultant to admit a patient, Ms Valerie Andrews (DOB 17/11/1988 – aged 23 years), who has been referred by her GP this morning with a fever and severe headache.

■ Please take a focussed diagnostic history with a view to presenting it to the Consultant. The patient is lying in a dimly lit side room on the MAU.

*You will be assessed on the following areas, as well as the content and diagnostic reasoning of your history – take them into account in your presentation.*

### Professionalism

- Professional appearance (NHS dress code) – including general appearance, hair and jewellery
- Maintains patient and personal safety
- Polite introduction; identifies patient or interviewee correctly; confirms patient's date of birth from name band or other source
- Obtains informal consent; maintains patient's privacy
- Displays empathetic and caring attitudes and behaviours throughout.

### Process

- Good organisation and structure; appropriate use of open and closed questions
- Appropriate fluency/rhythm/pace to the interview – this may change depending on environment and acute nature of the problem
- Appropriate time for the patient to respond/reply to questions
- Appropriate acknowledgement of difficult or emotional areas of the patient's history.

### Communication skills

- Demonstrates caring and sympathetic attitude
- Asks open questions
- Invites patient to ask questions and answers them appropriately
- Addresses patient's ideas, concerns and expectations.

SCENARIO 17

## Station 2

*Examination*              *10-minute station*

■ **After you have presented your history to the MAU Consultant, she asks you to perform a focussed clinical assessment of Ms Andrews with a view to confirming your diagnosis and presenting your findings.**
**(If you do not have a model, please read and present the information given on page 388.)**

*You will be assessed on the following areas, as well as the content and skills of your examination – take them into account in your presentation.*

### Professionalism

- Professional appearance; maintains infection control standards, including hand cleaning and appropriate use of gloves and aprons
- Maintains patient and personal safety
- Polite introduction; identifies patient and confirms date of birth from name band or other source
- Obtains informal consent; maintains patient privacy and dignity
- Displays empathetic and caring attitudes and behaviours throughout.

### Process

- Appropriate fluency/rhythm/pace to the examination – this may change depending on environment and acute nature of the problem
- Organisation and structure of examination; sensitive and empathetic approach
- Uses appropriate clinical techniques throughout
- Maintains privacy and dignity throughout.

### Clinical communication

- Explains proposed examination/procedure: explains examination/procedure as it proceeds
- Offers information in a clear, structured and fluent manner, avoiding jargon
- Listens to patient and responds appropriately
- Demonstrates appropriate body language.

## Station 3

*Procedural skills*                    *10-minute station*

### Procedure

Recognising how sick Ms Andrews is, the MAU Consultant asks you to draw up and give the benzylpenicillin that she has just prescribed on the drug chart shown below. She has also prescribed her some analgesia and anti-emetic, as shown.

| Allergies, sensitivities and adverse drug reactions | | | Patient details/addressograph | |
|---|---|---|---|---|
| No known allergies ✓ | | Initials AF | NHS/ Hospital No: 612321 | |
| Not possible to ascertain ☐ | | Date 7/05 | | |

| Medicine/substance | Reaction & Severity | Initials & Date | Gender M (F) | |
|---|---|---|---|---|
| | | | Weight (kg) 70kg | Date |
| | | | Surname: ANDREWS | |
| | | | Height 1.63m | First name: VALERIE |
| Alerts | | | Surface area (m²) | Date of birth: 17.11.88 |

### IN-PATIENT MEDICATION PRESCRIPTION AND ADMINISTRATION RECORD

PasTest HOSPITAL

| Consultant GAMBON | Trainee Dr. Name and Bleep no. FEATHER 007 | Date of admission 7/05/12 | Date chart reboarded | Estimated date of discharge |
|---|---|---|---|---|
| This chart is no. ......1...... of ......1...... | Transcribing Check by Pharmacy Sign .......... Date .......... | Ward 1. .......... | | 2. .......... |

Supplementary Medication charts in use:  Other (please specify): 1 .......... 2 ..........

| Epidural/PCA ☐ | Syringe driver ☐ | | TPN ☐ | | Chemotherapy ☐ | Insulin sliding scale ☐ |
|---|---|---|---|---|---|---|

Once only medications – loading doses, pre-medication, PGDs or surgical antibiotic propylaxis

| Date | Time to be given | Medicine (approved name) | Dose | Route | Signature and bleep no. | Pharmacy | Time given | Given by | Checked by |
|---|---|---|---|---|---|---|---|---|---|
| 7/05 | Stat | BENZYLPENICILLIN | 2.4g | IV | JG (007) | | | | |
| 7/05 | Stat | MORPHINE | 2.5mg | IV | JG (007) | | | | |
| 7/05 | Stat | CYCLIZINE | 50mg | IV | JG (007) | | | | |
| 7/05 | Stat | VITAMIN K | 2mg | IV | JG (007) | | | | |

### Equipment provided

- Dry powder preparations of benzylpenicillin or similar (to simulate benzylpenicillin)
- Box of 21 G needles, 5 ml and 10 ml syringes
- 100 ml 0.9% saline bag
- IV giving set
- Sticker for additive to saline bag
- Water for injection
- Manikin arm with cannula in situ, and patient name band with correct details added.

SCENARIO 17

## Station 4

*Prescribing skills*                    *10-minute station*

The MAU Consultant now asks you to complete the rest of Ms Andrews' charts.

- Using the appropriate drug and fluid charts please write up the management regime for this patient.

**Details**

- o Ms Valerie Andrews, DOB 17/11/1988, Hospital no. 612321, Ward: MAU, Consultant: Dr Gambon, FY1 bleep number 007
- o Height 1.63m, weight approximately 70 kg
- o U&Es: Na⁺ 145 mmol/l, K⁺ 3.5 mmol/l, urea 13.8 mmol/l, creatinine 101 μmol/l
- o Allergies: nil known.

---

**Remember: DRUG DRs Don't Forget Signing Off (page 396)**

---

## Station 5

*Clinical communication skills*        *10-minute station*

You have an additional 5-minute preparation time to read the following information sheet and prepare your discussion.

The MAU Consultant has decided that Ms Andrews should not undergo a lumbar puncture as she is very unwell, has disseminated intravascular coagulopathy (DIC) and has already had two doses of antibiotics. However, the Consultant would like you to explain the procedure to her as if she were a patient undergoing a lumbar puncture. She gives you 5 minutes to read the page she has prepared for patients (and their carers) prior to undergoing the procedure, to help you.

- Please read the information below regarding lumbar puncture and make notes. You may make notes and take these into the following station with you. Then explain the lumbar puncture to the Consultant, who is role-playing a patient, and address any concerns she may have regarding the procedure.

The procedure you are about to have is called a lumbar puncture (LP). It is a relatively straightforward and simple procedure that should take between 10 and 15 minutes to complete.

The equipment that will be used includes:

Wheeled trolley that all the equipment is placed on

Cleaning solution – iodine or other cleaning solutions; these will feel cold but are necessary to make the area sterile (clean) enough to proceed

Gauze swabs – to clean the area

Forceps – these look like large plastic tweezers and are used to hold the gauze

Local anaesthetic – this is injected into the area to numb it

LP needle – this is a long but very thin needle that will be inserted into your back to remove some fluid, called cerebro-spinal fluid (CSF)

Manometer – this is a plastic tube with a three-way tap attached; this allows the pressure inside the brain to be measured

Sterile bottles – these will be used to collect the fluid that comes out of the needle and are sent away to be processed in the laboratory.

Procedure:

The most important part of the procedure is positioning you, the patient, on the bed.

You must take off enough of your clothes to adequately expose the lower back. This often means removing your top (women may retain their bra) and lowering your trousers. Most often you will be in a hospital gown and this will need to be removed.

The doctor will then ask you to sit upright, leaning over a bedside table (this will have a pillow(s) on top), or will ask you to lie down on your left side with your back parallel to the edge of the bed facing away from the doctor and the equipment.

The doctor will then mark the area to be injected by feeling your lower back. They will then mark the area in the midline of your back by either pressing with the plastic cap of a pen or by using a marker.

They will then place sterile paper (drapes) into the top of your underpants to keep the lower area clean.

They will then clean the area using the cleaning solution and cover you with another clean drape.

Once the doctor is clear they have the right area (you will feel some pushing on the back) they will inject the area of skin (about 0.5 cm) with the local anaesthetic (this will sting a little).

They will then inject local anaesthetic into the deeper tissues until the area goes numb.

Once numb (30 seconds or so), they will then insert the lumbar puncture needle.

You will feel a little pushing but no pain.

The needle is well away from your spinal cord, so there is no need to worry that it will be damaged by the insertion of the needle.

Once the doctor has inserted the needle into the correct position, they will do two things:

(a) Measure the pressure (this may not always be done) using the manometer

(b) Take samples using the sterile bottles; only a few drops (3–10) of the fluid is usually placed in each bottle.

The doctor will then remove the needle and clean up the area and will then apply a dressing.

You will be asked to lie flat in bed for up to 4 hours; you will be given fluids via a cannula in the arm, painkillers, and injections to stop you feeling sick; you will be checked by a nurse every 30 minutes (or more).

Please report if you have any worsening pain, vomiting, drowsiness, confusion or blurring of your vision.

## Station 6

*Data interpretation*                    *10-minute station*

1. Ms Andrews had some emergency bloods taken on arrival in the MAU, and the Consultant has asked you to review the results (shown below), and record them in the patient's notes.

■ Please answer the questions below regarding Ms Andrews' results, indicating whether each of the statements is TRUE (T) or FALSE (F).

- ○ FBC: Hb 10.1 g/dl, MCV 77 fl, WCC 26.6 × 10⁹/l, neutrophils 22.7 × 10⁹/l, platelets 31 × 10⁹/l
- ○ U&Es: Na⁺ 145 mmol/l, K⁺ 3.5 mmol/l, urea 13.8 mmol/l, creatinine 101 μmol/l
- ○ RBG: 4.1 mmol/l
- ○ LFTs: TBil 4.7 mmol/l, ALT 14 iu/l, AST 18 iu/l, Alk phos 133 iu/l, Alb 27 g/l
- ○ Clotting: INR 2.1; APTT 57 s
- ○ ESR 89 mm/h; CRP 421 mg/l
- ○ Blood cultures × 2 sent (note – bleeding/bruising++ from both venepuncture sites with withdrawal of needle).

A   The haemoglobin (Hb) and mean corpuscular volume (MCV) are most likely explained by menstrual loss.

B   Similar Hb and MCV values are commonly found in hypothyroidism.

C   The white cell and differential are in keeping with viral meningitis.

D   The white cell and differential suggests she may have cryptococcal infection.

E   The urea : creatinine ratio is suggestive of pre-renal impairment.

F   In keeping with bacterial meningitis, one would expect the CSF glucose to be 2.0 mmol/l.

G   The hypoalbuminaemia is likely to be spurious in this case.

H   The erythrocyte sedimentation rate (ESR) is more in keeping with a vasculitis.

I   The coagulation screen and platelet count are suggestive of DIC.

J   The blood cultures are likely to be negative in this case.

2. The MAU Consultant draws up a chart of CSF results (shown below) from recent admissions to the MAU.
- Please complete the likely microbiological organism and the appropriate treatment in each of the cases.

| | Patient presentation | Gram stain/comment | Opening pressure/cm H$_2$O (6–18 cm H$_2$O) | White cells/mm$^3$ (<5 cells per mm$^3$) | Glucose mmol/l (2/3 blood glucose) | Protein normal (0.2–0.4 g/l) | Likely organism | Treatment |
|---|---|---|---|---|---|---|---|---|
| A | A 21-year-old nursery nurse is admitted with a 12-hour history of a severe global headache, photophobia and a high fever; in the last few hours she has developed a non-blanching purpuric rash | Gram-negative diplococci | 31 cm | 234 polymorphs, all neutrophils | CSF: 1.1 Blood: 4.1 | 4.8 | | |
| B | A 34-year-old male mature student is admitted with a 24-hour history of sore throat, severe headache, fever and meningism | Gram-positive cocci in chains | 27 cm | 277 polymorphs | CSF: 2.3 Blood: 5.1 | 3.9 | | |
| C | A 12-year-old Sudanese immigrant girl is admitted with severe headache and fever | Gram-negative cocco-bacilli | 24 cm | 212 polymorphs | CSF: 1.9 Blood 4.0 | 3.1 | | |
| D | An 83-year-old man is admitted with insidious worsening of confusion, headache and fevers for 2 days | Tumbling, motile Gram-positive bacilli | 24 cm | 223 polymorphs | CSF 1.4 Blood: 6.6 | 3.8 | | |
| E | A 27-year-old Polish man of no fixed abode is admitted with a 1-week history of worsening global headache, vomiting and fevers | No organisms identified | 25 cm | Mononuclear cells 239; polymorphs 99 | CSF: 1.7 Blood: 4.5 | 4.3 | | |

| | | | | | | | |
|---|---|---|---|---|---|---|---|
| F | A 22-year-old student with a 3-day history of shivering, aches and pains and a worsening headache | No organisms identified | 13 cm | Mononuclear cells 70; no polymorphs | CSF: 3.1<br><br>Blood: 4.6 | 0.7 | | |
| G | A 31-year-old woman with known systemic lupus erythematosus (SLE) is admitted with a 2-day history of worsening headache, mild fevers and chills | No organisms identified | 10 cm | Mononuclear cells 40; no polymorphs | CSF: 3.6<br><br>Blood: 4.2 | 0.2 | | |
| H | A 48-year-old man is admitted with long-standing poorly controlled type 2 diabetes melitus and 'offensive' leg ulcers | Gram positive cocci in clusters | 23 cm | Mononuclear cells 123; polymorphs 100 | CSF: 12.2<br><br>Blood: 48.6 | 3.3 | | |
| I | A 26-year-old known HIV-positive Ugandan man is admitted with a 10-day history of insidious worsening of confusion, headaches and fever | Gram-positive yeast-like cells with marked stippling | 29 cm | Monocytes 50; no polymorphs | CSF: 2.4<br><br>Blood: 4.9 | 1.1 | | |

# Answers

## Station 1 – History

**Patient script**

You are Ms Valerie Andrews (DOB 17 November 1988 – 23 years old), who works as a nursery nurse in a local nursery. You are normally very fit and well with no medical problems.

You started to come down with what you thought was 'flu' last night. You were really looking forward to a night out at the pub with your colleagues (it was one of the girls' birthdays) but you had to excuse yourself and went home at about 1830 h. You had been suffering with a sore throat all afternoon but in the pub you started to feel 'hot and shivery', 'aching all over' and 'really, really rough'.

You felt so poorly that you made yourself a hot toddy, drank it with two or three paracetamol tablets and took yourself off to bed. You must have been asleep about an hour or two when you woke shivering and 'sweating like crazy' – 'I was drenched'. It was then that you started to get a headache. At first it wasn't too bad and you took some Nurofen and managed to doze a bit but by midnight or so it started to get really bad. You took a few more paracetamol around 0100 h but vomited them back up. By this point your partner, Angie, had come back from work (she works as a solicitor in a local law firm and often gets home late when her work demands it). She wanted to call out the doctor then but you convinced her not to. By about 0530–0600 h you were really suffering, and this is when Angie called the doctor. He came at about 0630 h and sent you immediately in by ambulance, after first giving you an injection in the back of your hand. You think it was a shot of an antibiotic.

The headache is all over your head (global), with no radiation. It started slowly and got worse and worse over a few hours. It was poorly relieved with paracetamol and Nurofen. You have had no tablets for several hours.

Associated features:

- You can't bear to look into the light/have the lights on – really hurts your eyes
- You have vomited two or three times over the last few hours, including vomiting the second lot of paracetamol
- Your 'head feels heavy and like it's about to explode' – your neck is very stiff, you are unable to lift your head off the bed
- Fever – shivery and cold but sweating profusely
- Rash – don't know but you think the nurse who you first saw when you came in mentioned that you had a few spots on your arms and legs; these definitely weren't there yesterday morning
- Aching and painful muscles – feel battered and bruised.

No seizures (fits) or loss of consciousness; feel drowsy, and 'out of it a bit'.

No motor or sensory problems in your arms or legs.

You are a nursery nurse – kids always have coughs and colds but none of them have been seriously ill recently; no one has mentioned meningitis to you. Your colleagues are all well.

Previous medical history – nil of note; tonsillectomy – aged 15 years old; a few broken bones here and there as a kid (broke your right wrist twice) – falling off your bike and playing with your brothers.

You have no regular medicines and no known allergies.

You live with your female partner, Angie, in a third-floor flat (house conversion). You are a smoker – 10–20 cigarettes per day; you have the occasional joint with friends at parties but 'nothing stronger'; no intravenous drug use. You often have a glass or two of white wine with Angie in the evenings; you also have the occasional binge but not as often as you used to.

Ideas – 'I'm pretty sure I've got meningitis because I had to learn about it when I was doing my diploma.'

Concerns – 'I'm pretty seriously ill aren't I?'

Expectations – 'I just hope you can get me better with some antibiotics and things …'

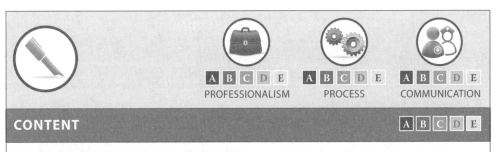

PROFESSIONALISM    PROCESS    COMMUNICATION

## CONTENT

A B C D E

**Identifies key information**
- Duration and progression of presenting complaint
- Headache (SOCRATES – defines sinister features of meningism, fever, rash).

**Includes important negatives, including system enquiry**
- Loss of consciousness, seizure, upper and lower limb weakness/sensory loss
- Systemic symptoms – including upper respiratory/ENT.

**Identifies key information from rest of history**
- Asks about contacts, occupation.

**Completing the patient history**
- Drug and allergy history: specifically asks about allergies to antibiotics
- Previous medical history: nil of note; usually very fit and well
- Social and occupational history: lives with partner (well); asks about occupation, as well as smoking and alcohol and illicit drug taking.

**Summarises important areas of the history back to the patient**

**Invites patient to ask questions and deals with them appropriately**

**Establishes patient's ideas, concerns and expectations**

## CLINICAL DIAGNOSTIC REASONING

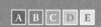

- **Please present your history**
  - Candidate offers a logical, well-structured account of the history.

- **Could you tell me the likely diagnoses in this case, and the likely causative organisms?**
  - Likely to be bacterial meningitis (could be viral but unlikely) – in a patient of this age group the likeliest causes are *Neisseria meningitidis* or *Streptococcus pneumoniae*. If she had any risk factors
  - Tuberculosis may be another cause (but only in given demographics); this is rather acute for tuberculous meningitis (TBM), which often presents more insidiously.

- **Could you tell me five essential interventions at this point?**
  - Nurse in high-dependency area BUT isolate and keep lights dimmed
  - Cool patient down – antipyretics and fanning
  - Intravenous fluids
  - Intravenous analgesia (avoid intramuscular injections until DIC excluded)
  - Intravenous antibiotics – empirical treatment with benzylpenicillin or cephalosporin, eg cefatoxime; chloramphenicol may be used in known severe penicillin allergy
  - Lumbar puncture – note: most patients will undergo CT head scan at this point but this may be unnecessary and wastes valuable time
  - Contact tracing – Public Health Team will need to be involved, especially in view of the patient's job.

**Demonstrates safe, sensible and appropriate management plan**

**Demonstrates clear and logical diagnostic reasoning**

## GLOBAL HISTORY MARK

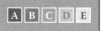

## Station 2 – Examination

**Patient script (see also page 388)**

You are a previously fit and well 24-year-old woman. You are very distressed, with a severe headache and photophobia. You are able to cooperate with the doctor but are not able to allow bright lights to be shone in your eyes or to complete complex actions, such as those involved with testing eye movements or limb power/sensation.

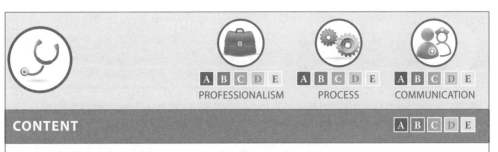

PROFESSIONALISM          PROCESS          COMMUNICATION

## CONTENT

**Exposes and positions patient correctly and maintains comfort**

**Comments on wellbeing of patient, ie well or unwell**

**'Feet to face'**
- Observes and comments on patient and surroundings from foot of bed
- Obvious rash, bleeding (DIC), photophobia.

**Asks for appropriate/relevant clinical observations**
- Observations: HR 123 bpm, BP 87/56 mmHg, RR 22 bpm, $O_2$ sats 95% on air, temperature 39.2 °C, CBG 4.3 mmol/l.

**Level of consciousness**
- GCS or AVPU.

**General/systemic examination**
- Hydration; rash
- Specifically assesses ear, nose and throat.

**Neurological assessment**
- Meningism and raised intracranial pressure
- Rash
- Acknowledges assessment limited by patient's clinical status but tries to be thorough, systematic and comprehensive
- Eyes – including attempt at ophthalmoscopy
- Cranial nerves V–XII
- Limbs – upper and lower; informal assessment of power and reflexes.

**Excludes other systemic sepsis and signs of organ failure**
- Assessing: chest; heart sounds (signs of endocarditis); abdomen; skin – ulcers and cellulitis; joints – arthritis; signs of vasculitis may also be present.

**Thanks patient, offers assistance, maintains patient's dignity and privacy until they are dressed**

**CLINICAL DIAGNOSTIC REASONING**

**Correctly identifies the relevant physical signs, including important negative findings**

- **Can you tell me five essential investigations at this time, with a reason for each?**
  - Blood tests:
  - FBC – Hb/MCV – haemolysis; WCC and differential – bacterial vs other organisms; platelets – ?DIC
  - U&Es – renal impairment – pre-(dehydration); renal (? nephritis)
  - Blood glucose – needed to compare against CSF glucose
  - Blood cultures – may be negative since GP (correctly) gave stat dose of IV antibiotics
  - Bags – often performed in such sick patients to exclude severe metabolic acidosis
  - Lumbar puncture – microscopy and culture; PCR (often performed now); protein and glucose
  - Radiology – chest radiograph and CT head scan are routinely performed on such patients but may waste valuable time in very sick patients who do not demonstrate signs of significantly raised intracranial pressure.

**Demonstrates safe, sensible and appropriate management plan**

**Demonstrates clear and logical diagnostic reasoning**

**GLOBAL EXAMINATION MARK**

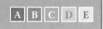

## Station 3 – Procedural skills

**Procedure**

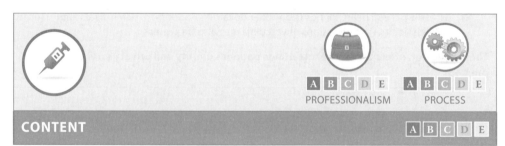

PROFESSIONALISM    PROCESS

**CONTENT**

**Exposes and positions patient correctly and maintains comfort**

**Identifies and sets out equipment correctly; maintains aseptic technique throughout**
- Reviews patient's drug chart to confirm correct, prescribed antibiotic – type and dose
- Verifies correct patient – both verbally and against name band; confirms no allergies to prescribed antibiotic
- Checks prescribed ampoules and fluid bag for discoloration, particles/tampering and broken seal/leaking
- Checks antibiotic ampoule and fluid bag - correct drug; expiry date.

**Correctly performs the procedure**
- Washes hands; puts on sterile gloves – uses non-touch technique throughout drawing up antibiotic
- Inspects cannula site and aseptically delivers saline flush to observe for pain and features of tissue infiltration
- Draws up diluting into 10 ml syringe using aseptic technique; changes needle
- Breaks seal on ampoule of antibiotic powder and cleans surface with alcohol wipe
- Slowly injects diluting into antibiotic powder and mixes gently to dissolve powder; adds enough diluting to dissolve all the powder
- Withdraws antibiotic solution ensuring ALL powder and fluid withdrawn; mixes gently in the syringe; expels any air bubbles
- Adds antibiotic solution to 100 ml bag of saline; gently mixes
- Writes and attaches label to 100 ml saline bag with patient details and description of prescription
- Attaches infusion set to saline bag and purges line
- Observes for air bubbles in line and eliminates as necessary
- Cleans cannula ports with alcohol wipe and then connects line to cannula
- Starts infusion at an appropriate drip rate, so infusion lasts 30–60 minutes
- Signs off prescription on chart.

**Obtains an acceptable/appropriate result**

**Disposes of all sharps and other items correctly**

**Ensures patient receives correct advice about what to do next and follow-up**

**Ensures nursing staff or other healthcare professionals receive correct information about the consequences/outcome of the procedure/task and any observations that may be required**

**Thanks patient, offers assistance, maintains patient's dignity and privacy until they are dressed**

**GLOBAL PROCEDURE MARK**

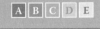

## Station 4 – Prescribing skills

**Thromboprophylaxis please prescribe treatment regimens in the regular medications section**

| Choice of mechanical prophylaxis and leg(s) to be applied to | | | | | | Enter Time | Enter details below | | | | | | | |
|---|---|---|---|---|---|---|---|---|---|---|---|---|---|---|
| Graduated elastic compression stockings | Intermittent pneumatic compression device (IPC) | Leg | | | | | | | | | | | | |
| | | | Left | Right | Both | | | | | | | | | |
| ☑ | ☐ | Signature and Bleep No. | ☐ | ☐ | ☑ | | | | | | | | | |
| Start Date: | End Date: | | | | | | | | | | | | | |
| ☐ | ☐ | Signature and Bleep No. AF | ☐ | ☐ | ☐ | | | | | | | | | |
| Start Date: | End Date: | | | | | | | | | | | | | |

| Medication NOT FOR HEPARIN D.I.C | | Dose | | Dose Change | Enter Time | Enter details below | | | | | | | |
|---|---|---|---|---|---|---|---|---|---|---|---|---|---|
| Please ensure you have completed the VTE risk assessment form | Date | | | | | | | | | | | | |
| | Route | | | | | | | | | | | | |
| | Signature | AF | | | Instructions | | | | | | Pharmacy | | ☐ |
| | Bleep no. | 007 | | | | | | | | | | | |

**Regular prescriptions continued**

**Anti-infectives prescription**  *prescribe long term prophylaxis and anti-tuberculosis medications in regular medications section*

| FOR 7 DAYS | Dose | | | Date | 7 | 8 | 9 | 10 | 11 | 12 | 13 | | | |
|---|---|---|---|---|---|---|---|---|---|---|---|---|---|---|
| Date | 7/05 | | | Medication BENZYLPENICILLIN (4 HOURLY) | | | | Indication MENINGITIS | | | | Signature and bleep no. AF 007 | | Pharmacy ☐ |
| Route | IV | | | | | | | | | | | | | |
| Signature | | | | | | | | | | | | | | |
| (06) | 2.4g | | | | | | | | | | | | | |
| (10) | 2.4g | | | | | | | | | | | | | |
| (14) | 2.4g | | | | | | | | | | | | | |
| (18) | 2.4g | | | | | | | | | | | | | |
| (22) | 2.4g | | | | | | | | | | | | | |
| (02) | 2.4g | | | | | | | | | | | | | |

**Regular prescriptions continued**

| | Dose | | | Date | 7 | 8 | 9 | 10 | 11 | 12 | 13 | | | |
|---|---|---|---|---|---|---|---|---|---|---|---|---|---|---|
| Date | 7/05 | | | Medication CODEINE PHOSPHATE | | | | Indication | | | | Signature and bleep no. AF 007 | | Pharmacy ☐ |
| Route | PO | | | | | | | | | | | | | |
| Signature | | | | | | | | | | | | | | |
| 06 | | | | | | | | | | | | | | |
| (09) | 60mg | | | | | | | | | | | | | |
| (12) | 60mg | | | | | | | | | | | | | |
| (18) | 60mg | | | | | | | | | | | | | |
| (22) | 60mg | | | | | | | | | | | | | |
| 24 | | | | | | | | | | | | | | |

## Regular prescriptions continued

| | Dose | | | Date | | | | | | | | | | | | | |
|---|---|---|---|---|---|---|---|---|---|---|---|---|---|---|---|---|---|
| Date | 7/05 | | | Medication | | | Indication | | | | | Signature and bleep no. | | | Pharmacy | | |
| Route | PO | | | PARACETAMOL | | | | | | | | AF 007 | | | ☐ | | |
| Signature | | | | | | | | | | | | | | | | | |
| 06 | | | | | | | | | | | | | | | | | |
| ⑨ | 1g | | | | | | | | | | | | | | | | |
| ⑫ | 1g | | | | | | | | | | | | | | | | |
| ⑱ | 1g | | | | | | | | | | | | | | | | |
| ㉒ | 1g | | | | | | | | | | | | | | | | |
| 24 | | | | | | | | | | | | | | | | | |

## Infusion prescriptions continued

SC = subcutaneous    IVC = intravenous central    IVP = intravenous peripheral

| Date & time | Route | Infusion Fluid Name & strength | Volume | Medication Approved name with expiry / unit number | Dose | Duration | Rate | Prescriber's signature & bleep no. | Date given | Given by / Added by | Check by | Start time | Finish time | Pharmacy |
|---|---|---|---|---|---|---|---|---|---|---|---|---|---|---|
| 7/05 | IV | 0.9% Saline Exp: Batch/unit no: | 1l | | | | 30 MINS | AF 007 | | | | | | |
| 7/05 | IV | 0.9% Saline Exp: Batch/unit no: | 1l | + 20mmol KCL | | | 1 HOUR | AF 007 | | | | | | |
| 7/05 | IV | 0.9% Saline Exp: Batch/unit no: | 1l | | | | 2 HOURS | AF 007 | | | | | | |
| 7/05 | IV | 0.9% Saline Exp: Batch/unit no: | 1l | + 20mmol KCL | | | 4 HOURS | AF 007 | | | | | | |
| 7/05 | IV | 0.9% Saline Exp: Batch/unit no: | 1l | | | | 4 HOURS | AF 007 | | | | | | |
| 7/05 | IV | 0.9% Saline Exp: Batch/unit no: | 1l | + 20mmol KCL | | | 6 HOURS | AF 007 | | | | | | |
| | | TITRATE FLUID AGAINST U.O. > 35ml/HR; BP > 100 Systolic; HR < 100 bpm Exp: Batch/unit no: | | | | | | | | | | | | |
| | | Exp: Batch/unit no: | | | | | | | | | | | | |
| | | Exp: Batch/unit no: | | | | | | | | | | | | |
| | | | | | | | | | | | | | | |
| | | | | | | | | | | | | | | |

'A LITTLE RASH'

| As required medications | | | | | | | | | | | | | | | | | | | | | | |
|---|---|---|---|---|---|---|---|---|---|---|---|---|---|---|---|---|---|---|---|---|---|---|
| **Medication** MORPHINE | | | **Date** | | | | | | | | | | | | | | | | | | | | |
| **Indication** | | | **Time** | | | | | | | | | | | | | | | | | | | | |
| **Dose** 2.5 - 5mg | **Route** SC/ IV | **Maximum frequency / dose** As Required | **Start date** 7/05 | **Dose** | | | | | | | | | | | | | | | | | | | | |
| | | | **Stop date** | **Route** | | | | | | | | | | | | | | | | | | | | |
| **Signature** AF 007 | | | **Bleep no.** | **Given** | | | | | | | | | | | | | | | | | | | | |
| **Additional instructions:** | | | | | | | | | | | | | **Pharmacy** | | | | | | | | | | |

| As required medications | | | | | | | | | | | | | | | | | | | | | | |
|---|---|---|---|---|---|---|---|---|---|---|---|---|---|---|---|---|---|---|---|---|---|---|
| **Medication** METOCLOPRAMIDE | | | **Date** | | | | | | | | | | | | | | | | | | | | |
| **Indication** | | | **Time** | | | | | | | | | | | | | | | | | | | | |
| **Dose** 10 mg | **Route** IV/ SC | **Maximum frequency / dose** 8° | **Start date** | **Dose** | | | | | | | | | | | | | | | | | | | | |
| | | | **Stop date** | **Route** | | | | | | | | | | | | | | | | | | | | |
| **Signature** AF 007 | | | **Bleep no.** | **Given** | | | | | | | | | | | | | | | | | | | | |
| **Additional instructions:** | | | | | | | | | | | | | **Pharmacy** | | | | | | | | | | |

## GLOBAL PRESCRIBING MARK

A B C D E

## Station 5 – Clinical communication skills

**Patient script**

You are the MAU Consultant acting as the patient. You should act accordingly.

Despite the painkillers you still have a pretty severe headache, and are not really in the mood to talk very much. However you are happy to listen to the doctor's explanation.

You have seen people on *ER* and *Holby City* have the 'needle in the back' but don't really know much about it. No one has explained it to you on this admission.

If the doctor is reassuring and provides an adequate explanation, you should be agreeable to have the procedure. If they are unsympathetic, unable to address your concerns, or provide a poor explanation you should refuse the procedure.

Ideas and concerns – You are frightened that the needle will cause damage to your spine and that this will leave you paralysed.

Expectations – 'None really'; you just want to get it over and done with if it needs to be done at all!

SCENARIO 17

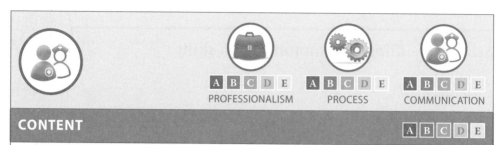

A B C D E
PROFESSIONALISM

A B C D E
PROCESS

A B C D E
COMMUNICATION

## CONTENT

A B C D E

**Confirms reason for discussion**
- To talk to patient about an LP.

**Establishes what the patient wishes to know; gains agreement/informal consent to participate in the discussion**

**Investigates patient's present level of understanding of scenario**

**Summarises and confirms what has happened so far**

**Establishes patient's ideas, concerns and expectations**

**Explains the key, important information**
- Indication and urgency to perform the LP
- The equipment used, including reassurance about the diameter of the needle
- Positioning the patient, including removing their clothes to expose the lower back
- The key steps involved in the procedure, including:
  - Exposing the patient's lower back
  - Pushing on the back and marking the correct location – lower spine; midline
  - Draping the patient with sterile paper drapes
  - Cleaning the back with cold solution
  - Injecting, first the skin, and then the deeper tissues with local anaesthetic; mentions LA will sting a little
  - Inserting LP needle through the injected area; patient will only feel some pushing
  - Taking samples using sterile specimen bottles; mentions the small volume of fluid removed (about 3–5 ml)
  - Removal of needle; cleaning area and then placing a dressing over wound site.
- Patient then expected to lie flat in bed for several hours (up to 4 hours); probably won't feel like getting up anyway!
- Will be given pain relief and fluids (IV), and will be checked by nurses regularly
- Should notify staff if worsening headache, vomiting, confusion or drowsiness.

**Explains further management**
- Depending on what the fluid shows, the doctors may change the antibiotics
- Rest, fluids and antibiotics will continue until patient better; this should be 24–48 hours; may take several days to complete adequate course of antibiotics.

**Invites patient to ask questions and is able to deal with them appropriately**

**Summarises important areas of the consultation back to the patient**

**Formally ends the consultation and ensures appropriate follow-up has been discussed**

**GLOBAL COMMUNICATION MARK**  A B C D E

## Station 6 – Data interpretation

**1.**

**A**    True – menstruating women often run a mild microcytic anaemia due to their periods. This may be significant in women suffering with menorrhagia. However, this is the diagnosis of exclusion and must be confirmed by the patient history.

**B**    False – hypothyroidism is associated with a macrocytosis and may also be associated with pernicious anaemia, causing a macrocytic anaemia.

**C**    False – this patient has a neutrophilic leucocytosis implying a bacterial infection. Patients with overwhelming, serious sepsis may present with a normal, or even low, white cell count.

**D**    False – *Cryptococcus* is a yeast and is rarely seen in immunocompetent patients in the UK. It is most commonly associated with immunocompromised patients such as those undergoing chemotherapy, or most commonly poorly controlled HIV/AIDS. These patients often have normal or low white cell counts.

**E**    True – the urea (13.8) represents an approx 3–5 fold increase: creatinine (101) represents approx 1.5 fold increase (ratio = 3.5 : 1.5), and thus is highly suggestive of pre-renal impairment.

**F**    True – the CSF glucose is routinely less than 50% of the blood glucose in bacterial meningitis but may be much lower.

**G**    False – this is a sinister sign and may be consistent with acute, severe sepsis.

**H**    False – although a vasculitis may occur in severe sepsis and is a cause of a highly raised ESR, the ESR in this case is most likely due to the overwhelming, severe sepsis.

**I**    True – DIC is relatively common in patients with bacterial meningitis, especially meningococcal and streptococcal disease. The blood markers include thrombocytopenia and deranged clotting.

**J**    True – when patients with suspected meningitis are this ill, they should receive rapid, empirical antibiotic cover. The GP rightly gave the patient a stat dose of antibiotic before sending them into hospital and it is most likely that such a presentation in an Emergency Department would precipitate further empirical treatment prior to any bloods or CSF being collected. Thus the blood cultures will often be negative. However, in untreated cases blood and CSF culture is positive in between 70–90% of cases and is therefore considered essential.

**2.**

**A**        Given this young woman's presentation it is very likely that she has bacterial meningitis. Her LP results support this diagnosis with a high opening pressure of 31 cm of $H_2O$, and a CSF : blood glucose ratio of 1.1 : 4.1 = 0.27. There are Gram-negative diplococci that are characteristic of *Neisseria meningitidis*. Treatment: benzylpenicillin or cefotaxime (ceftriaxone may also be used). Chloramphenicol is suggested for severe penicillin-allergic patients.

**B**        This patient has features suggestive of streptococcal meningitis. This is confirmed on the CSF results. He has a high opening pressure, and a low CSF : blood glucose ratio (2.3 : 5.1 = 0.45). There are high numbers of polymorphs (neutrophils) and the Gram stain shows Gram-positive cocci in chains, characteristic of streptococcus. Treatment: cefotaxime or ceftriaxone is recommended; if cultures show the organism to be penicillin-sensitive, then the patient should be changed to benzylpenicillin. If the organism is highly cephalosporin- and penicillin-resistant, then one should add vancomycin (see BNF). As well as antibiotic therapy, patients with suspected streptococcal meningitis should be treated with dexamethasone. However, dexamethasone should be avoided in patients with septic shock, meningococcal sepsis, or if immunocompromised.

**C**        This young immigrant from Africa has signs and a CSF result consistent with *Haemophilus influenzae* infection. This is rare in developed countries in indigenous populations as it is now routinely vaccinated against. It is a disease of babies, young children and teens who have not been vaccinated against the organism. Treatment: cefotaxime, ceftriaxone, or in allergic patients, chloramphenicol. Dexamethasone is also recommended.

**D**        This elderly man has presented with *Listeria meningitis*. The insidious headache and confusion, common in many elderly presentations, should always make one think of possible *Listeria* infection. Although classically a disease of the elderly, it may also present in neonates, pregnant women and the immunocompromised. The organism, a Gram-positive bacillus, is classically described as having 'tumbling' motility. Treatment: prolonged course of penicillin (21 days), usually amoxicillin and gentamicin (7 days).

**E**        This Polish man of no fixed abode has presented with symptoms and CSF results consistent with TBM. As in this case, there are often more mononuclear cells (lymphocytes), than neutrophils in the CSF. Treatment: 6–12-month course of anti-tubercular treatment, including rifampicin, isoniazid, pyrizinamide and ethambutol for the first 4 months, and then rifampicin, isoniazid and pyrizinamide for a further 2–8 months. Dexamethasone should be started with the antibiotic therapy, especially in cases where there is evidence of very high intracranial pressure. Note: this man is a public health hazard if he is allowed to go back on the street and will invariably be non-adherent to his treatment. He should be placed in a suitable home and his therapy should be supervised. Any direct contacts he may have had should be traced and tested for TB infection. This of course may prove very challenging!

**F**        This young adult has symptoms and CSF results suggestive of viral meningitis. The CSF has normal opening pressure, mononuclear cells (lymphocytes) and a CSF : blood glucose of 3.1 : 4.6 = 0.67. The protein is mildly elevated. Treatment: principally symptomatic – IV fluids, analgesia and bed rest; until the diagnosis is confirmed the patient should remain in isolation.

**G**    This young woman has 'aseptic' meningitis. This may be infectious in nature, causes including viral, bacterial and fungal organisms but is classically non-infectious, caused by drugs (nonsteroidal anti-inflammatory drugs and antibiotics), vaccines, sarcoidosis and vasculitides such as SLE. In non-infectious causes the treatment is supportive (as in 1J above) and treatment of the underlying disorder.

**H**    This gentleman has 'offensive' (and, by implication, infected) leg ulcers. This is a presentation common to staphylococcal meningitis. Other associations include alcohol excess and recent neurosurgical intervention. Of note in the CSF there are Gram-positive cocci in clusters (compared with chains seen with *Streptococcus*) and the common features of bacterial infection, including high opening pressures, a very low CSF : blood glucose ratio and high protein levels. The mixed leucocyte picture is common in staphylococcal and TB infections. Treatment: if staphylococcal infection is suspected (or indeed proven), flucloxacillin should be included in the treatment regime, alongside benzylpenicillin or a cephalosporin. Vancomycin may be used in pencillin-allergic individuals.

**I**    This gentleman has an insidious 10-day history of worsening headache and confusion. Given his HIV status this should alert the clinician to several possible diagnoses, including intracerebral abscess, lymphoma, tuberculosis and cryptococcal meningitis. Given the diverse nature of this differential, he should have a CT scan of the brain (possibly with contrast) to exclude the other diagnoses. His CSF results are highly suggestive of cryptococcal meningitis and a cryptococcal antigen (CRAG) test should be sent, alongside the other routine CSF items. Treatment: it is recommended that cryptococcal infection be treated with intravenous amphotericin B 0.7– 1.0 mg/kg and flucytosine 100 mg/kg for 2 weeks, followed by an 8-week course of fluconazole 200 mg (orally) once a day.

NOTE: Other CSF indices differentiating bacterial meningitis from other causes include raised levels of lactate (>6.0 mmol/l) and lactate dehydrogenase (LDH).

Poor prognostic factors in patients presenting with meningitis include:

Age >60 years old

Diabetes mellitus

Malignancy

Seizures

Severe neurological deficit at presentation

Gram-negative bacilli

High white cell count in the CSF

Positive bacteraemia.

**GLOBAL DATA INTERPRETATION MARK**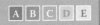

## Scenario 17: Reflection and consolidation

### History

Ms Valerie Andrews is a 23-year-old woman who works as a nursery nurse in a local nursery. She is normally very fit and well with no medical problems.

She became unwell yesterday afternoon with a sore throat, and later, in the early evening, started to complain of feeling 'hot and shivery' and 'aching all over'. On arriving home from work (about 1900 h) she took some paracetamol tablets and went to bed. She awoke about an hour or two later shivering, and sweating profusely.

She then developed a headache that slowly worsened over the next few hours. By the early morning (0530 h) she was 'really suffering' and it was then that she called the local GP service out. They saw her and sent her in to the MAU after giving her a stat dose of IV antibiotics.

The headache is global with no radiation. It has been poorly relieved with paracetamol and Nurofen.

Of note: Ms Andrews has marked photophobia and a rash that has developed over her arms and legs, and she has vomited two to three times over the last few hours. She has aching, painful muscles and a fever, with possible rigours. She feels very unwell and drowsy.

There have been no seizures (fits) or loss of consciousness and she denies any focal neurological deficit in her upper or lower limbs.

Ms Andrews is a nursery nurse, but the children and her colleagues have all been fine recently. She takes no regular medications and has no known allergies. She lives with her partner, Angie, who is a solicitor in a local law firm. She has been well. She smokes 10–20 cigarettes per day and the occasional joint with friends at parties but 'nothing stronger'; there is no intravenous drug use. She drinks a glass or two of white wine most evenings and has the occasional binge.

### Examination

Examination of this patient revealed a thin, acutely unwell-looking young woman. She was in obvious distress with a severe headache, lying in a dimly lit side room because of photophobia.

She had marked meningism and a non-blanching purpuric rash over upper and lower limbs. She was responding appropriately to voice commands and conversation but was distressed.

Her observations showed that she was tachycardic (HR 123 bpm), hypotensive (BP 87/56 mmHg) and pyrexial (temperature 39.2 °C). Her $O_2$ sats were 95% on air, RR was 22 bpm, and her CBG was 4.3 mmol/l.

General examination revealed her to be clinically dehydrated and limited assessment of her ears, nose and throat was remarkable for an erythematous but non-pustular throat.

Neurological assessment was limited by the patient's clinical status but did not reveal any focal neurological deficit. She was able to move all four limbs to command, and her plantars were bilaterally downgoing.

Chest, cardiovascular, abdominal, skin and joint assessments were likewise unremarkable.

In summary – this young woman has signs consistent with probable bacterial meningitis with fever, septic shock, marked meningism, photophobia and a non-blanching purpuric rash.

### Investigations

Patients presenting with signs and symptoms of bacterial meningitis need rapid assessment and investigation and these should not delay empirical antibiotic therapy. Blood tests should include FBC, U&Es, RBG, CRP, VBGs and blood cultures. A CT head scan may help exclude significantly raised intracranial pressure and other, differential diagnoses, but must not delay treatment of the seriously ill patient. CT head scan is not indicated for patients who do not have features of significantly raised intracranial pressure – see guidelines (although it is still routinely performed in most hospitals).

Lumbar puncture should be attempted but is not always technically very easy in such distressed and unwell patients. This too should not delay therapy.

## Management

Until the causative microbiological organism is confirmed and definitive therapy initiated, patients need to be isolated. Supportive therapy should be started immediately, including fluid resuscitation, analgesia and anti-pyretics.

Empirical antibiotic therapy should be started after discussion with a microbiologist and/or consultation of local antibiotic protocols.

In similar cases to Ms Andrews', contact tracing is imperative and the Public Health Team should be notified as soon as is possible. Strictly, only intimate contacts really require antibiotic prophylaxis, but in cases where young babies/children are involved, it is common to offer classmates (children and colleagues) prophylactic antibiotic therapy with rifampicin or similar.

### Further reading and web links

*NICE guidelines - meningitis in the young*:
http://guidance.nice.org.uk/CG102/QuickRefGuide/pdf/English
*Excellent review with clear and important messages (2004)*:
www.uphs.upenn.edu/bugdrug/antibiotic_manual/idsameningitisNov04.pdf
*This is part of the NEJM's excellent video series on practical procedures*:
www.nejm.org/doi/full/10.1056/NEJMvcm054952
*Guidelines for CT head scan prior to LP – see also review above (2004)*:
http://neurology.jwatch.org/cgi/content/full/2002/124/1

# Scenario 18: 'Drunk and disorderly'

## Station 1

*History*                                   *10-minute station*

You are the FY1 on the Medical Admissions Unit (MAU). The next patient is Mr Charles Lamb (DOB 06/10/1956 – 55 years old), who has been referred by his GP with 'falls and weight loss'.

■ Please take a focussed, diagnostic history with a view to presenting it to the MAU Consultant.

*You will be assessed on the following areas, as well as the content and diagnostic reasoning of your history – take them into account in your presentation.*

### Professionalism

- Professional appearance (NHS dress code) – including general appearance, hair and jewellery
- Maintains patient and personal safety
- Polite introduction; identifies patient or interviewee correctly; confirms patient's date of birth from name band or other source
- Obtains informal consent; maintains patient's privacy
- Displays empathetic and caring attitudes and behaviours throughout.

### Process

- Good organisation and structure; appropriate use of open and closed questions
- Appropriate fluency/rhythm/pace to the interview – this may change depending on environment and acute nature of the problem
- Appropriate time for the patient to respond/reply to questions
- Appropriate acknowledgement of difficult or emotional areas of the patient's history.

### Communication skills

- Demonstrates caring and sympathetic attitude
- Asks open questions
- Invites patient to ask questions and answers them appropriately
- Addresses patient's ideas, concerns and expectations.

## Station 2

*Examination*                    *10-minute station*

■ After presenting your history to the Consultant, please perform a focussed clinical assessment of Mr Lamb, to include:
  1.  An assessment of his cerebellar function and balance
  2.  An assessment of his gait
  3.  A holistic assessment of a patient with suspected metastatic lung cancer.
(If you do not have a model, please read and present the information given on page 389.)

*You will be assessed on the following areas, as well as the content and skills of your examination – take them into account in your presentation.*

### Professionalism

- Professional appearance; maintains infection control standards, including hand cleaning and appropriate use of gloves and aprons
- Maintains patient and personal safety
- Polite introduction; identifies patient and confirms date of birth from name band or other source
- Obtains informal consent; maintains patient privacy and dignity
- Displays empathetic and caring attitudes and behaviours throughout.

### Process

- Appropriate fluency/rhythm/pace to the examination – this may change depending on environment and acute nature of the problem
- Organisation and structure of examination; sensitive and empathetic approach
- Uses appropriate clinical techniques throughout
- Maintains privacy and dignity throughout.

### Communication skills

- Explains proposed examination/procedure: explains examination/procedure as it proceeds
- Offers information in a clear, structured and fluent manner, avoiding jargon
- Listens to patient and responds appropriately
- Demonstrates appropriate body language.

## Station 3

*Data interpretation*                    *10-minute station*

1. The grand round at your local hospital is being run by the Professor of Oncology. His first slide is a jumbled list of paraneoplastic neurological conditions, a description of their main neuro-disability, their commonly associated antibodies, and the commonly associated malignancy with each of the conditions. He requests the audience get into teams and try to rearrange the lists correctly.

- Please try to match the list of the paraneoplastic neurological conditions with the correct description of their major neuro-disability, the commonly associated auto-antibody and the commonly associated malignancy. You can match more than one malignancy, and antibody, to each of the syndromes and their disabilities.

| Paraneoplastic neurological condition | Neuro-disability | Paraneoplastic antibody | Commonly associated malignancy |
|---|---|---|---|
| Limbic and brainstem encephalomyelitis | Progressive rigidity and stiffness principally affecting the axial muscles | Anti-voltage gated calcium channel (VGCC) | Breast cancer |
| Cerebellar degeneration | Rapid, involuntary eye movements | Anti-Hu (ANNA-1) | Ovarian carcinoma |
| Stiff person syndrome | Proximal lower limb, and upper limb weakness | Anti-Yo (APCA-1) | Testicular germ cell tumours |
| Opsoclonus | Ataxia, dysdiadokokinesia and staccato speech | Anti-Ta | Lymphoma |
| Lambert–Eaton myasthenic syndrome | Loss of distal sensation in the limbs | Anti-GAD and anti-ampiphysin antibodies | Small cell lung cancer |
| Subacute peripheral sensory neuropathy | Short-term memory loss; seizures, confusion; features of parkinsonism, motor weakness, ataxia | Anti-Ri (ANNA-2) | Prostate cancer |

2. The next slide from the Professor's grand round is an extended matching question (EMQ) based on cerebellar disease.

- Please match the patient vignettes with the correct item from the list below. You may use the items once, more than once or not at all.
  - A. Alcohol excess
  - B. Arnold-Chiari malformation
  - C. Basal skull metastases
  - D. Cerebellar haemorrhage
  - E. Cerebellar metastases
  - F. Cerebellar-pontine angle tumour
  - G. Demyelination
  - H. Freidrich's ataxia

I. Paraneoplastic syndrome

J. Phenytoin toxicity

K. Wallenberg's syndrome

1. A 63-year-old man who had a craniotomy for excision of a large meningioma several years ago presents to his GP with increasing unsteadiness and falls. On examination he has bilateral nystagmus, past pointing and slurred speech, and has marked ataxia on walking. On arrival in the Emergency Department he has some routine bloods that show FBC: Hb 8.9 g/dl, MCV 112 fl, WCC 5.7 × 10⁹/l, platelets 332 × 0⁹/l; a CT head scan is similar to one he had a few years ago, with no acute changes noted.

2. A 39-year-old man is seen in the Emergency Department after a fall in the street. He is unable to give any coherent history. Examination reveals him to have bilateral Dupuytren's contracture, multiple spider naevi and gynaecomastia. Routine blood tests reveal FBC: Hb 7.9 g/dl, MCV 105 fl, WCC 5.7 × 10⁹/l, platelets 82 × 10⁹/l; U&Es Na⁺ 126 mmol/l, K⁺ 3.9 mmol/l, urea 1.1 mmol/l, creatinine 67 μmol/l, INR 1.6, APTT 58 s.

3. A 61-year-old man presents to his GP with a 3-month history of worsening tinnitus, unsteadiness on walking, and a 'droopy right side of the face'. On examination he has past pointing and nystagmus to the right, a right-sided facial palsy, and signs of a right-sided trigeminal nerve lesion.

4. A 57-year-old man with a previous history of type 2 diabetes mellitus and hypertension presents in the Emergency Department with sudden onset of vomiting, severe dizziness, unsteadiness on walking, and a droopy right eye. Examination reveals a BP = 210/130 mmHg, HR 99 bpm regular. Neurological assessment reveals a right-sided Horner's syndrome and right-sided trigeminal lesions, with loss of pain and temperature sensation on the left side of his face, and nystagmus, dysdiadokokinesia and past pointing on the right.

5. A 23-year-old woman presents to her GP with several recent episodes of visual blurring and loss, now associated with a 24-hour history of increasing unsteadiness on walking. Examination of her eyes, including ophthalmoscopy, is normal but she has several features of a cerebellar syndrome.

## Station 4

*Clinical communication skills*          *10-minute station*

Post-take you return to the Respiratory Team as the FY1. Several days later you are asked by your Consultant to role play telling Mr Lamb the results of his tests, including the blood tests, bronchoscopy biopsy, the CT chest and the MRI brain scan reports, shown below.

■ With your Consultant acting as the patient, please explain the results and address any concerns that 'Mr Lamb' may have.

Before meeting the Consultant you have an additional 5 minutes to study the following results.

FBC: Hb 9.9 g/dl, MCV 78 fl, WCC $11.7 \times 10^9$/l, platelets $512 \times 10^9$/l

U&Es: Na$^+$ 127 mmol/l, K$^+$ 3.6 mmol/l, urea 4.7 mmol/l, creatinine 123 μmol/l

RBG: 5.8 mmol/l

LFTs: TBil 58 μmol/l, AST 87 iu/l, ALT 65 iu/l, Alk phos 774 iu/l, albumin 29 g/l, CCa$^{2+}$ 2.87 mmol/l, PO$_4^{2-}$ 0.76 mmol/l

Auto-antibodies: Anti-Hu, Anti-CV2 and Anti-zic4 antibodies identified – consistent with a paraneoplastic cerebellar syndrome most likely due to small cell lung cancer.

### Radiology reports

CXR – large left-sided pleural effusion; several 'ragged' ribs on the right and left consistent with probable metastatic deposits. Soft tissue shadowing in the neck and supraclavicular fossa noted, probably due to associated lymphadenopathy.

CT chest – there is a large bronchogenic carcinoma arising from the fist division of the left main bronchus measuring $4 \times 3.2$ cm. There is evidence of collapse of several segments of the left upper lobe with associated bilateral hilar and paratracheal lymphadenopathy, more marked on the left than the right. There is also a large left-sided pleural effusion. Several, presumed metastatic, lesions are seen through posterior sections of ribs 4, 5 and 7 on the left and ribs 3, 7 and 8 on the right.

CT abdomen – several lesions seen within the liver consistent with secondary malignant deposits. Para-aortic lymphadenopathy noted.

Summary: changes are consistent with metastatic carcinoma of the left lung.

MRI brain – There are no acute bleeds, infarcts or space occupying lesions identified. Marked bilateral cerebellar degeneration is noted but no focal lesions are identified.

### Bronchoscopy biopsy

'Section shows mainly necrotic tissue; several preserved 'islands' show changes consistent with small cell carcinoma.'

Summary – Histological changes consistent with small cell carcinoma.

## Station 5

*Clinical communication skills* *10-minute station*

**Several months later whilst doing a taster day in General Practice you are asked to accompany the GP to see a patient with metastatic lung cancer. The patient is Mr Charles Lamb. Mr Lamb is pleased to see you but has called the GP out because he and his wife are struggling to cope. Up until this point he has refused outside support, insisting that he and his wife could manage. As you know the patient, the GP asks you to assess his present condition and his palliative care needs.**

- **Please assess Mr Lamb with a view to improving his present care.**

## Station 6

*Prescribing skills* *10-minute station*

**Mr Lamb deteriorates and is admitted to the local hospice.**

- **Using the drug and fluid charts provided please write up an appropriate set of medications to cover Mr Lamb's symptoms.**

**Patient Details:**

**Mr Charles Lamb; DOB 06.10.1956; Number 888432; Consultant Dr Philips; Ward Marley; Dr Feather: Bleep 622.**

- **Present medications include:**
  - **MST 20 mg bd**
  - **Oromorph – last 36 hours – 5 mg, 2.5 mg, 2.5 mg, 5 mg, 5 mg, 5 mg, 5 mg.**
  - **Paracetamol 1 g qds**
  - **Ibuprofen 600 mg bd**
  - **Nystatin pastilles (one) – qds**
  - **Temazepam 20 mg nocte**
  - **Metoclopramide 10 mg SC tds**
  - **Cyclizine 50 mg prn**
  - **Laxido (macrogols) 1 sachet bd**
  - **Senna 2 tablets bd**
  - **Docusate 200 mg bd**
  - **Phosphate enema – prn**
- **Main symptoms:**
  - **All over 'gnawing' pain – 'it just won't go away'**
  - **Occasional pains in his ribs and thigh, where he has metastatic deposits**
  - **Severe oral candidiasis**
  - **Nausea (occasional dry retching)**
  - **Poor appetite**
  - **Poor sleep – 'mainly due to pain and 'worry'.**

**Remember: DRUG DRs** **D**on't **F**orget **S**igning **O**ff (page 396)

# Answers

## Station 1 – History

**Patient script**

You are Mr Charles Lamb (DOB 06/10/1956 – 55 years old), a previously fit and well HGV driver. You went to see your GP this morning after several recent falls, the last one on the way home from the pub last night. 'I know what you're thinking doc, but its not like that at all'. You have been off work for the last 1–2 weeks as you've been feeling 'right queer'. You've been feeling increasingly unsteady and dizzy, 'like I was drunk and disorderly' but haven't had a 'proper drink' in weeks.

Looking back now you've been unwell for about 3 or 4 months but haven't been 'really right' since this dizziness started. Initially you noticed that you were coughing up a bit of blackened spit in the mornings and then occasionally bits of fresh red blood and bits of clotted blood would come up into your mouth as you were driving. It was about this time that you noticed you were losing weight. It wasn't much initially but since then people have been commenting and you've had to make up stories about how you are training to do a run for charity. Your wife was getting increasingly concerned and has been begging you to see the GP for weeks.

Previously 'fighting weight' about 15 stone (95 kg), now down to 10 stone (62.5 kg) (height – used to be 6ft 2in (1.83 m)). You've lost your appetite 'right off my food', 'just don't feel like it'. No nausea, vomiting or dysphagia. No active dieting – 'What, at my age?' Bowels – a bit constipated recently – normally BO x once or twice per day, recently once every 3 days – 'really hard and have to strain to get them out'.

Over the last few weeks (about 1–2) you have become increasingly unsteady and dizzy, so much so that you had to stop driving, 'there's no way I could drive like this... I mean I can't even walk to the pub and back without falling over!' You've had three or four 'proper falls' where you've just lost balance and 'smack, I was on the floor' but also 'loads and loads' of near misses where you've grabbed onto something or someone, and that's stopped you falling. You've had no loss of consciousness and no pre-warning symptoms but are feeling 'totally unable to carry on like this'.

During the last few weeks, your children and wife have commented that you 'look and sound drunk – my speech is all slurred'.

You've not had any headaches but your vision has been blurry and you're finding it increasingly difficult to watch the TV – 'I certainly couldn't drive like this'. You've also noticed that you've been a bit clumsy when reaching for things and have dropped/knocked things over during the last week.

No hearing problems/no tinnitus/no other facial or limb weakness or sensory changes.

During the last few weeks – increasing cough, mainly dry but occasional episodes of fresh red blood (which you've not told your wife about). Severe left-sided chest pain 'catches me when I take a deep breath in or cough' relieved with the increasing numbers of ibuprofen you're taking.

Short of breath when lying down and now having to sleep with three pillows; no wheeze, no paroxysmal nocturnal dyspnoea (PND), no oedema.

Of note: your father and his brother (your uncle) both died of lung cancer in their 50s – both were heavy smokers. Your mother died with 'liver problems' when you were in your teens. You have been a smoker since you were 16 years old; you smoke roll-ups –about 2 oz tobacco per week. You like the occasional 'drink up' at get-togethers but rarely drink week to week because of your driving job. You have been a HGV driver all your working life; no history of asbestos exposure.

You normally don't take any medications but over the last few weeks have been 'eating handfuls of paracetamol and brufen tablets because of the pains'. You have no known allergies.

You are married, and your wife is a 'diamond' – 'brought up our lovely children almost on her own (I was away driving for long periods)'. You have five children: one 27 years old, married with two children; one 25 years old, Royal Marine, in Afghanistan at the moment; one 21 years old, at university ('I have no idea where he came from – at Cambridge studying to be a vet'); one 19 years old, training to be a fireman; one 18 years old, doing A levels at college – wants to be a lawyer.

Ideas – 'I have no idea what's going on but I know it ain't good – I'm falling apart.'

Concerns – 'I'm not stupid doc, I'm pretty sure it's something really serious.'

Expectations – 'I just hope you can do something about it – and quick.'

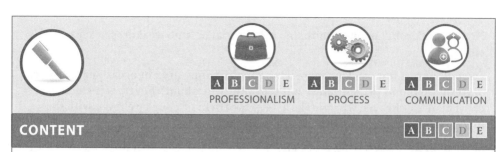

PROFESSIONALISM  PROCESS  COMMUNICATION

**SCENARIO 18**

## CONTENT

### Identifies key information
- History of presenting complaint
- Duration and progression
- Neurological symptoms: unsteadiness 'like being drunk', dizziness, blurring of vision, slurred speech.

### Includes important negatives, including systemic enquiry
- Loss of consciousness, headaches, upper and lower limb weakness/sensory loss, hearing problems and tinnitus.

### Identifies key information from rest of history
- Falls: number, character including pre-, intra- and post-fall symptoms
- Respiratory symptoms: cough, sputum, haemoptysis (defines), dyspnoea, exercise tolerance, orthopnoea, wheeze
- Weight loss: previous and present weight; height; appetite, dysphagia, nausea/vomiting, upper and lower abdominal pain
- Bowel habit.

### Completing the patient history
- Drug and allergy history: previously no meds – now taking 'handfuls' of paracetamol and ibuprofen; no known allergies
- Malignancy risk: family history, smoking history, occupation – HGV driver
- Alcohol: occasional binge but week to week very little due to job as a driver
- Social and occupational history: married with five children.

### Summarises important areas of the history back to the patient

### Invites patient to ask questions and deals with them appropriately

### Establishes patient's ideas, concerns and expectations

## CLINICAL DIAGNOSTIC REASONING

- **Please present your history**
  - Candidate offers a logical, well-structured account of the history.

- **Could you tell me the likely diagnoses in this case, and how you derived these diagnoses?**
  - Probable lung cancer – lifelong heavy smoker, cough with haemoptysis; severe, unplanned weight loss
  - Cerebellar symptoms – slurred speech, dizziness/unsteadiness, multiple falls, clumsiness
  - Differential: metastatic disease; paraneoplastic disease.

- **Apart from malignancy, can you tell me three other causes of cerebellar syndromes?**
  - Alcohol
  - Drugs – especially anti-epileptics
  - Congenital causes – Freidrich's ataxia, Arnold-Chiari malformation
  - NOTE: stroke disease, demyelination and space-occupying lesions most often cause unilateral cerebellar deficits, but may on occasion cause bilateral disease and therefore a syndrome.

**Demonstrates safe, sensible and appropriate management plan**

**Demonstrates clear and logical diagnostic reasoning**

## GLOBAL HISTORY MARK

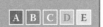

## Station 2 – Examination

**Patient script (also see page 389)**

You are a previously fit and well 55-year-old man who has now been unwell for several months; you are anxious and concerned and know something is seriously wrong with you. On examination you have bilateral signs of cerebellar disease and are very unsteady on sitting, standing and walking.

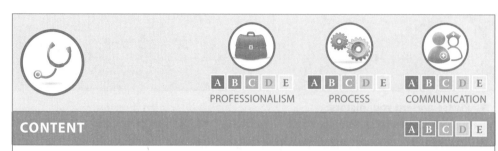

PROFESSIONALISM    PROCESS    COMMUNICATION

## CONTENT

**Exposes and positions patient correctly and maintains comfort**

**Comments on wellbeing of patient, ie well or unwell**

**'Feet to face'**
- Observes and comments on patient and surroundings from foot of bed
- Evidence of obvious neurological deficit, mobility aids.

**Asks for appropriate/relevant clinical observations**
- Observations: HR 96 bpm, BP 134/86 mmHg, height 1.83 m, weight 62.5 kg, BMI 19.1.

**General/systemic examination**
- Signs of cerebellar disease – assesses both LEFT and RIGHT
- Hands – past pointing and dysdiadokokinesia
- Upper limbs – tone and reflexes
- Face – nystagmus; speech – slow, staccato, slurred
- Truncal ataxia – assesses by sitting patient on edge of bed unsupported (or comments on whilst examining patient)
- Balance/gait – candidate is attentive and close to patient (in case they lose balance/fall) at all times
- Romberg's test – comments on positive/negative result
- Standing heel to toe with eyes open/then closed (arms by side)
- Gait/walking – comments on general pattern, eg ataxic or waddling, specifically comments on gait cadence, legs swing through, foot plant.

**Holistic assessment for suspected metastatic lung cancer**
- General appearance – cachectic, unwell, pale, obvious lymphadenopathy, jaundiced
- Hands – nails: tar staining, clubbing; general: wasting, signs of Pancoast syndrome (wasting of the first interosseal space)
- Upper limbs – bruising, wasting
- Face – Horner's syndrome; oral candidiasis; speech – comments of presence/absence of hoarseness
- Neck and SCF – full assessment of local lymph node groups
- Chest – full respiratory examination – anterior and posterior
- Abdomen – specifically assesses for hepatomegaly and ascites
- Bones – specifically assesses for spinal, ribs and long bone tenderness.

**Thanks patient, offers assistance, maintains patient's dignity and privacy until they are dressed**

**CLINICAL DIAGNOSTIC REASONING**

A B C D E

**Correctly identifies the relevant physical signs, including important negative findings**

■ **Can you tell me three pathologies you might expect to demonstrate clinically on assessment of the chest of a patient with lung cancer?**
  - Pleural effusion(s)
  - Consolidation
  - Lobar collapse.

■ **Can you tell me five blood tests and five other investigations that would be important in the diagnosis and management of this patient?**
  - Blood tests – FBC (anaemia), U&Es (hydration, renal involvement, eg glomerulonephritis), LFTs (metastases), clotting profile (liver metastases), calcium/phosphate (bony metastases, paraneoplastic antibodies (see station 3)
  - Radiology – CXR, staging CT chest, abdomen and pelvis; MRI brain (in view of cerebellar symptoms)
  - Sputum – cytology
  - Bronchoscopy and biopsy
  - Bone scan – if bony metastases were suspected/confirmed on history and radiology.

**Demonstrates safe, sensible and appropriate management plan**

**Demonstrates clear and logical diagnostic reasoning**

**SCENARIO 18**

**GLOBAL EXAMINATION MARK**

A B C D E

## Station 3 – Data interpretation

1. This station is included not to punish the reader (as it may have felt!) but more to demonstrate how rapidly modern medicine is evolving. Doctors and medical students of the future will have to have a keen understanding of molecular biology and be able to relate this knowledge to the patient sitting in front of them. At present the paraneoplastic antibodies remain sensitive but are in the main poorly specific to given neurological syndromes; they are produced in a relatively small number of malignancies, and remain rare. Malignancies more commonly associated with these antibodies include small cell and (less commonly) non-small cell lung cancer, breast, gynaecological, testicular, prostate, lymphomas and colonic cancers. In a similar manner to the massive explosion in the production and utilisation of monoclonal antibody therapies, these poorly understood markers will become increasingly useful in oncological screening, diagnosis, prognosis and evaluating the success of oncological interventions. Until such time, watch this space!

| Paraneoplastic neurological condition | Neuro-disability | Paraneoplastic antibody | Commonly associated malignancy |
|---|---|---|---|
| Limbic and brainstem encephalomyelitis | Short-term memory loss; seizures, confusion; features of parkinsonism, motor weakness, ataxia | Anti-Ta | Testicular germ cell tumours |
| Cerebellar degeneration | Ataxia, dysdiadokokinesia and staccato speech | Anti-Yo (APCA-1) | Ovarian carcinoma |
| Stiff person syndrome | Progressive rigidity and stiffness principally affecting the axial muscles | Anti-GAD and Anti-Ampiphysin antibodies | Breast cancer |
| Opsoclonus | Rapid, involuntary eye movements | Anti-Ri (ANNA-2) | Breast and ovarian cancer |
| Lambert–Eaton myasthenic syndrome | Proximal lower limb, and upper limb weakness | Anti-Voltage gated calcium channel (VGCC) | Small cell lung cancer |
| Subacute peripheral sensory neuropathy | Loss of distal sensation in the limbs | Anti-Hu (ANNA-1) | Small cell lung cancer<br><br>Prostate cancer |

## Other paraneoplastic antibodies associated with neurological syndromes

| Auto-antibody | Associated paraneoplastic syndrome | Malignancy |
|---|---|---|
| Anti-Yo (APCA-1)<br><br>(Anti-Purkinje cell Antibody) | Cerebellar degeneration | Gynaecological and breast<br><br>(thus is a marker predominantly found in women) |
| Anti-Tr | Cerebellar degeneration | Lymphoma |
| Anti-Zic4 | Cerebellar degeneration<br><br>(zic proteins are essential for normal maturation of the neurones of the CNS) | Very strong association with SCLC |
| Anti-voltage gated Potassium channels<br><br>(aVGKC) | Peripheral nerve hyperexcitability<br><br>(VGKC are responsible for controlling membrane excitability) | SCLC and Thymoma |
| Anti-Ma2 | Limbic and brain stem encephalitis; several other neurological syndromes | Testicular tumours; several other tumours – middle-aged men and women |
| Anti-CV2 – aCRMP5 | Cerebellar degeneration; peripheral sensory neuropathy; several other neurological syndromes | SCLS and thymoma; found in association with aHu |
| Anti-ampiphysin | Breast – stiff person syndrome<br><br>SCLC – similar spectrum to a-Hu | Breast (strong association)<br><br>SCLC |

**2.**

**1.       J**

Phenytoin is often used in post-craniotomy patients, as it has relatively rapid onset of action and is very effective. Unfortunately, phenytoin has a narrow therapeutic window and has several significant side effects, including a cerebellar syndrome. Many of the drugs that cause peripheral sensory neuropathy (including phenytoin) also cause cerebellar degeneration. These include amiodarone, cyclosporin, isoniazid, metronidazole and lithium.

**2.       A**

This man's clinical signs and his blood results suggest he has chronic alcohol-related liver disease. He has bilateral Dupuytren's contracture, multiple spider naevi and gynaecomastia, a macrocytic anaemia (Hb 7.9 g/dl, MCV 105 fl), thrombocytopenia (platelets $82 \times 10^9$/l), hyponatraemia(Na$^+$ 126 mmol/l), low urea (urea 1.1 mmol/l) and deranged clotting (INR 1.6, APTT 58 s).

**3.       F**

This man has signs and symptoms suggestive of a cerebellar-pontine angle (CPA) tumour. The duration and the progression of the condition exclude a stroke syndrome. Patients with CPA disease present with ipsilateral cerebellar signs associated with lesions of the ipsilateral pontine cranial nerves, ie V, VII, VII and VIII. Common CPA tumours include acoustic neuroma, meningioma, metastases from lung and breast tumours and cerebellar tumours.

**4.       K**

Wallenberg's syndrome (lateral medullary syndrome or posterior inferior cerebellar artery (PICA) syndrome) – this patient has signs and symptoms suggestive of a stroke syndrome. He has features of unilateral cerebellar disease, ipsilateral V and VII nerve palsies and contralateral loss of pain and temperature in the limbs. This ipsilateral loss of pain and temperature in the face and contralateral loss in the limbs is pathognomonic of lateral medullary syndrome. Adolf Wallenberg (German Neurologist, 1862–1949).

**5.       G**

This young woman has clinical features suggestive of demyelination. In younger patients congenital disease and demyelination are the common causes of cerebellar disease, although this would be late onset for congenital disease, eg Freidrich's ataxia, Dandy-Walker syndrome or Arnold-Chiari malformation.

**GLOBAL DATA INTERPRETATION MARK**

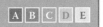

SCENARIO 18

## Station 4 – Clinical communication skills

**Patient script**

You are the Consultant, playing Mr Charles Lamb.

You are quite anxious and scared, as you have worked out that you probably haven't got too long to live; you should be frank and open with the doctor and want to be told 'all the gory details' – 'I've got to be able to tell my wife and children'.

You have been told that you have a 'shadow on the lung' – that is probably something serious – 'you understood this to mean a cancer'. You've also gathered from conversations with the doctors and nurses that the dizziness and unsteadiness you've been experiencing is due to spread of the cancer to your brain. You have also been told that the cancer may have spread to your liver and bones.

Ideas – you know it's really bad and probably not curable but want to be told what can be done.

Concerns – you are worried that you've only got a few weeks left and that you won't see your son graduate from Cambridge.

Expectations – you are just hoping that you could be given something (medicines or radiotherapy) to make you live with not too many symptoms for a few years until he graduates.

Question: 'How long do you think I've got left doc?'

Question: 'Is there any treatment I can have to make this all go away?'

Question: 'Will I suffer a lot towards the end?'

NOTE: This is a complex case with multiple, complex investigation results to explain. It is really important in such cases that you don't try to explain every result, as this will lead to information overload, a diminution of the important messages, and will create uncertainty and confusion for the patient.

There are three important 'take-home messages' for Mr Lamb to understand:

- He does have a lung cancer that has spread to his liver and bones
- The dizziness is caused as a result of the cancer but is not directly due to it spreading to the brain
- He will need to be reviewed by an oncologist (cancer specialist) who may be able to offer some treatments to improve his quality of life (eg radiotherapy to the bones) and other possible interventions, but there are no curative treatments.

If you don't know the treatments or the prognosis in a given case, you should be open and truthful with the patient. Senior members of your team and the oncologists will be able to give much better insight into prognosis and possible interventions. You may be able to direct the patient to web-based information that may help them better understand their condition but always quality assure these, as they may be full of misinformation. The Mayo Clinic, and other leading centres, have produced extensive web-based patient materials.

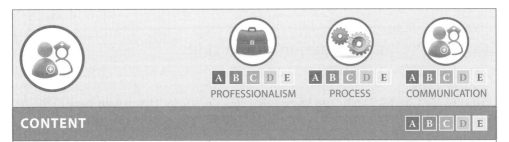

PROFESSIONALISM · PROCESS · COMMUNICATION

## CONTENT

**Confirms reason for discussion**
- To talk to the patient about the investigation results and to answer any questions he may have.

**Establishes what patient wishes to know; gains agreement/informal consent to participate in the discussion**

**Investigates patient's present level of understanding of scenario and what he's been told by other healthcare professionals**

**Establishes patient's ideas, concerns and expectations**

**Explains the key, important information**
- The diagnosis of lung cancer – implied by the CXR and CT chest scan; confirmed by the biopsy results taken at the bronchoscopy
- Metastases – the cancer has spread to the liver and bones (ribs) as seen on the CT scan
- Dizziness – resultant of the cancer, but not due to direct spread; if challenged – the cancer produces proteins (antibodies) that attack the back of the brain (cerebellum), causing it not to work properly; this part of the brain controls balance and movement, hence the dizziness and unsteadiness; it is the part of the brain commonly affected by alcohol, hence you feel drunk.

**Explains further management**
- Review by cancer MDT - including specialist cancer doctors and nurses
- No curative treatment but possible palliative interventions – 'treatments to make you feel better and stop any suffering'.

**Invites patient to ask questions and is able to deal with them appropriately**
- Prognosis – probable weeks to months
- No curative treatments
- Follow-up with oncology and palliative care should mean that any symptoms are dealt with speedily and appropriately.

**Summarises important areas of the consultation back to the patient**

**Formally ends the consultation and ensures appropriate follow-up has been discussed**

## Station 5 – Clinical communication skills

**Patient script**

You are Mr Charles Lamb. You know the young doctor well from your time in the hospital and are happy to talk to him/her about your present problems.

On leaving the hospital you were pretty sure that you and your wife would be able to cope, especially with the input of your family and friends. 'They've all been superb and are really keeping my spirits up… even though we all know it's not long to go.'

Your main problems are:
- Shortness of breath – increasing shortness of breath (just like when I came into the hospital); orthopnoea, occasional episodes of haemoptysis (fresh and red)
- Pain – you've got several types; the main one is an all over 'gnawing' pain – 'It just won't go away' – eased with the morphine but always there day and night; occasional pains in your ribs and ibuprofen
- Nasty taste in your mouth; lost all your appetite and just don't feel like eating at all
- Nausea (occasional dry retching); no dysphagia
- Constipation – only opening your bowels with enemas from the chemist; causing you to have griping pains in your tummy
- Drinking poorly – poor urine output (like treacle)
- Poor sleep – lie awake worrying about your wife and children and what they'll do without you
- Mood – find yourself very tearful and crying when you're alone – nothing in particular causes it, just feeling generally sad
- Dizziness/unsteadiness – still a major problem but no worse than before; 'learnt to live with it really' – wife helps you to walk and get you up and down the stairs; find it difficult to go to the toilet, and to get washed because of the dizziness.

Activities of daily living (ADLs) – need the help of at least one person to transfer, mobilise, dress, wash, shave, go to the toilet.

Haven't been out the house in weeks – too dizzy and weak.

'How do I occupy my day?' – friends come round, watch the TV, doze in armchair in the conservatory.

Ideas – 'Just want to feel a little bit better and stronger – can't be that hard can it doc?'

Concerns – 'Don't want to be a burden on the family all the time.'

Expectations – 'You must be able to give me a little shot of something and I'll be better.'

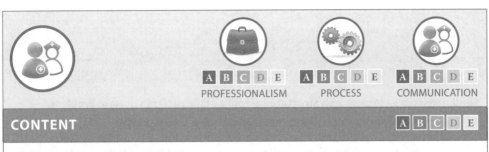

PROFESSIONALISM     PROCESS     COMMUNICATION

## CONTENT

A B C D E

**Confirms reason for discussion**
- To talk to patient about his present state of health, specific symptoms and possible solutions.

**Establishes what patient wishes to know; gains agreement/informal consent to participate in the discussion**

**Confirms the major symptoms causing concern for the patient**
- Local (chest problems) – asks about chest pains, shortness of breath, haemoptysis
- Metastatic problems – asks about bone pain; abdominal pains, abdominal swelling
- Other – dizziness and unsteadiness, falls
- Specifically asks about:
- Pain – invites patient to describe different types of pain (SOCRATES)
- GI symptoms - Appetite; upper and lower GI symptoms
- UG symptoms - Hydration and micturition
- Mood and sleep
- Asks about ADLs – transfers, mobility, washing and dressing, shaving, continence and toileting, getting out of the house, how he occupies his day.

**Establishes patient's ideas, concerns and expectations**

**Invites patient to ask questions and is able to deal with them appropriately**

**Summarises important areas of the consultation back to the patient**

**Formally ends the consultation and ensures appropriate follow-up has been discussed**

## CLINICAL DIAGNOSTIC REASONING

**Candidate offers a logical, well-structured account of the patient's present problems**

- **Could you tell me five interventions you might suggest in this case?**
  - General – family and patient need increased level of support – would benefit from nursing and occupational therapy input, Macmillan team review, possible need for brief hospice admission for symptom control
  - Specific therapeutic inputs:
    - Review of analgesia – may require subcutaneous pump with morphine, anti-emetic and possible anxiolytic; increase NSAIDs; ?further radiotherapy to bony metastases
    - Anti-emetic – see above
    - Addition of oral steroids – dexamethasone 4 mg tds – improves mood and stimulates appetite
    - Regular laxatives and enemas until bowels improve
    - Investigate 'nasty taste in mouth': ?candidiasis; ?secondary to morphine (bitter taste)
    - Mood – consider anti-depressants (may also help with appetite)
    - Sleep – consider sleeping tablets
    - Shortness of breath – may be due to new pleural effusion or possibly pulmonary embolism; these may be demonstrated by clinical assessment.

**Demonstrates safe, sensible and appropriate management plan**

**Demonstrates clear and logical diagnostic reasoning**

## GLOBAL COMMUNICATION MARK

## Station 6 – Prescribing skills

| Allergies, sensitivities and adverse drug reactions | | | | | Patient details/addressograph | |
|---|---|---|---|---|---|---|
| No known allergies ✓ | | Initials  AF | Gender  (M)/ F | | NHS/ Hospital No:  888432 | |
| Not possible to ascertain ☐ | | Date  2/05 | Weight (kg) | Date | | |
| Medicine/substance | Reaction & Severity | Initials & Date | 62.5kg | | Surname:  LAMB | |
| | | | Height | | First name:  CHARLES | |
| | | | 1.83m | | | |
| Alerts | | | Surface area (m²) | | Date of birth:  06.10.56 | |

### IN-PATIENT MEDICATION PRESCRIPTION AND ADMINISTRATION RECORD

PasTest HOSPITAL

| Consultant  PHILLIPS | Trainee Dr. Name and Bleep no.  FEATHER 622 | Date of admission  2/05/12 | Date chart reboarded | Estimated date of discharge |
|---|---|---|---|---|
| This chart is no.  ......1...... of ......1...... | Transcribing Check by Pharmacy  Sign ............ Date ............ | Ward  1. ....MARLEY......  2. ............ | | |

Supplementary Medication charts in use:  Other (please specify): 1 ............................................ 2 ............................................

| Epidural/PCA ☐ | Syringe driver ☐ | | TPN ☐ | Chemotherapy ☐ | Insulin sliding scale ☐ |
|---|---|---|---|---|---|

Once only medications – loading doses, pre-medication, PGDs  or surgical antibiotic propylaxis

| Date | Time to be given | Medicine (approved name) | Dose | Route | Signature and bleep no. | Pharmacy | Time given | Given by | Checked by |
|---|---|---|---|---|---|---|---|---|---|
| 2/05 | Stat | FLUCLONAZOLE | 150mg | PO | AF 622 | | | | |
| | | | | | | | | | |
| | | | | | | | | | |
| | | | | | | | | | |

| Regular prescriptions continued | | | | | | | | | | |
|---|---|---|---|---|---|---|---|---|---|---|
| Anti-infectives prescription    *prescribe long term prophylaxis and anti-tuberculosis medications in regular medications section* | | | | | | | | | | |
| | Dose | | | Date | 2 | 3 | 4 | 5 | 6 | |
| Date 2/05 | PO – TO SUCK | | | Medication  NYSTATIN PASTILLES | | Indication | | | Signature and bleep no.  AF 622 | Pharmacy ☐ |
| Route | | | | | | | | | | |
| Signature | | | | | | | | | | |
| 06 | | | | | | | | | | |
| (10) | ○ T | | | | | | | | | |
| (14) | ○ T | | | | | | | | | |
| (18) | ○ T | | | | | | | | | |
| (22) | ○ T | | | | | | | | | |
| 02 | | | | | | | | | | |

| | Dose | | | Date | | | | | | | | | | | | | | | |
|---|---|---|---|---|---|---|---|---|---|---|---|---|---|---|---|---|---|---|---|
| Date | 2/05 | | | Medication | | | | Instructions | | | | Signature and bleep no. | | | | Pharmacy | | | |
| Route | PO | | | IBUPROFEN | | | | | | | | AF 622 | | | | | | | |
| Signature | | | | | | | | | | | | | | | | | | | |
| 06 | | | | | | | | | | | | | | | | | | | |
| (09) | 600mg | | | | | | | | | | | | | | | | | | |
| (14) | 600mg | | | | | | | | | | | | | | | | | | |
| 18 | 600mg | | | | | | | | | | | | | | | | | | |
| (22) | 600mg | | | | | | | | | | | | | | | | | | |
| 24 | | | | | | | | | | | | | | | | | | | |

**Regular prescriptions continued**

| | Dose | | | Date | | | | | | | | | | | | | | | |
|---|---|---|---|---|---|---|---|---|---|---|---|---|---|---|---|---|---|---|---|
| Date | 2/05 | | | Medication | | | | Indication | | | | Signature and bleep no. | | | | Pharmacy | | | |
| Route | PO/IM/SC | | | CYCLIZINE | | | | | | | | AF 622 | | | | | | | |
| Signature | | | | | | | | | | | | | | | | | | | |
| 06 | | | | | | | | | | | | | | | | | | | |
| (09) | 50mg | | | | | | | | | | | | | | | | | | |
| (14) | 50mg | | | | | | | | | | | | | | | | | | |
| 18 | | | | | | | | | | | | | | | | | | | |
| (22) | 50mg | | | | | | | | | | | | | | | | | | |
| 24 | | | | | | | | | | | | | | | | | | | |

**Regular prescriptions continued**

| | Dose | | | Date | | | | | | | | | | | | | | | |
|---|---|---|---|---|---|---|---|---|---|---|---|---|---|---|---|---|---|---|---|
| Date | 2/05 | | | Medication | | | | Instructions | | | | Signature and bleep no. | | | | Pharmacy | | | |
| Route | PO | | | DEXAMETHASONE | | | | FOR MOOD/ | | | | AF 622 | | | | | | | |
| Signature | | | | | | | | APPETITE | | | | | | | | | | | |
| 06 | | | | | | | | | | | | | | | | | | | |
| (08) | 4mg | | | | | | | | | | | | | | | | | | |
| (12) | 4mg | | | | | | | | | | | | | | | | | | |
| 18 | | | | | | | | | | | | | | | | | | | |
| (20) | 4mg | | | | | | | | | | | | | | | | | | |
| 24 | | | | | | | | | | | | | | | | | | | |

**Regular prescriptions continued**

| | Dose | | | Date | | | | | | | | | | | | | | | |
|---|---|---|---|---|---|---|---|---|---|---|---|---|---|---|---|---|---|---|---|
| Date | 2/05 | | | Medication | | | | Indication | | | | Signature and bleep no. | | | | Pharmacy | | | |
| Route | PO | | | DOCUSATE | | | | | | | | AF 622 | | | | | | | |
| Signature | | | | | | | | | | | | | | | | | | | |
| 06 | | | | | | | | | | | | | | | | | | | |
| (09) | 200mg | | | | | | | | | | | | | | | | | | |
| 14 | | | | | | | | | | | | | | | | | | | |
| (18) | 200mg | | | | | | | | | | | | | | | | | | |
| 22 | | | | | | | | | | | | | | | | | | | |
| 24 | | | | | | | | | | | | | | | | | | | |

**Regular prescriptions continued**

| | Dose | | | Date | | | | | | | | | | | | | | | |
|---|---|---|---|---|---|---|---|---|---|---|---|---|---|---|---|---|---|---|---|
| Date | 2/05 | | | Medication | | | Indication | | | Signature and bleep no. | | | Pharmacy | |
| Route | PO | | | SENNA | | | | | | AF 622 | | | ☐ | |
| Signature | | | | | | | | | | | | | | |
| 06 | | | | | | | | | | | | | | |
| (09) | ᵒᵒ↑↑ | | | | | | | | | | | | | |
| 14 | | | | | | | | | | | | | | |
| (18) | ᵒᵒ↑↑ | | | | | | | | | | | | | |
| 22 | | | | | | | | | | | | | | |
| 24 | | | | | | | | | | | | | | |

**Regular prescriptions continued**

| | Dose | | | Date | | | | | | | | | | | | | | | |
|---|---|---|---|---|---|---|---|---|---|---|---|---|---|---|---|---|---|---|---|
| Date | 2/05 | | | Medication | | | Indication | | | Signature and bleep no. | | | Pharmacy | |
| Route | PO | | | LACTULOSE | | | | | | AF 622 | | | ☐ | |
| Signature | | | | | | | | | | | | | | |
| 06 | | | | | | | | | | | | | | |
| (09) | 10ml | | | | | | | | | | | | | |
| 14 | | | | | | | | | | | | | | |
| (18) | 10ml | | | | | | | | | | | | | |
| 22 | | | | | | | | | | | | | | |
| 24 | | | | | | | | | | | | | | |

**Regular prescriptions continued**

| | Dose | | | Date | | | | | | | | | | | | | | | |
|---|---|---|---|---|---|---|---|---|---|---|---|---|---|---|---|---|---|---|---|
| Date | 2/05 | | | Medication | | | Indication | | | Signature and bleep no. | | | Pharmacy | |
| Route | MOUTH/TOP | | | REGULAR MOUTHCARE | | | | | | AF 622 | | | ☐ | |
| Signature | | | | | | | | | | | | | | |
| 06 | | | | | | | | | | | | | | |
| (09) | ✓ | | | | | | | | | | | | | |
| (14) | ✓ | | | | | | | | | | | | | |
| (18) | ✓ | | | | | | | | | | | | | |
| (22) | ✓ | | | | | | | | | | | | | |
| 24 | | | | | | | | | | | | | | |

**SCENARIO 18**

### As required medications

| Medication | | | | | Date | | | | | | | | | | | | | | | | | | | |
|---|---|---|---|---|---|---|---|---|---|---|---|---|---|---|---|---|---|---|---|---|---|---|---|---|
| PARACETAMOL | | | | | | | | | | | | | | | | | | | | | | | | |
| **Indication** | | | | | Time | | | | | | | | | | | | | | | | | | | |
| **Dose** 1g | **Route** PO | **Maximum frequency / dose** QDS | **Start date** 2/05 | | Dose | | | | | | | | | | | | | | | | | | | |
| | | | **Stop date** | | Route | | | | | | | | | | | | | | | | | | | |
| **Signature** AF 622 | | | | | | | | | | | | | | | | | | | | | | | | |
| | | | **Bleep no.** | | Given | | | | | | | | | | | | | | | | | | | |
| **Additional instructions:** | | | | | | | | | | | | | | | Pharmacy | | | | | | | | | |

### As required medications

| Medication | | | | | Date | | | | | | | | | | | | | | | | | | | |
|---|---|---|---|---|---|---|---|---|---|---|---|---|---|---|---|---|---|---|---|---|---|---|---|---|
| OROMORPH | | | | | | | | | | | | | | | | | | | | | | | | |
| **Indication** BREAKTHROUGH PAIN | | | | | Time | | | | | | | | | | | | | | | | | | | |
| **Dose** 20 mg | **Route** PO | **Maximum frequency / dose** as req. | **Start date** 2/05 | | Dose | | | | | | | | | | | | | | | | | | | |
| | | | **Stop date** | | Route | | | | | | | | | | | | | | | | | | | |
| **Signature** AF 622 | | | | | | | | | | | | | | | | | | | | | | | | |
| | | | **Bleep no.** | | Given | | | | | | | | | | | | | | | | | | | |
| **Additional instructions:** | | | | | | | | | | | | | | | Pharmacy | | | | | | | | | |

### As required medications

| Medication | | | | | Date | | | | | | | | | | | | | | | | | | | |
|---|---|---|---|---|---|---|---|---|---|---|---|---|---|---|---|---|---|---|---|---|---|---|---|---|
| TEMAZEPAM | | | | | | | | | | | | | | | | | | | | | | | | |
| **Indication** | | | | | Time | | | | | | | | | | | | | | | | | | | |
| **Dose** 20 mg | **Route** PO | **Maximum frequency / dose** nocte | **Start date** 2/05 | | Dose | | | | | | | | | | | | | | | | | | | |
| | | | **Stop date** | | Route | | | | | | | | | | | | | | | | | | | |
| **Signature** AF 622 | | | | | | | | | | | | | | | | | | | | | | | | |
| | | | **Bleep no.** | | Given | | | | | | | | | | | | | | | | | | | |
| **Additional instructions:** | | | | | | | | | | | | | | | Pharmacy | | | | | | | | | |

## GLOBAL PRESCRIBING MARK

A B C D E

# Scenario 18: Reflection and consolidation

## History

Mr Charles Lamb is a previously fit and well 55-year-old HGV driver. He was referred in by his GP with weight loss and falls, the last being on the way home from the pub last night.

He was well until about 3 or 4 months ago, when he first noticed episodes of haemoptysis. Initially this was a bit of blackened spit in the mornings but then occasionally he would cough up bits of fresh red blood and bits of clotted blood.

At this time he also began to lose weight. His previous 'fighting weight' was about 95 kg, but over this period he has gone down to 62.5 kg (height used to be 1.83 m). He has lost his appetite and is eating poorly. He denies nausea, vomiting or dysphagia but does admit to recent constipation; normally his bowels opened once or twice per day but recently once every 3 days, and he is straining at stool.

Over the last few weeks (about 1–2) he has become increasingly unsteady and dizzy; so much so, that he had to stop driving. He has had three or four 'actual falls', where he loses his balance and falls to the floor but is feeling very unsteady and has, on numerous occasions, had to grab onto something or someone to stop himself falling. He denies loss of consciousness, pre-warning symptoms or any residual deficit after he falls. During the last few weeks his wife and children have commented that he looked and sounded drunk, with slurred speech. He denies any headaches, but his vision has been blurred; so much so, that he is finding it increasingly difficult to watch the TV. He has also noticed that he's been a bit clumsy when reaching for things and has dropped/knocked things over. There has been no hearing problem, tinnitus, or facial or limb weakness or sensory changes.

Over the last few weeks he has suffered with a dry cough, and occasional episodes of fresh red haemoptysis. He has had increasing, severe left-sided pleuritic chest pain and orthopnoea. He is sleeping with three pillows.

Of note – his father and uncle both died of lung cancer in their 50s – they were both heavy smokers. Mr Lamb is a lifelong smoker (since 16 years of age) and smokes roll-ups – about 2 oz tobacco per week. He has been an HGV driver all his working life and has no history of asbestos exposure.

He has the occasional alcohol binge but week to week drinks little because of his job.

He normally doesn't take any medications, but over the last few weeks has been 'eating handfuls of paracetamol and brufen tablets because of the pains'. He has no known allergies.

Mr Lamb is married and has five grown-up children – the youngest two living at home.

## Examination

On examination, this was a chronically unwell, pale, thin-looking man; he was unsteady on transfers and walking and had to be helped on and off the bed. He was alert and orientated in time, place and person. Mr Lamb had signs consistent with a cerebellar syndrome, as evidenced by bilateral past pointing, dysdiadokokinesia, hyporeflexia, nystagmus, and cerebellar speech. He had signs of metastatic lung cancer, with clubbing of his fingernails, hard fixed lymphadenopathy of the neck and signs of left-sided pleural effusion. He also had 4 cm hepatomegaly.

### Investigations

When patients present with complex signs and symptoms it is easy for the novice clinician to get lost in this complexity. As with all patients, you should concentrate on doing the simple things well.
In this case the patient requires helpful, diagnostic and prognostic investigations to be considered.

- Helpful/managerial – blood tests are in the main simply helpful; Mr Lamb will require FBC, U&Es, glucose, LFTs, calcium, clotting screen and perhaps a group and save. The paraneoplastic auto-antibodies should be discussed with seniors, and may not be processed for weeks. A CXR is essential but is not diagnostic.
- Diagnostic – bronchoscopy and biopsy; an MRI of his brain is essential to exclude stroke and metastatic disease, and confirm cerebellar degeneration.
- Prognostic – staging CT chest, abdomen and pelvis; bone scan.

### Management

This man has presented late with evidence of metastatic and paraneoplastic disease. His prognosis is poor and would be measured in weeks to months.
Management should be aimed at palliation and ensuring he has as good a quality of life as possible. Palliative radiotherapy may improve his bone pain and his haemoptysis.
Multiple agencies may be involved, including Oncology, Palliative Care services (doctors, nurses, occupational therapist and social worker), his GP and the community healthcare team, and his family and friends.

### Further reading and web links

*Excellent and comprehensive site dealing with all aspects of palliative care*:
www.palliativecareguidelines.scot.nhs.uk/
*Website dedicated to palliative care matters*:
www.pallcare.info/index.php?menu=1
*Website describing all the major paraneoplastic neurological syndromes and antibodies*:
www.pnseuronet.org/index.php
*The excellent patient resources of the Mayo Clinic*:
www.mayoclinic.com/health/DiseasesIndex/DiseasesIndex

# Scenario 19: 'Blood in the pan'

## Station 1

*History*                                    *10-minute station*

**You are a FY1 doctor in the General Surgical Clinic with your Consultant and Registrar. Your Consultant would like to observe you assessing a patient, Henry Hatcher.**

■ **Please take a history from the patient and present it to the Consultant.**

*You will be assessed on the following areas, as well as the content and diagnostic reasoning of your history – take them into account in your presentation.*

### Professionalism

- Professional appearance (NHS dress code) – including general appearance, hair and jewellery
- Maintains patient and personal safety
- Polite introduction; identifies patient or interviewee correctly; confirms patient's date of birth from name band or other source
- Obtains informal consent; maintains patient's privacy
- Displays empathetic and caring attitudes and behaviours throughout.

### Process

- Good organisation and structure; appropriate use of open and closed questions
- Appropriate fluency/rhythm/pace to the interview – this may change depending on environment and acute nature of the problem
- Appropriate time for the patient to respond/reply to questions
- Appropriate acknowledgement of difficult or emotional areas of the patient's history.

### Communication skills

- Demonstrates caring and sympathetic attitude
- Asks open questions
- Invites patient to ask questions and answers them appropriately
- Addresses patient's ideas, concerns and expectations.

## Station 2

*Examination*                                     *10-minute station*

Your Consultant now wishes to observe you performing a focussed abdominal examination, including a digital rectal examination (on the mannequin provided). A set of observations were performed by the clinic nurse earlier and are available to you.

■ After you have performed the examination, you should present your findings to the Consultant, who may have some questions.

(If you do not have a model, please read and present the information given on page 390.)

*You will be assessed on the following areas, as well as the content and skills of your examination – take them into account in your presentation.*

### Professionalism

- Professional appearance; maintains infection control standards, including hand cleaning and appropriate use of gloves and aprons
- Maintains patient and personal safety
- Polite introduction; identifies patient and confirms date of birth from name band or other source
- Obtains informal consent; maintains patient privacy and dignity
- Displays empathetic and caring attitudes and behaviours throughout.

### Process

- Appropriate fluency/rhythm/pace to the examination – this may change depending on environment and acute nature of the problem
- Organisation and structure of examination; sensitive and empathetic approach
- Uses appropriate clinical techniques throughout
- Maintains privacy and dignity throughout.

### Clinical communication

- Explains proposed examination/procedure: explains examination/procedure as it proceeds
- Offers information in a clear, structured and fluent manner, avoiding jargon
- Listens to patient and responds appropriately
- Demonstrates appropriate body language.

SCENARIO 19

## Station 3

*Prescribing skills*                    *5-minute station*

Mr Hatcher is admitted one week later for colonoscopy and further investigation. He has been admitted to Silvertown ward under the care of Mr Jones, colorectal surgeon.

Hospital Number 433543; DOB 29.08.49; weight 71Kg; height 1.94M; allergies: nil known

■ Please prescribe sodium picosulphate bowel preparation (a BNF is available for you to use) which he is to have at 18:00 on the day of his admission, for a colonoscopy the next day.

> **Remember: DRUG DRs Don't Forget Signing Off (page 396)**

## Station 4

*Data interpretation*                    *10-minute station*

1. This procedure confirms the presence of a large colonic tumour, and biopsy confirms that this is adenocarcinoma. Mr Hatcher is then sent for a staging CT scan. Pictured below is a slice from his abdominal CT scan. Please label A–G.

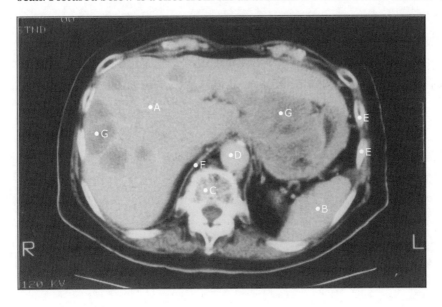

SCENARIO 19

2. You discuss this case with your Registrar on the ward, who would now like you to look at the following contrast studies, all of which have been taken from patients that presented with rectal bleeding. Please look at the statements that accompany each image, and indicate whether they are TRUE (T) or FALSE (F).

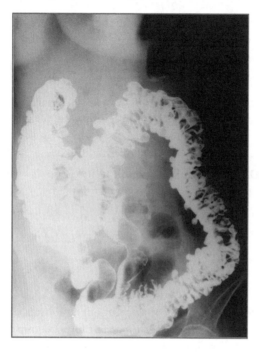

A
a) This is a barium enema.
b) There has been poor bowel preparation.
c) This is a decubitus view.
d) The disorder shown is more common in Black Africans.
e) This disorder is a complication of inflammatory bowel disease.

**B**

a) This is a single contrast barium study.
b) The loss of haustral pattern in the descending colon is termed 'lead piping'.
c) There is evidence of diverticulae.
d) The disorder shown is more common in women.
e) The patient is at increased risk of colonic carcinoma.

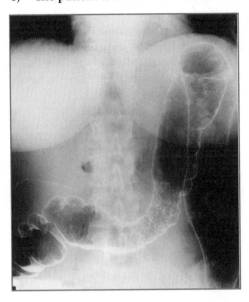

**C**

a) This is a double contrast study.
b) It shows a benign stricture of the transverse colon.
c) The stricture is sited in the distal transverse colon.
d) This stricture is almost certainly related to inflammatory bowel disease (IBD).
e) This patient is probably in their 6th to 7th decade.

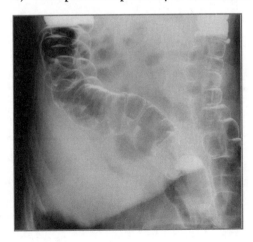

## Station 5

*Clinical communication skills*            *10-minute station*

Two weeks later Mr Hatcher is admitted for surgery scheduled for the following morning. He is due to have an 'open left hemicolectomy with resection of tumour ± stoma formation' and has commenced taking bowel preparation. The nurses bleep you as Mr Hatcher has asked if he can speak to somebody about the operation.

■ Mr Hatcher is anxious to know what the separation entails and realized this may involve the positioning of a temporary or permanent stoma. Please discuss this with him and answer the questions he has on stoma managment.

# Answers

## Station 1 – History

**Patient script**

Your name is Henry Hatcher, DOB 29 August 1949. You have been referred to the clinic by your GP.

For the past 3 or 4 months you have been passing blood-stained stool. The blood generally seems to be mixed in with the stool rather than separate, although sometimes you feel it is fresh blood as well. You have not had any abdominal pain or anal pain. You feel the stool seems to be a bit 'sticky' and 'like mucus' as well. You still open your bowels most days, but sometimes may go 24 hours without passing stool. You used to open your bowels regularly every morning.

You have not had any nausea or vomiting, and otherwise feel 'alright', although you have felt more tired recently but had put that down to your recent retirement. You have noticed that you have been losing quite a lot of weight in the past 6 months or so, and have dropped three trouser sizes. You feel like you are eating OK so are not sure why this has been happening.

You have no medical history really other than high blood pressure and an occasional migraine.

You take amlodipine 5 mg od and have no allergies.

You are married and live with your wife and youngest son. You used to work as an accountant for the local council. You have been a lifelong smoker, 20/day since age 16. You used to be a moderate drinker when you were younger, but only have one or two pints of beer in a typical week now.

Your father died of some sort of cancer, which you believe had spread to the lung but don't know any more about it. You are not aware of any other family history.

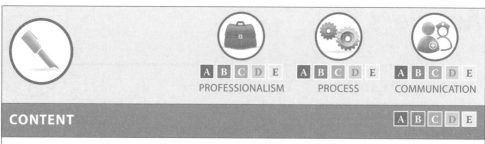

PROFESSIONALISM    PROCESS    COMMUNICATION

## CONTENT

**Identifies key information**
- Blood in stool for last 3 or 4 months
- Blood mixed with stool, and also fresh
- 'Sticky' stool with mucus
- Altered bowel habit – reduced frequency of stool
- Weight loss over 6 months – dropped several trouser sizes.

**Includes important negatives, including systemic enquiry**
- No nausea or vomiting
- Normal appetite.

**Identifies key information from rest of history**
- Increasingly tired.

**Relevant factors from employment, housing, social support**
- Recent retirement.

**Completing the patient history**
- Drug and allergy history: amlodipine 5 mg od; no allergies
- Previous medical history: hypertension
- Social and occupational history: smoked 20/day since age 16 (approx 50 pack years); moderate alcohol intake; retired accountant; married with children
- Family history: paternal history of cancer – unspecified.

**Summarises important areas of the history back to the patient**

**Invites patient to ask questions and deals with them appropriately**

**Establishes patient's ideas, concerns and expectations**

SCENARIO 19

**CLINICAL DIAGNOSTIC REASONING**

A B C D E

- **Please present your history**
    - Candidate offers a logical, well-structured account of the history
    - Summarises the history and correctly identifies key areas of the history that support the correct diagnosis.

- **What do you suspect is the cause of this patient's symptoms?**
    - Candidate offers the correct diagnosis and appropriate differentials
    - Symptoms of persistent rectal bleeding with mucus, altered bowel habit and weight loss all point to a diagnosis of colorectal cancer
    - Differential diagnoses of rectal bleeding include:
    - Inflammatory bowel disease (ulcerative colitis/Crohn's disease)
    - Diverticular disease
    - Haemorrhoids
    - Angiodysplasia
    - Coagulopathies.

- **What risk factors for colorectal cancer do you know?**
    - Diet rich in fat and cholesterol
    - Adenomatous polyps
    - Ulcerative colitis
    - Previous colorectal cancer
    - Familial predisposition of colorectal cancer or familial adenomatous polyposis.

**GLOBAL HISTORY MARK**

A B C D E

## Station 2 – Examination

> **Patient script (see also page 390)**
>
> You are a 63 year-old-gentleman who is largely comfortable at rest. You have lost a large amount of weight recently. On examination of your abdomen you have a large left-sided mass, which is not tender.

SCENARIO 19

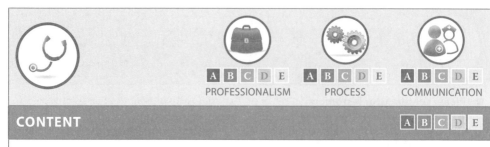

## CONTENT

**Exposes and positions patient correctly and maintains comfort**
- Supine position for abdominal examination; left lateral position for digital rectal examination (on mannequin).

**Comments on wellbeing of patient, ie well or unwell**

**'Feet to face'**
- Thin gentleman with evidence of weight loss; pale; height 194 cm, weight 71 kg, BMI 18.9.

**Asks for appropriate/relevant clinical observations**
- Observations: HR 74 bpm, BP 131/89 mmHg, RR 16 bpm, $O_2$ sats 96% on air, temperature 36.9 °C, CBG 7.9 mmol/l.

**Focussed abdominal examination**
- Inspection
  - Inspects for scars and asymmetry, fullness, and pulsations.
- Palpation
  - Systematic palpation – asks patient if areas of tenderness and begins examination remote to any areas of pain
  - Light followed by deep palpation
  - Identifies mass lesion and characterises by examining for pulsatility, texture and relationship to other structures
  - Palpates all areas of abdomen
  - Examines liver, spleen and ballots for kidneys; palpates liver edge at costal margin, timed with patients respiratory pattern.
- Percussion
  - Percusses for shifting dullness, and at costal margin for upper border of liver.

**Digital rectal examination (on mannequin)**
- Explains to patient what is to be done, and explains will be uncomfortable but should not be painful
- Positions appropriately on left lateral position with knees drawn up to chest
- Examines for external features: haemorrhoids, skin tags, fissures or fistulae
- Applies lubricating jelly to gloved finger and gently inserts index finger into rectum
- Examines both lateral, anterior and posterior walls of rectum systematically by sweeping rotation of finger
- Comments on size and consistency of prostate gland
- Asks patient to gently squeeze on finger by contracting anal sphincter, noting any weakness of sphincter contraction.

**Completes examination by asking to perform full systemic examination, including respiratory examination for evidence of pulmonary metastatic disease (pleural effusion, collapse)**

**Thanks patient, offers assistance, maintains patient's dignity and privacy until they are dressed**

## CLINICAL DIAGNOSTIC REASONING

**Correctly identifies the relevant physical signs, including important negative findings**

■ **Mr Hatcher has features in his history and examination findings that are concerning for a colorectal malignancy. How would you like to investigate him further?**
- Blood tests:
  - FBC: anaemia, infection
  - U&E: baseline, electrolyte imbalance in cachexia
  - LFTs and clotting screen: irregular liver edge raises suspicion of liver metastasis, albumin may be low in malnutrition
  - Carcinoembryonic antigen (CEA): important in following response to treatment and detecting recurrence.
- Imaging tests:
  - Chest X-ray: rule out pleural effusion and lung metastases
  - Endoscopy: rigid sigmoidoscopy/flexible sigmoidoscopy/colonoscopy
  - Contrast study: double contrast barium enema
  - CT scan: of chest, abdomen and pelvis for staging of disease.

■ **What system is used to stage Dukes – and how is each stage classified?**
- Dukes' classification (devised in 1932 by British pathologist Cuthbert Dukes)
  - Stage A: carcinoma in situ limited to mucosa or submucosa
  - Stage B1: cancer extends into the muscularis
  - Stage B2: cancer extends into or beyond the serosa
  - Stage C: cancer extends to regional lymph nodes
  - Stage D: cancer has metastasised to remote sites.

■ **By what routes can colorectal metastasise?**
  - Lymphatic: firstly to regional nodes, then to para-aortic nodes and the thoracic duct
  - Haematogenous: mainly via portal vein to the liver, but often to lungs, kidneys, adrenal glands and bones
  - Trans-coelomic: peritoneal seeding.

**Demonstrates safe, sensible and appropriate management plan**

**Demonstrates clear and logical diagnostic reasoning**

## GLOBAL EXAMINATION MARK

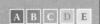

SCENARIO 19

## Station 3 – Prescribing skills

| Allergies, sensitivities and adverse drug reactions | | | | | Patient details/addressograph | |
|---|---|---|---|---|---|---|
| No known allergies ✓ | | Initials AF | Gender Ⓜ F | | NHS/ Hospital No: 433543 | |
| Not possible to ascertain ☐ | | Date 22/06 | Weight (kg) | Date | | |
| Medicine/substance | Reaction & Severity | Initials & Date | 71kg | | Surname: HATCHER | |
| | | | Height | | First name: HENRY | |
| | | | 1.94m | | | |
| Alerts | | | Surface area (m²) | | Date of birth: 29.08.1949 | |

**IN-PATIENT MEDICATION PRESCRIPTION
AND ADMINISTRATION RECORD**

PasTest HOSPITAL

| Consultant MR JONES | Trainee Dr. Name and Bleep no. FEATHER 007 | Date of admission 22/06/12 | Date chart reboarded | Estimated date of discharge |
|---|---|---|---|---|
| This chart is no. ........1........ of ........1........ | Transcribing Check by Pharmacy Sign .......... Date .......... | Ward SILVERTOWN 1. ................................................ 2. ................................................ | | |

Supplementary Medication charts in use:  Other (please specify): 1 .................................................... 2 ....................................

| Epidural/PCA ☐ | Syringe driver ☐ | | TPN ☐ | Chemotherapy ☐ | Insulin sliding scale ☐ | | |
|---|---|---|---|---|---|---|---|

Once only medications – loading doses, pre-medication, PGDs or surgical antibiotic propylaxis

| Date | Time to be given | Medicine (approved name) | Dose | Route | Signature and bleep no. | Pharmacy | Time given | Given by | Checked by |
|---|---|---|---|---|---|---|---|---|---|
| 22/06 | 18.00 | SODIUM PICOSULPHATE | 1 X 10mg sachet | PO | AF 007 | | | | |
| | | | | | | | | | |
| | | | | | | | | | |
| | | | | | | | | | |

**GLOBAL PRESCRIBING MARK**

A  B  C  D  E

## Station 4 – Data interpretation

1

    A  Liver

    B  Spleen

    C  Lumbar vertebra

    D  Abdominal aorta

    E  Ribs

    F  Right crus of diaphragm

    G  Liver metastases

2

A

a) True

b) False

c) True

d) False

e) False

This is a barium enema taken with the patient lying on their right, as witnessed by the fluid levels. The study shows multiple diverticulae throughout the colon. Diverticular disease is related to a poor fibre and Western diet, and is rarely seen in Black Africans. The disorder is unrelated to IBD.

B

a) False

b) True

c) False

d) False

e) True

This is a double contrast barium study showing loss of the haustral pattern in the distal two-thirds of the transverse colon and the descending colon. This appearance is termed 'lead piping' and is a feature of ulcerative colitis. The small indentations are pseudopolyps and not diverticulae. The incidence of IBD is similar in the two sexes. The incidence of colonic carcinoma is greatly increased in patients with ulcerative colitis for 10 years or more and they should be under colonoscopic surveillance.

**C**

a) True

b) False

c) True

d) False

e) True

This is a double contrast study showing a classical 'apple core' stricture of the transverse colon (see below). This appearance is classical of colonic cancer. Patients present with weight loss, change in bowel habit and bleeding and mucus per rectum. Colonic carcomoma usually presents in the 6th to 7th decade.

**GLOBAL DATA INTERPRETATION MARK**

A B C D E

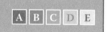

## Station 5 – Clinical communication skills

**Patient script**

You understand that the surgery you are due to have is to remove the cancer, but you do not really understand what is involved and would like some more information. You have been taking 'liquids only' for the last 2 days, as instructed, in order to prepare your bowel for the surgery, and you have also been given a laxative.

Your main anxiety is about the possibility of having a stoma. You are worried about what other people might think because you are concerned about a stoma being smelly and also that the bag may be cumbersome. You are anxious that you wont be able to manage very well with changing the bag, and you feel embarrassed about the prospect of your wife or son having to help you too much with it.

You are worried that it will take you a very long time to recover from this, and that because you have already lost a lot of weight, your body will not be strong enough to deal with this major surgery.

Question: 'Do you think I am likely to need a stoma?'

Question: 'If I have a stoma, how often does the bag need to be changed?'

Question: 'Will I need to change my diet if I have a stoma?'

Question: 'I don't want to burden my family – what other sort of help is available?'

A B **C** D E    A B **C** D E    **A** B **C** D E

PROFESSIONALISM    PROCESS    COMMUNICATION

## CONTENT

A B **C** D E

**Confirms reason for discussion**

**Establishes what patient wishes to know; gains agreement/informal consent to participate in the discussion**

**Investigates patient's present level of understanding of scenario**
- Patient understands the surgery is necessary to remove the cancer
- He has been taking bowel prep as is routine before bowel surgery of this nature.

**Summarises and confirms what has happened so far**

**Establishes patient's ideas, concerns and expectations**
- Anxious about needing a stoma
- Concerned about smell and unsightliness of stoma bag
- Concerned about managing at home and not wanting to burden his family
- Worried about changing the bag.

**Explains the key, important information**
- Explains that the operation is a left hemicolectomy to remove his cancer
- A stoma is not normally necessary with a left hemicolectomy, but it is important to discuss in case it becomes necessary at the time of surgery
- Stoma formation may be necessary if there is a high risk of anastomotic breakdown; it is also performed routinely if the primary anastomosis is close to the anal verge, or in non-elective cases
- Stomas are usually reversible, especially if performed in order to allow bowel rest (usually reversed at 6 weeks)
- In the event of a stoma:
  - A clinical nurse specialist (CNS) in stoma care will be able to talk to him about the practicalities of managing a stoma
  - Clinical nurse specialist will also be able to discuss psychological and psychosexual support
  - Community (district) nursing services will also be available to help him if he is finding it difficult to manage once he is discharged
  - However, stoma bags are well designed and tidy, and the bag tends only to need changing once or twice per day
- His diet should be normal post-operatively.
- Encourages him to allow himself to rely on his family for support as he will be feeling weak for several weeks and they are likely to want to help him through his recovery.

**Invites patient to ask questions and is able to deal with them appropriately**

SCENARIO 19

375

Summarises important areas of the consultation back to the patient

Formally ends the consultation and ensures appropriate follow-up has been discussed

- Explains that the Consultant or Registrar will also be coming to talk through the procedure and take consent – and he will be able to ask them further questions that may arise
- You will ask the stoma clinical nurse specialist to come and speak to him.

## GLOBAL COMMUNICATION MARK

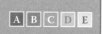

SCENARIO 19

# Scenario 19: Reflection and consolidation

### History

Mr Hatcher is a 63 year old retired accountant, who presents with a three to four month history of passing blood-stained stool. He describes the blood as mixed with stool, and occasionally has episodes of fresh blood as well as some mucus in the stool. He does not report any abdominal pain. His stool frequency has also possibly reduced, but he opens his bowels daily. He also reports feeling tired recently but denies other symptoms including nausea and vomiting. He has lost significant weight over the past six months, and has dropped three trouser sizes in spite of a reasonable appetite.

Mr Hatcher has hypertension and suffers from occasional migraines. His only regular medication is Amlodipine 5mg daily. He reports no allergies. He lives with his wife and son, and smokes 20 cigarettes per day since childhood. He drinks approximately 2 to 3 pints per week (approximately 5 units), although reports being a heavier drinker in the past. Of note, his father died of cancer, the nature of which is not known other than that it is likely he had lung metastases.

### Examination

This gentleman is comfortable at rest, although examination from the foot of the bed suggests significant recent weight loss as well as pale skin. His observations are all within normal limits. Examination of his abdomen reveals a fullness at the left iliac fossa which on palpation reveals a firm mass which is deep to the abdominal musculature, and is non-tender. The liver is also enlarged on palpation, and displays an irregular edge. Percussion and auscultation are unrevealing. Digital rectal examination was performed, demonstrating soft brown, mildly blood-stained stool, but no mass lesion was palpable within the rectum or at the anus.

### Investigations

**Blood tests**: FBC (anaemia, infection); U&E (baseline, electrolyte imbalance in cachexia); LFT (hepatomegaly suggestive of metastatic disease, hypoalbuminaemia in malnutrition; Carcinoembryonic antigen ((CEA), useful in monitoring response to treatment and in detecting recurrent disease).
**Endoscopy**: Rigid sigmoidoscopy / flexible sigmoidoscopy / colonoscopy
**Further imaging tests:**
Chest x-ray (consider pleural effusion or pulmonary metastasis); CT Abdomen, Chest, Pelvis for staging of disease. Contrast study: double contrast barium enema.

## Management

Curative resection demands that the primary tumour is removed with its lymphatic field, and a clearance margin is also resected (usually 5 cm) in order to ensure adequate resection. Laparoscopic resection is becoming increasingly commonplace.

Adjuvant therapy with chemotherapy or radiotherapy are also commonly used for the management of colorectal cancer. Radiotherapy is used in rectal cancer and can be given pre- or post-operatively to prevent recurrence. It is most successful when used in conjunction with chemotherapy. Radiotherapy is avoided in colon cancer owing to a high rate of post-irradiation adhesions.

Chemotherapy is used in rectal and colon cancer to eradicate micro-metastases and reduce the chance of future relapse. It has not been shown to improve outcomes in Dukes' A tumours, and there is only a limited survival benefit in Dukes' B cancer; however, in Dukes' C and D there is a marked benefit. 5-Fluorouracil tends to used in conjunction with oxaliplatin and folinic acid.

### Further reading and web links

Scottish Intercollegiate Guidelines Network (SIGN), guidance on diagnosis and management of colorectal cancer
www.sign.ac.uk/guidelines/fulltext/126/index.html
Excellent patient-friendly resource
www.patient.co.uk/health/Cancer-of-the-Bowel.htm

SCENARIO 19

## Clinical findings

These clinical examination findings are to be read by a model, together with the patient history, and they should then act-out the findings, presenting them to the candidate at appropriate times in the examination.

If no model is available, the candidate should read the information very carefully to be sure that he/she understands the examination findings and is in a position to present and discuss the patient with an examiner. Although this is not the usual sequence in clinical diagnosis, reading and acquiring information from patient notes is an essential clinical skill that must be mastered. As the time needed varies with experience, no set time is given, but by finals you should be able to organise and present this amount of information in 2 to 3 minutes.

## Scenario 1 (page 2)
## No post today

- o  Patient is a middle-aged, obese Asián man; looks unwell, pale and clammy; still has slight chest discomfort
- o  Observations – HR 104 bpm, BP 183/98 mmHg (large cuff required), RR 18 bpm, $O_2$ sats 87% on air, temperature 36.5 °C, CBG 16.4 mmol/l
- o  Feet to face – very overweight but nil else of note
- o  General examination – fingers of right hand heavily tar stained; no anaemia; no stigmata of hyperlipidaemia
- o  CV examinations – pulse 100 regular, low volume, normal character; no carotid or other bruits heard; BP 190/100, JVP not seen; heart sounds 1 + 2 + ? 3rd heart sound
- o  Focused examination – no ankle oedema; all peripheral pulses palpable; no ulcers or scars
- o  RS examination: bibasal crackles to the midzones.

## Scenario 2 (page 24)
## Collapse

- o Patient is tall and slim and looks well; appears breathless at rest; able to complete sentences
- o Observations – HR 103 bpm, BP 115/75 mmHg, RR 20 bpm, $O_2$ sats 94% on air, temperature 37.1 °C
- o General examination –patient is well perfused; capillary refill time is less than 2 seconds; no cyanosis; trachea not deviated
- o RS examination – inspection: visibly reduced chest expansion; palpation: reduced chest expansion on the right, anteriorly and posteriorly; percussion: hyper-resonant percussion note on right side of chest; auscultation: reduced breath sounds on the right side, normal vesicular breath sounds on the left side.

## Scenario 3 (page 37)
## One too many

- o Patient is drowsy, with a Glasgow coma score (GCS) of (12)E3V3M5, maintaining his airway, pupils equal and reactive
- o Observations – HR 110 bpm, BP 115/65 mmHg, RR 10 bpm, $O_2$ sats 95% on air, temperature 37.1 °C, BM 5.2
- o General examination – patient icteric with distended abdomen; scratch marks over skin
- o Focussed examination:
  - o Hands – leuconychia; palmer erythema; unable to assess asterixis; no Dupuytren's contracture
  - o Face – deep jaundice of skin and conjunctivae
  - o Chest – gynaecomastia and multiple spider naevi
  - o Abdomen – caput medusa and gross distension, no palpable liver edge or spleen, shifting dullness present, no peritonism; bowel sounds present; rectal examination (requested).

## Scenario 4 (page 54)
## Lost for words

- o Patient looks well
- o Observations – HR 98 bpm, BP 187/120 mmHg, RR 16 bpm, $O_2$ sats 93% on air, temperature 38.5 °C, CBG 6.1 mmol/l
- o Feet to face – no stigmata of CV disease
- o Height 1.78 m, weight 94 kg, BMI $94/(1.78)^2 = 29.7$ kg/m$^2$
- o General examination – fingers of right hand heavily tar-stained, no anaemia, no tendon xanthoma
- o Focussed examination – abdomen no bruits; no AAA; legs: no peripheral oedema; all PPP
- o CV examinations – pulse 98 regular; JVP not seen, AB forceful/undisplaced, HS 1 + 2 + soft ESM in aortic area – no radiation
- o RS examination – nil of note
- o Neurological examination – I: NFA; V/A, able to read large newspaper print both eyes; eyes: fields, ?right homonymous hemianopia ?inattention to the right; EOM: full; no nystagmus; PERL(A); CNs V, VII, XII: nil of note; UL and LL – all movements: right, grade 3–4/5; left, grade 5/5; no cerebellar signs; gait not assessed; all reflexes: right 0–1/2, left 2/2; plantars: right, equivocally, extensor; left, flexor; sensation: grossly intact
- o Ophthalmoscopy – poor view in both eyes
- o Speech – understands and follows three-stage command; expression: some dysnomia and reduced fluency
- o Swallowing – coughs and splutters when assessed.

## Scenario 5 (page 76)
## Breast lump

- o Patient looks generally well
- o Observations – HR 58 bpm, BP 108/71 mmHg, RR 14 bpm, $O_2$ sats 100% on air
- o Height 163 cm, weight 65 kg, BMI 24.5
- o Focussed examination:
    - o Symmetrical appearances on inspection
    - o Right breast examination – unremarkable; no masses palpated within breast tissue or regional lymph nodes
    - o Left breast – approximately 3 cm firm, non-tender lesion palpated within upper outer quadrant, not fixed to skin.; no changes to skin of breast; no nipple retraction or discharge; no axillary or supraclavicular lymphadenopathy.

## Scenario 6 (page 89)
## Terrible legs

- o Patient is overweight and looks unwell and clammy to the touch
- o Observations – HR 104 bpm, BP 156/96 mmHg, temperature 38.1 °C, CBG 16.3 mmol/l
- o General examination – no jaundice, anaemia, clubbing, cyanosis, lymphadenopathy
- o Focussed examination – assessment of the lower limbs
  - o Varicosities of the short and long saphenous veins (left and right); bilaterally oedematous legs
  - o Right – chronic venous changes of the calf, including haemosiderosis and lipodermatosclerosis; healed ? previous ulcerated area over the medial and anterior shin, approx 4.5 cm
  - o Left – chronic venous changes of the calf, including marked lipodermatosclerosis of the remaining, normal areas of skin; offensive-smelling, large circumferential, ulcerated area extending over most of the left shin; maximum width – approximately 8–10 cm minimum width approx 4–5 cm; base – very sloughy and pusy; occasional areas of granulation seen; ragged, uneven edges
  - o Sensation – LT/JPS/VIB sensation – normal left = right
  - o Arterial – popliteal, DP and PT pulses – easily palpable left = right.
- o Patient is a late-middle-aged woman; looks well
- o Chronic venous changes of both shins with haemosdierosis and lipodermatosclerosis. Small healing leg ulcer lateral and anterior aspect of mid left shin; left and right thigh – varicosities of long saphenous vein extending down medial aspect of thighs; right – varicosities of short saphenous vein extending over posterior aspect of calf; right – oedema extending to mid calf; left – no oedema, bandaging marks
- o Cough test – with fingers placed over sapheno-femoral junction (S-FJ):
  - o Right – positive thrill
  - o Left – positive thrill.
- o Tap test:
  - o Right – positive in long saphenous vein
  - o Left – positive in long saphenous vein.
- o Trendelenburg's test:
  - o Right – long saphenous vein did not refill with tourniquet placed 5 cm below the S-FJ
  - o Left – long saphenous vein did not refill with tourniquet placed 5 cm below the S-FJ.

- o Perthe's test:
  - o Right – superficial veins remain dilated and filled after standing and rocking onto balls of feet 10 times
  - o Left – superficial veins remain dilated and filled after standing and rocking onto balls of feet 10 times.

## Scenario 7 (page 111)
## Heart broken

- o Patient appears comfortable at rest; not sweaty or dyspnoeic, able to complete sentences
- o Observations – HR 94 bpm, BP 182/102 mmHg, RR 16 bpm, $O_2$ sats 95% on room air, temperature 36.2 °C, BM 5.2
- o General examination – pitting oedema to the knees; hands well perfused; pulse regular in rhythm and normal in volume at the carotid; no cyanosis or conjunctival pallor; JVP elevated at 5 cm above the sternum
- o Focussed examination – inspection: chest wall normal, no visible heaves; palpation: apex beat displaced to the anterior axillary line; percussion: normal percussion note throughout; auscultation: heart sounds normal, bibasal crackles on auscultation.

## Scenario 8 (page 126)
## Running on empty

- o Patient appears comfortable at rest; not sweaty or dyspnoeic, able to complete sentences
- o Observations – HR 102 bpm, BP 110/65 mmHg, RR 12 bpm, $O_2$ sats 96% on air, temperature 37.0 °C
- o Feet to face – patient appears pale from the end of the bed
- o General examination – patient is not icteric and her abdomen is not distended; hands: no palmar erythema, no koilonychia or leuconychia, pulse rate raised but regular; face: pallor of conjunctiva and angular stomatitis present, tongue normal, no palpable lymphadenopathy or central cyanosis
- o Abdomen – inspection: not distended, no scars visible; palpation: no guarding or tenderness, fullness in right iliac fossa but no discrete mass, 2 cm hepatomegaly with a nodular edge, no splenomegaly; percussion: normal percussion note; auscultation: bowel sounds present.

## Scenario 9 (page 141)
## Frequent and profuse

o Patient is a thin man; clinically anaemic
o Observations – HR 110 bpm, BP 105/66 mmHg, RR 20 bpm, $O_2$ sats 97% on air, temperature 38.2 °C, CBG 4.9 mmol/l
o Height 1.78 m, weight 62.3 kg, BMI 19.7 kg/m$^2$
o Feet to face – in obvious distress lying on the examination couch; APVU – Alert and orientated in time, place and person; midline laparotomy scar
o General examination – looks clinically dehydrated; mouth: multiple aphthous ulcers of the buccal mucosa; nil else; clubbing of fingernails; no jaundice, cyanosis, oedema or lymphadenopathy
o Abdomen – thin; midline laparotomy scar and several drain site scars; RIF appendicectomy scar; moderately tender all over abdomen: guarding+, no rigidity; no organomegaly; no masses; DRE – deferred at request of consultant
o Stigmata of acute/chronic disease – abdomen: as above; no signs of chronic liver disease; eyes: no signs of uveitis/conjunctivitis; joints: unable to assess lumbar spine/sacro-iliac joints because of patient's acute clinical status; small joints of hands very tender with some swelling, but no obvious erythema or heat; skin: no rashes over upper or lower limbs
o CV examinations – otherwise unremarkable
o RS examination – otherwise unremarkable.

## Scenario 10 (page 167)
## All very confusing

o Patient is elderly, thin, slightly unkempt; looks unwell and 'flushed'
o Observations – HR 123 bpm, BP 93/65 mmHg, RR 26 bpm, $O_2$ sats 92% on air, temperature 39.1 °C, CBG 16.1 mmol/l, GCS 13/15; AVPU, AMTS 1/10
o Urinalysis – blood ++, protein ++, leuc ++, nitrite +
o Feet to face – alert, agitated and mumbling to herself; heavily bruised from ?multiple falls; no obvious fractures; no obvious signs of systemic illness
o General examination – fingernails of right hand caked in faeces; hot and vasodilated peripheries; no jaundice, anaemia, clubbing, cyanosis, oedema or lymphadenopathy
o Focussed examination:
  o Abdomen – soft, non-tender, no organomegaly, no masses, BS – normal, DRE: hard, pellet-like stools, no blood or melaena
  o Legs – no peripheral oedema, all PPP

o Hips and pelvis – F.R.O.M. (active movement) both hips; no shortening or external rotation of lower limbs; Pelvis - Spring test negative
o CV examinations – pulse 130 irregular; JVP not seen, AB not palpable; HS 1 + 2 + loud 4/6 PSM at apex, and at lower left sternal edge
o RS examination – chest clear
o Neurological examination – no meningism, no cranial nerve lesions; moving all four limbs normally; bilateral flexor plantars

---

# Scenario 11 (page 191)
## Hyper, Hyper

o Patient is a well-looking, middle-aged gentleman
o Observations – BP 130/78 mmHg sitting and 128/76 mmHg standing; HR 68 bpm, regular, good volume
o Feet to face – no obvious signs of systemic illness
o Urinalysis – blood: protein +, glucose +, leuc –, nitrite –
o Weight 81.5 kg; height 1 m 81 cm
o General examination – nil of note; no stigmata of hyperlipidaemia; no tar staining of fingers
o CV examinations – all peripheral pulses were easily palpated; no evidence of an abdominal aortic aneurysm; no bruits, carotid, renal or aortic; no signs of peripheral vascular disease; no ulcers; no signs of heart failure – JVP not raised; no pulmonary oedema or effusions; no peripheral oedema; AB – undisplaced; heart sounds – 1 + 2 + nil added
o Eyes – no stigmata of hyperlipidaemia; no obvious cranial nerve lesions; no cataracts; V/A 6/12 (R); 6/18 (L) – no change since last year
o Ophthalmoscopy – R: disc and macula, normal; retina few dot and blot haemorrhages
o Ophthalmoscopy – L: disc and macula, normal; retina few dot and blot haemorrhages
o Peripheral neurology – PP/LT/JPS/vibration sense, normal; upper and lower limbs (R) = (L)
o No stigmata of peripheral sensory neuropathy; no ulcers or signs of trauma
o Feet – well cared for, no ulcers, calluses or signs of trauma; toe webs, NAD

## Scenario 12 (page 213)
## All fall down

- o Patient is a well, thin-looking elderly Asian woman
- o Observations – HR 46 bpm, BP 122/73 mmHg, RR 14 bpm, $O_2$ sats 95% on air, temperature 36.4 °C, CBG 4.9 mmol/l
- o AVPU – alert; AMTS – 10/10
- o Feet to face – independently mobile; able to get on and off the bed unassisted
- o General examination – well, euthyroid; no signs of jaundice, anaemia, clubbing, cyanosis, oedema or lymphadenopathy
- o CV examinations – pulse 44 bpm, regular; BP 122/73 mmHg sitting and 125/80 mmHg standing (2 minutes); JVP not seen; carotid pulse normal in character; HS: 1 + 2 + nil added; no peripheral oedema
- o Respiratory and abdominal examination – nil of note
- o Neurological assessment – CNs I–XII – intact L = R; PNS: UL and LL, bulk/tone/power/coordination/reflexes – L = R = normal
- o Plantars – downgoing L = R
- o No features of cerebellar disease; no features of Parkinsonism
- o Romberg's – slightly unsteady with eyes shut but not definitive
- o Gait – slightly slow but normal.

## Scenario 13 (page 235)
## Lose my breath

- o Patient appears comfortable at rest; not sweaty or dyspnoeic, able to complete sentences
- o Observations – HR 60 bpm, BP 115/60 mmHg, RR 12 bpm, O2 sats 94% on room air, temperature 36.7 °C
- o General examination – patient has clubbing of the fingernails; no palmer erythema or sclerodactyly; no central cyanosis; no evidence of anaemia or lymphadenopathy
- o Chest examination – no scars over the chest, no asymmetry; chest expansion reduced bilaterally; normal percussion note in all areas anteriorly and posteriorly; bilateral fine end inspiratory crackles at both bases, no change on coughing
- o Heart sounds normal
- o No evidence of peripheral oedema.

## Scenario 14 (page 249)
## Abdominal agony

- o Patient is overweight and appears unwell and in moderate to severe pain
- o Observations – HR 108 bpm, BP 89/48 mmHg, RR 22 bpm, O$_2$ sats 96% on air, temperature 37.9 °C, CBG 11.1 mmol/l
- o Height 1.62 m, weight 81 kg, BMI = 30.9
- o General examination – cool hands, clammy skin, dry mucous membranes; no evidence of jaundice
- o Focussed abdominal examination – Inspection: appendicectomy scar noted, no asymmetry, no masses, no visible pulsations seen, no flank, periumbilical or inguinal ecchymosis seen; palpation: marked tenderness at epigastrium with rebound tenderness and guarding suggesting localised peritonitis, rest of abdomen generally tender but soft, not suggestive of generalised peritonitis, liver edge palpated, gall bladder not palpated, Murphy's sign negative; percussion: percussion tenderness at epigastrium, otherwise normal percussion findings; auscultation: bowel sounds heard, normal pitch and frequency; no evidence of paralytic ileus
- o Digital rectal examination (requested).

## Scenario 15 (page 265)
## Weaker and Weaker

- o Patient is unwell and terminally ill.
- o Observations – HR 58 bpm irregularly irregular, BP 95/48 mmHg, RR 20 bpm, O2 sats 97% on air, temperature 35.9 °C, CBG 7.9 mmol/l
- o Height 1.78 m, weight 59 kg, BMI 18.6
- o General examination – marked cachexia, pale skin colour; dry tongue and other mucous membranes, reduced skin turgor; JVP not seen
- o CV examinations – normal other than pulses irregularly irregular
- o Chest – equal, vesicular breath sounds, percussion tenderness at ribs of lateral chest margins bilaterally
- o Abdomen – irregular liver edge, 3 cm hepatomegaly, nil else of note
- o Back – bony tenderness on palpation of spinous processes at lumbar spine (L2/3), no crepitus or deformity on palpation; no other long-bone pains (humerus/femur) elicited
- o Digital rectal examination (requested).

## Scenario 16 (page 279)
## The pit of despair

- o Patient is an acutely unwell-looking Chinese man
- o Observations – HR 119 bpm, BP 87/56 mmHg (lying), 68/44 mmHg (sitting to 90 degrees); $O_2$ sats 95% on 2l/min, RR 26 bpm, temperature 39.6 °C, CBG 2.4 mmol/l (treated in the ambulance)
- o Feet to face – not overtly panhypopituitary; no obvious hormone excess or deficiency
- o General examination – pale and clammy; drowsy but easily rousable; AVPU – responding to voice
- o Peripheries – cold and shut down
- o Hormone replacement assessment: normal facies; hair: normal; skin: no hyper- or hypopigmentation; thyroid status: no features of thyrotoxicosis or hypothyroidism; steroid status: no overt features of Addison's or Cushing's BUT has features of Addisonian crisis, including hypotension and postural drop, and hypoglycaemia; testosterone: normal distribution of adult male hair; evidence of a few days facial growth; penis and testes normal
- o RS examination – trachea: midline; expansion: difficult to assess formally but appears normal and symmetrical; percussion note: dull left base; TVF/VF: normal; breath sounds: coarse crackles left base.

## Scenario 17 (page 312)
## A little rash

- o Patient is a thin, acutely unwell-looking young woman; in obvious distress (severe headache) lying in a dimly lit room due to photophobia
- o Observations – HR 123 bpm, BP 87/56 mmHg, RR 22 bpm, $O_2$ sats 95% on air, temperature 39.2 °C, CBG 4.3 mmol/l
- o Feet to face – AVPU: responding appropriately to voice commands and conversation but distressed
- o General examination – clinically dehydrated; non-blanching purpuric rash over upper and lower limbs; ear: unable to assess; nose: nostrils clear; throat: erythematous++; no pus; signs of meningism and raised intracranial pressure: neck stiffness++; unable to touch chin to chest; photophobia+++; unable to visualise optic discs; rash – as above
- o Neurological assessment – limited by patient's clinical status; eyes: pupils appear equal and react to light; fields not assessed; unable to visualise retina (left or right); EOM – not able to assess due to photophobia and distress
    - o V– sensation appears intact L = R
    - o VII – face symmetrical

- o IX/X – not assessed
- o XII – tongue dry; movement looks normal
- o UL and LL – moving all four limbs to command
- o Plantars – downgoing (flexor) L = R.
- o Chest – clear; abdomen – soft, non-tender; BS – normal; urinalysis: NAD
- o Joints – no arthritis noted
- o Skin – rash as above; no ulcers, no cellulitis
- o CV examinations – no stigmata of endocarditis; tachycardic, hypotensive; otherwise unremarkable.

## Scenario 18 (page 337)
## Drunk and disorderly

- o Patient is a chronically unwell, pale, thin-looking man
- o Observations – HR 96 bpm, BP 134/86 mmHg, RR 18 bpm, $O_2$ sats 94% on air, temperature 36.6 °C, CBG 5.4 mmol/l
- o Height 1.83 m, weight 62.5 kg
- o Feet to face – thin, unsteady on walking and getting on and off the bed
- o APVU – alert and orientated in time, place and person
- o General examination – heavy tar staining of fingers of right hand, marked clubbing of fingernails; pale ?anaemic; no signs of candidiasis in mouth; hard, fixed lymph nodes in the anterior cervical chain (left and right) and left supraclavicular fossa; no jaundice, cyanosis, oedema
- o Neurological examination: cerebellar – past pointing and dysdiadokokinesia (left and right); reflexes: reduced left and right upper limbs; tone: normal; bilateral nystagmus; speech: slurred and staccato; balance: ?Romberg's positive, very unsteady in both directions with eyes closed; unable to stand heel to toe with eyes open; evidence of truncal ataxia when sat on the edge of the bed; gait: markedly ataxic; needed support of one when walking
- o Assessment for signs of metastatic lung cancer: heavy tar staining of fingers of right hand, marked clubbing of fingernails; no signs of Horner's or Pancoast's syndrome; speech: cerebellar; no hoarseness; hard fixed lymphadenopathy in anterior cervical chain (L=R) and left SCF; trachea: midline; expansion: reduced left side; percussion note: dull left base; TVF/VF: reduced left base; breath sounds: reduced left base; abdomen: 4 cm hepatomegaly (hard and craggy) below right costal margin; no ascites; spine and long bones: no obvious tenderness; pupils: unable to visualise discs clearly but venous pulsation noted in both retina.

## Scenario 19 (page 362)
## Blood in the pan

- Patient is a very thin gentleman with loose skin suggestive of marked recent weight loss; pale skin
- Observations – HR 74 bpm, BP 131/89 mmHg, RR 16 bpm, O2 sats 96% on air, temperature 36.9 °C, CBG 7.9 mmol/l
- Height 194 cm, weight 71 kg, BMI 18.9
- Focussed examination – no scars seen, slight fullness at left flank/left iliac fossa; no pulsations seen; no abdominal tenderness on palpation; firm mass palpated at left iliac fossa, deep to abdominal musculature, non-tender; non-tender hepatomegaly, with irregular liver edge
- Percussion and auscultation unrevealing
- Digital rectal examination (requested) – no external signs: no tags, haemorrhoids or fissures identified; soft stool on glove, slightly blood-stained; no rectal lesion palpated; prostate gland not enlarged.

# Prescription charts

<table>
<tr><td colspan="3">Allergies, sensitivities and adverse drug reactions</td><td colspan="2">Patient details/addressograph</td></tr>
<tr><td colspan="2">No known allergies ☐</td><td>Initials</td><td colspan="2" rowspan="2">Gender M / F</td><td>NHS/ Hospital No:</td></tr>
<tr><td colspan="2">Not possible to ascertain ☐</td><td>Date</td><td></td></tr>
<tr><td>Medicine/substance</td><td>Reaction & Severity</td><td>Initials & Date</td><td>Weight (kg)</td><td>Date</td><td>Surname:</td></tr>
</table>

| Allergies, sensitivities and adverse drug reactions | | | | Patient details/addressograph |
|---|---|---|---|---|
| No known allergies ☐ | | Initials | Gender M / F | NHS/ Hospital No: |
| Not possible to ascertain ☐ | | Date | Weight (kg)    Date | |
| Medicine/substance | Reaction & Severity | Initials & Date | | Surname: |
| | | | Height | First name: |
| Alerts | | | Surface area (m²) | Date of birth: |

---

**IN-PATIENT MEDICATION PRESCRIPTION
AND ADMINISTRATION RECORD**

PasTest HOSPITAL

| Consultant | Trainee Dr. Name and Bleep no. | Date of admission | Date chart reboarded | Estimated date of discharge |
|---|---|---|---|---|
| This chart is no. ................. of ............................ | Transcribing Check by Pharmacy Sign .................... Date ............... | Ward 1. ........................................................................ | 2. ........................................................................ | |

---

Supplementary Medication charts in use: Other (please specify): 1 .................................................................. 2 ..................................................................

| Epidural/PCA ☐ | Syringe driver ☐ | | TPN ☐ | Chemotherapy ☐ | Insulin sliding scale ☐ |

Once only medications – loading doses, pre-medication, PGDs or surgical antibiotic propylaxis

| Date | Time to be given | Medicine (approved name) | Dose | Route | Signature and bleep no. | Pharmacy | Time given | Given by | Checked by |
|---|---|---|---|---|---|---|---|---|---|
| | | | | | | | | | |
| | | | | | | | | | |
| | | | | | | | | | |
| | | | | | | | | | |

## Regular prescriptions

### Oral anticoagulation follow the anticoagulation guidelines available on the intranet

| Indication | Target INR | Baseline INR (if applicable) | Duration of therapy / Date therapy started | Date of anticoagulation follow-up appointment (clinic or other)* | Anticoagulant record book given or updated. Sign and date | Date patient counselled and sign |
|---|---|---|---|---|---|---|
| | | | | | | |

\* A follow-up appointment must be booked with the anti-coagulant clinic or enhanced provider of primary care services. If not, the TTA will not be dispensed

| Initiating warfarin | Perform baseline coagulation screen, LFTs, U&Es and FBC | Prescribe initiation dose as per guidelines | CHECK INR ON DAY 3 | FOLLOW DOSING ALGORITHM IN GUIDELINE |
|---|---|---|---|---|
| Continuing warfarin | Maintenance therapy | FOLLOW MAINTENANCE DOSING ALGORITHM IN GUIDELINE | | |

Do not use the initiation protocol for patients already on warfarin. More frequent INR monitoring may be required for patients on interacting drug(s)

| Medication | | | | Date | | | | | | | | | | | | | | |
|---|---|---|---|---|---|---|---|---|---|---|---|---|---|---|---|---|---|---|
| 1 | | | | INR | | | | | | | | | | | | | | |
| Route | Frequency OD | Time 18.00 | Start | Dose | | | | | | | | | | | | | | |
| | | | Stop | Dr sign | | | | | | | | | | | | | | |
| Signature | | Bleep no. | Pharmacy | Given | | | | | | | | | | | | | | |

### Initiating warfarin – Reduced dosing regimen in red. Refer to anticoagulation policy

| Day | One | Two | Three | | | | | | | Four and above | | | | | | | | |
|---|---|---|---|---|---|---|---|---|---|---|---|---|---|---|---|---|---|---|
| INR | <1.4 | No test | <2.0 | 2.0-2.1 | 2.2-2.5 | 2.6-2.9 | 3.0-3.3 | 3.4-4.0 | >4.0 | <1.4 | 1.4-1.5 | 1.6-1.7 | 1.8-1.9 | 2.0-2.3 | 2.4-3.0 | 3.1-4.0 | 4.1-4.5 | >4.5 |
| Dose mg | 10 5 | 10 5 | 10 | 5 | 4 | 3 | 2 | 1 | 0 | 9 | 8 | 7 | 6 | 5 | 4 | 3 | Miss 1 day | Miss 2 day |

### Thromboprophylaxis please prescribe treatment regimens in the regular medications section

| Choice of mechanical prophylaxis and leg(s) to be applied to | | | | | | Enter Time | Enter details below | | | | | | | | | | |
|---|---|---|---|---|---|---|---|---|---|---|---|---|---|---|---|---|---|
| Graduated elastic compression stockings | Intermittend pneumatic compression device (IPC) | | Leg | | | | | | | | | | | | | | |
| | | | Left | Right | Both | | | | | | | | | | | | |
| Start Date: | End Date: | Signature and Bleep No. | ☐ | ☐ | ☐ | | | | | | | | | | | | |
| Start Date: | End Date: | Signature and Bleep No. AF | ☐ | ☐ | ☐ | | | | | | | | | | | | |

| Medication | | Dose | Dose Change | Enter Time | Enter details below | | | | | | | | | | | |
|---|---|---|---|---|---|---|---|---|---|---|---|---|---|---|---|---|
| Please ensure you have completed the VTE risk assessment form | Date | | | | | | | | | | | | | | | |
| | Route | | | | | | | | | | | | | | | |
| | Signature | | | Instructions | | | | | | Pharmacy | | | | | ☐ | |
| | Bleep no. | | | | | | | | | | | | | | | |

## Oxygen  ☐   ☐

| Target Saturation | 88-92% | 94/98% | If oxygen saturation falls below target range on prescribed oxygen, patient needs urgent clinical review. If oxygen saturation is above targent range on prescribed oxygen, ask for review. |
|---|---|---|---|
| Other specify) | | | *Device: N= nasal cannula, SM = simple face mask, V = venturi, H = humidified, RM = reservoir mask, OTHER = other eg. NCPAP/NIPPV   Pharmacy ☐ |
| Target Saturation not applicable | | ☐ | |

| | Date Changed | Date Changed | Enter Time | Enter details below | | | | | | | | | | | | |
|---|---|---|---|---|---|---|---|---|---|---|---|---|---|---|---|---|
| Device | | | | | | | | | | | | | | | | |
| % or L/min (specify a range eg 1-21 L/min) | | | | | | | | | | | | | | | | |
| Signature and Bleep no. | | | | | | | | | | | | | | | | |

## Regular prescriptions continued

### Regular medications

| | Dose | | | Date | | | | | | | | | | | | | | | |
|---|---|---|---|---|---|---|---|---|---|---|---|---|---|---|---|---|---|---|---|

| Date | | | | Medication | | Instructions | | Signature and bleep no. | | Pharmacy | |
|---|---|---|---|---|---|---|---|---|---|---|---|
| Route | | | | | | | | | | | |
| Signature | | | | | | | | | | | |
| 06 | | | | | | | | | | | |
| 09 | | | | | | | | | | | |
| 12 | | | | | | | | | | | |
| 18 | | | | | | | | | | | |
| 22 | | | | | | | | | | | |
| 24 | | | | | | | | | | | |

## Regular prescriptions continued

### Regular medications

| | Dose | | | Date | | | | | | | | | | | | | | | |
|---|---|---|---|---|---|---|---|---|---|---|---|---|---|---|---|---|---|---|---|

| Date | | | | Medication | | Instructions | | Signature and bleep no. | | Pharmacy | |
|---|---|---|---|---|---|---|---|---|---|---|---|
| Route | | | | | | | | | | | |
| Signature | | | | | | | | | | | |
| 06 | | | | | | | | | | | |
| 09 | | | | | | | | | | | |
| 12 | | | | | | | | | | | |
| 18 | | | | | | | | | | | |
| 22 | | | | | | | | | | | |
| 24 | | | | | | | | | | | |

## Infusion prescriptions continued

SC = subcutaneous  IVC = intravenous central  IVP = intravenous peripheral

| Date & time | Route | Infusion Fluid | | | Medication | | | Duration | Rate | Prescriber's signature & bleep no. | Date given | Given by / Added by | Check by | Start time | Finish time | Pharmacy |
|---|---|---|---|---|---|---|---|---|---|---|---|---|---|---|---|---|
| | | Name & strength | Volume | | Approved name with expiry / unit number | | Dose | | | | | | | | | |
| | | Exp: Batch/unit no: | | | | | | | | | | | | | | |
| | | Exp: Batch/unit no: | | | | | | | | | | | | | | |
| | | Exp: Batch/unit no: | | | | | | | | | | | | | | |
| | | Exp: Batch/unit no: | | | | | | | | | | | | | | |
| | | Exp: Batch/unit no: | | | | | | | | | | | | | | |
| | | Exp: Batch/unit no: | | | | | | | | | | | | | | |
| | | Exp: Batch/unit no: | | | | | | | | | | | | | | |
| | | Exp: Batch/unit no: | | | | | | | | | | | | | | |
| | | Exp: Batch/unit no: | | | | | | | | | | | | | | |
| | | | | | | | | | | | | | | | | |
| | | | | | | | | | | | | | | | | |

| As required medications | | | | | | | | | | | | | | | | | | | | | | | | | | | | |
|---|---|---|---|---|---|---|---|---|---|---|---|---|---|---|---|---|---|---|---|---|---|---|---|---|---|---|---|---|
| Medication | | | | Date | | | | | | | | | | | | | | | | | | | | | | | | |
| Indication | | | | Time | | | | | | | | | | | | | | | | | | | | | | | | |
| Dose | Route | Maximum frequency / dose | Start date | Dose | | | | | | | | | | | | | | | | | | | | | | | | |
| | | | Stop date | Route | | | | | | | | | | | | | | | | | | | | | | | | |
| Signature | | | Bleep no. | Given | | | | | | | | | | | | | | | | | | | | | | | | |
| Additional instructions: | | | | | | | | | | | | | | | Pharmacy | | | | | | | | | | | | | |

| As required medications | | | | | | | | | | | | | | | | | | | | | | | | | | | | |
|---|---|---|---|---|---|---|---|---|---|---|---|---|---|---|---|---|---|---|---|---|---|---|---|---|---|---|---|---|
| Medication | | | | Date | | | | | | | | | | | | | | | | | | | | | | | | |
| Indication | | | | Time | | | | | | | | | | | | | | | | | | | | | | | | |
| Dose | Route | Maximum frequency / dose | Start date | Dose | | | | | | | | | | | | | | | | | | | | | | | | |
| | | | Stop date | Route | | | | | | | | | | | | | | | | | | | | | | | | |
| Signature | | | Bleep no. | Given | | | | | | | | | | | | | | | | | | | | | | | | |
| Additional instructions: | | | | | | | | | | | | | | | Pharmacy | | | | | | | | | | | | | |

# FP10

| Pharmacy stamp | Age | Title, Forename, Surname & Address |
| --- | --- | --- |
| | DOB | |

Please don't stamp over age box

Number of days' treatment
NB: Ensure dose is stated

| Signature of prescriber | Date |
| --- | --- |

For dispenser
No. of prescns

FP10NC02.08

# Drug chart

**Generic Prescribing: The following details were completed and correct:**
- Patient's name, DOB, age, weight, height
- The ward, consultant, responsible junior doctor and bleep number.

**The drug chart is legible**

**For each of the drugs prescribed the following details are correctly completed:**

(**DRUG DR**s **D**on't **F**orget **S**igning **O**ff)

**DRUG** - name (generic)
**Dose**
**Route of administration**
**Signature**
**Dose**
**Frequency**
**Signature**
**Others – duration, gated, maximum dose per 24 hours, levels**

**As it is written – the drug can be dispensed**

# Station Index

# Subject Index